ON CALL
Principles and Protocols

7th Edition

ON CALL

Principles and Protocols

Shane A. Marshall
MD, FRCPC
Director and Consultant Cardiologist,
The Cardiac Echo Lab, Paget, Bermuda

John Ruedy
MDCM, FRCPC, LLD (HON), DMED (HON)
Professor (Emeritus) of Pharmacology, Faculty of Medicine,
Dalhousie University, Halifax, Nova Scotia, Canada

ELSEVIER

Elsevier
1600 John F. Kennedy Blvd.
Ste 1800
Philadelphia, PA 19103-2899

ON CALL PRINCIPLES AND PROTOCOLS   ISBN: 978-0-443-11104-4

Previous editions copyrighted 2017, 2011, 2004, 2000, 1993, and 1989.

Senior Content Strategist: Marybeth Thiel
Senior Content Development Specialist: Sneha Kashyap
Content Development Manager: Somodatta Roy Choudhury
Publishing Services Manager: Shereen Jameel
Project Manager: Haritha Dharmarajan
Design Direction: Amy Buxton

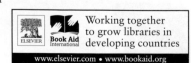

Printed in India

Last digit is the print number: 9 8 7 6 5 4 3 2 1

To our families in
Bermuda and Canada

Preface

Taking calls at night is one of the traditional duties of medical students and residents in teaching hospitals. *On Call Principles and Protocols* facilitates the transition of medical students and residents from the classroom to the hospital setting. We believe that the initiation of the medical student to hospital practice needn't be one of trial and error and needn't be recalled as a time of stress and uncertainty.

The seventh edition of *On Call Principles and Protocols* provides referenced updates for the assessment and management of common problems for which medical students and residents are called at night. The popular On Call Formulary, a quick reference of commonly prescribed medications, has also been expanded and updated.

We have been careful to maintain an approach that provides both instruction and reference while emphasizing the rational thought processes required for optimal patient care in specific clinical situations. In this edition of *On Call Principles and Protocols*, medications are in blue type and, where appropriate, the thought processes behind management decisions and instructions are indented.

It is our belief that this structured approach deserves greater emphasis in the undergraduate years, and we are hopeful that it will help students in their introduction to clinical medicine.

Acknowledgments

We are grateful to the physicians and allied health care workers who provided helpful and detailed comments on individual chapters, and to Marybeth Thiel, Sneha Kashyap, and Baljinder Kaur for their patience and encouragement during the preparation of the seventh edition of this book.

Shane A. Marshall
John Ruedy

Structure of the Book

The book is divided into four sections: Introduction, Patient-Related Problems, Laboratory-Related Problems, and Appendices.

Introduction

The first section covers introductory material in four chapters:
- Chapter 1, Approach to the Diagnosis and Management of On-Call Problems
- Chapter 2, Documentation of On-Call Problems
- Chapter 3, Assessment and Management of Volume Status
- Chapter 4, Viruses and the House Officer.

Volume status is discussed in the introductory section because assessment of volume status is essential for the proper management of many problems in hospitalized patients. Statements on transmissible viruses are included in Chapter 4 because of the small risk that infected patients pose to healthcare workers.

Patient-Related Problems

The second section contains the common calls associated with patient-related problems. Each problem is approached from its inception, beginning with the relevant questions that should be asked over the phone, the temporary orders that should be given, and the major life-threatening problems to be considered as one approaches the bedside. The names and doses of medication are in green for easy location and reference. The rationales behind questions that are asked are preceded by a book symbol 📖.

Each chapter in the second section is divided as follows:

PHONE CALL

Questions

Pertinent questions that should be asked to assess the urgency of the situation.

Orders

Urgent orders to be carried out before you arrive at the bedside.

Inform RN

The time you anticipate arriving at the bedside.

ELEVATOR THOUGHTS

The differential diagnosis that should be considered while you are on the way to assess the patient (i.e., while in the elevator).

MAJOR THREAT TO LIFE

Identification of the major threat to life is essential in providing a focus for the effective management of the patient.

BEDSIDE

Quick-Look Test

A rapid visual assessment to place the patient in one of three categories: well, sick, or critical. This helps determine the necessity for immediate intervention.

Airway and Vital Signs

Selective History

Selective Physical Examination

Management

LABORATORY-RELATED PROBLEMS

The third section contains the common calls associated with laboratory-related problems. Each problem is addressed by its causes, manifestations, and management.

APPENDICES

Appendices A–E consist of reference items that are useful in managing calls. The On Call Formulary is a compendium of commonly used medications that are likely to be prescribed by the student or resident on call. The alphabetically arranged formulary serves as a quick reference for drug dosages, routes of administration, side effects, contraindications, and modes of action.

Commonly Used Abbreviations

ABD	Abdomen
ABG	Arterial blood gas
AC	*Ante cibum* (before meals)
ACE	Angiotensin-converting enzyme
ACLS	Advanced cardiac life support
ACS	Acute coronary syndrome
ACTH	Adrenocorticotropic hormone
ADH	Antidiuretic hormone
AED	Automated external defibrillator
AFB	Acid-fast bacillus
AIDS	Acquired immunodeficiency syndrome
AMI	Acute myocardial infarction
AMP	Adenosine monophosphate
ANA	Antinuclear antibody
AP	Anteroposterior
aPTT	Activated partial thromboplastin time
ARB	Angiotensin receptor blocker
ARDS	Adult respiratory distress syndrome
ASD	Atrial septal defect
AV	Atrioventricular
BBB	Bundle branch block
BID	Twice a day
BLS	Basic life support
BNP	Brain natriuretic peptide
BP	Blood pressure
BPH	Benign prostatic hypertrophy
C+S	Culture and sensitivity
Ca	Calcium
CABG	Coronary artery bypass graft
CBC	Complete blood (cell) count
CCU	Cardiac care unit
CGL	Chronic granulocytic leukemia
CHF	Congestive heart failure
CLL	Chronic lymphocytic leukemia
CMV	Cytomegalovirus

CNS	Central nervous system
CO	Cardiac output
CO_2	Carbon dioxide
COPD	Chronic obstructive pulmonary disease
CPK	Creatine phosphokinase
CPR	Cardiopulmonary resuscitation
CrCl	Creatinine clearance
CSF	Cerebrospinal fluid
CT	Computed tomography
CTPA	Computed tomography pulmonary angiogram
CVS	Cardiovascular system
CXR	Chest x-ray
D5NS	5% dextrose in normal saline
D5W	5% dextrose in water
D10W	10% dextrose in water
D20W	20% dextrose in water
D50W	50% dextrose in water
DC	Direct current
DIC	Disseminated intravascular coagulation
DKA	Diabetic ketoacidosis
DOAC	Direct-acting oral anticoagulant
DPP-4	Dipeptidyl peptidase
DRESS	Drug reaction with eosinophilia and systemic symptoms
DSRS	Distal splenorenal shunt
DVT	Deep venous (vein) thrombosis
ECF	Extracellular fluid
ECG	Electrocardiogram
EDTA	Edetate disodium
EF	Ejection fraction
EHT	Endoscopic hemostatic therapy
ELISA	Enzyme-linked immunosorbent assay
EMT	Emergency medical technician
ENDO	Endocrine
ENT	Ears, nose, and throat
ESR	Erythrocyte sedimentation rate
ET	Endotracheal
Ext	Extremities
FDA	Food and Drug Administration
FDP	Fibrin degradation product
FEV_1	Forced expiratory volume in 1 second
FFP	Fresh frozen plasma
Fio_2	Fraction of inspired oxygen
FPBG	Finger-prick blood glucose
FTA-ABS	Fluorescent treponemal antibody absorption
FUO	Fever of unknown origin
G-6-PD	Glucose-6-phosphate dehydrogenase

GERD	Gastroesophageal reflux disease
GI	Gastrointestinal
GLP-1	Glucagon-like peptide
GTT	Glucose tolerance test
GU	Genitourinary
Hb	Hemoglobin
HBV	Hepatitis B virus
HCV	Hepatitis C virus
HEENT	Head, eyes, ears, nose, throat
HFpEF	Heart failure with preserved ejection fraction
HFrEF	Heart failure with reduced ejection fraction
HIV	Human immunodeficiency virus
HJR	Hepatojugular reflux
HPI	History of present illness
HR	Heart rate
HS	*Hora somni* (at bedtime)
IBW	Ideal body weight
ICD	Implantable cardioverter-defibrillator
ICF	Intracellular fluid
ICU	Intensive care unit
ICU/CCU	Intensive care unit/cardiac care unit
Ig	Immunoglobulin
IM	Intramuscular
INR	International normalized ratio
IO	Interosseous
IP	Intraperitoneally
ISI	International Sensitivity Index
ITP	Idiopathic thrombocytopenic purpura
IV	Intravenous
IVP	Intravenous pyelogram
J	Joule
JVP	Jugular venous pressure
K	Potassium
L	Liter
LDH	Lactate dehydrogenase
LLL	Left lower lobe
LLQ	Left lower quadrant
LMWH	Low-molecular-weight heparin
LOC	Level of consciousness
LP	Lumbar puncture
LUQ	Left upper quadrant
LV	Left ventricle (ventricular)
LVH	Left ventricular hypertrophy
MAO	Monoamine oxidase
MAOI	Monoamine oxidase inhibitor
MCV	Mean corpuscular volume

MD	Doctor of medicine
MERS	Middle East respiratory syndrome
MHA-TP	Microhemagglutinin assay—*Treponema pallidum*
MI	Myocardial infarction
Misc	Miscellaneous
MRI	Magnetic resonance imaging
MSS	Musculoskeletal system
MVP	Mitral valve prolapse
NA	Sodium
NAAT	Nucleic acid amplification test
Neuro	Neurologic system
NG	Nasogastric
NMR	Nuclear magnetic resonance (scan)
NNRTI	Non-nucleoside reverse transcriptase inhibitor
NPH	Neutral protamine Hagedorn (insulin)
NPO	*Nil per os* (nothing by mouth)
NRTI	Nucleoside/nucleotide reverse transcriptase inhibitor
NS	Normal saline (0.9% saline in water)
NSAID	Nonsteroidal anti-inflammatory drug
NSTEMI	Non–ST-elevation myocardial infarction
NT-pro BNP	N-terminal pro brain natriuretic peptide
NYD	Not yet diagnosed
P_2	Pulmonic second sound
PA	Posteroanterior
PAo_2	Calculated partial pressure of oxygen
Pao_2	Measured partial pressure of oxygen
PAC	Premature atrial contraction
PAT	Paroxysmal atrial tachycardia
PB	Barometric pressure
PC	*Post cibum* (after meals)
PCI	Percutaneous coronary intervention
Pco_2	Partial pressure of carbon dioxide
PEA	Pulseless electrical activity
PEEP	Positive end-expiratory pressure
PEFR	Peak expiratory flow rate
PH_2O	Partial pressure of water vapor in the lung
PI	Protease inhibitor
PMN	Polymorphonuclear cell
PND	Paroxysmal nocturnal dyspnea
PO	*Per os* (by mouth)
Po_2	Partial pressure of oxygen
PR	Per rectum
PRN	*Pro re nata* (as needed)
PSVT	Paroxysmal supraventricular tachycardia
Psych	Psychiatric
PT	Prothrombin time

PTH	Parathyroid hormone
PVC	Premature ventricular contraction
QD	Every day
QHS	*Quaque hora somnia* (every "hour of sleep," i.e., each night)
QID	Four times a day
R	Respiratory quotient
RA	Rheumatoid arthritis
RAD	Right axis deviation
RBBB	Right bundle branch block
RBC	Red blood cell (count)
Resp	Respiratory system
RLL	Right lower lobe
RLQ	Right lower quadrant
RN	Registered nurse
ROM	Range of motion
RR	Respiratory rate
RTA	Renal tubular acidosis
RUQ	Right upper quadrant
RV	Right ventricle (ventricular)
S_3	Third heart sound
SA	Sternal angle
SAH	Subarachnoid hemorrhage
SARS	Severe acute respiratory syndrome
SBE	Subacute bacterial endocarditis
SC	Subcutaneous
SGLT2	Sodium-glucose cotransporter-2
SI	International System of Units
SIADH	Syndrome of inappropriate antidiuretic hormone (secretion)
SL	Sublingual
SLE	Systemic lupus erythematosus
SOB	Shortness of breath
SNRI	Serotonin-norepinephrine reuptake inhibitor
SSRI	Selective serotonin reuptake inhibitor
SSS	Sick sinus syndrome
stat	*Statim* (immediately)
STEMI	ST-elevation myocardial infarction
STS	Serological test for syphilis
SV	Stroke volume
SVT	Supraventricular tachycardia
T_3	Triiodothyronine
T_4	Thyroxine
TACO	Transfusion associated circulatory overload
TAVR	Transcatheter aortic valve replacement
TB	Tuberculosis
TBW	Total body water
Temp	Temperature

TIA	Transient ischemic attack
TID	Three times a day
TIPS	Transjugular intrahepatic portosystemic shunt
TKVO	To keep the vein open
tPA	Tissue plasminogen activator
TPN	Total parenteral nutrition
TPR	Total peripheral resistance
TRALI	Transfusion related acute lung injury
TSH	Thyroid-stimulating hormone
TTP	Thrombotic thrombocytopenic purpura
UFH	Unfractionated heparin
URTI	Upper respiratory tract infection
UTI	Urinary tract infection
V/Q	Ventilation-perfusion
VF	Ventricular fibrillation
VIPoma	Vasoactive intestinal polypeptide-secreting tumor
VP	Ventriculoperitoneal
VSD	Ventricular septal defect
VT	Ventricular tachycardia
WBC	White blood cell (count)
WPW	Wolff-Parkinson-White
ZN	Ziehl-Neelsen

Dosage Notice

Extraordinary efforts have been made by the authors and the publisher of this book to ensure that dosage recommendations are precise and in agreement with the highest standards of practice. (The drug dosage recommendations are those for adults).

Dosage schedules are changed from time to time in the light of accumulating clinical experience and continued laboratory studies. These changes are most likely to occur in the case of recently introduced products.

We urge, therefore, that you check your hospital's formulary and/or the manufacturer's recommended dosage. In addition, there are some quite serious situations, each encountered only rarely, in which drug therapy must be individualized, and expert judgment advises the use of a higher dosage or administration by a different route than is included in the manufacturer's recommendations.

Contents

LABORATORY-RELATED PROBLEMS: THE COMMON CALLS

APPENDIXES

Introduction

Approach to the Diagnosis and Management of On-Call Problems

Clinical problem solving is an important skill for the physician on call. Traditionally, a physician approaches the diagnosis and management of a patient's problems with an ordered, structured system (e.g., history taking, physical examination, and review of available investigations) before formulating the provisional and differential diagnoses and the management plan. The history taking and physical examination may take 30 to 40 minutes for a patient with a single problem who is visiting a family physician for the first time, and longer still for a patient with multiple complaints. Clearly, if the patient arrives at the emergency department unconscious, having been found on the street, the chief issue is coma, and the history of current illness may be limited to the information provided by the ambulance attendants or by the contents of the patient's wallet or purse. In this situation, physicians must proceed concurrently with examination, investigation, and treatment. How this should be achieved is not always clear, although there is agreement on the steps that should be completed within the initial 5 to 10 minutes.

The physician first confronts on-call problem solving in the final years of medical school. At this stage, the structured history taking and physical examination direct the student's approach to patient evaluation. When on call, the medical student is faced with well-defined problems (e.g., fall out of bed, fever, chest pain) and yet may feel ill equipped to begin clinical problem solving unless a *complete history and physical examination* are obtained. However, every on-call problem can't involve 60 or more minutes of the physician's time, because unnecessary time spent on relatively minor complaints may preclude adequate treatment time for patients who are very ill.

The approach recommended in this book is based on a system that is structured but can be logically adapted to most situations. It is intended as a practical guide to assist in efficient clinical problem solving when on call. The clinical chapters are divided into four parts:

1. Phone call
2. Elevator thoughts
3. Major threat to life
4. Bedside

PHONE CALL

Most problems confronting the on-call physician are first communicated by telephone. The physician must determine the severity of the problem on the basis of this information because it is not always possible to assess the patient at the bedside immediately. Patients must be evaluated in order of priority. The phone call section of each chapter is divided into three parts:

1. Questions
2. Orders
3. Informing the registered nurse (RN)

The questions are intended to assist in determining the problem's urgency. Orders that expedite the investigation and management of urgent situations are suggested. Finally, the RN is informed of the physician's anticipated arrival time at the bedside and the interim responsibilities of the nurse.

ELEVATOR THOUGHTS

The on-call physician isn't always in the immediate vicinity when they're informed of a problem that necessitates assessment, but the time spent traveling to the ward (up to 10 minutes in some large hospitals) can be used efficiently to consider the differential diagnosis of the problem. Because travel time is often spent in elevators, the term *elevator thoughts* has been coined to summarize the directed differential diagnosis. The lists of differential diagnosis that are presented are not exhaustive; rather, they focus on the most common or most serious (life-threatening) causes that should be considered in hospitalized patients.

MAJOR THREAT TO LIFE

To identify each problem's major threat to life, physicians must consider the differential diagnosis, which provides a focus for the subsequent investigation and management of the patient. Rather than arriving at the bedside with a memorized list of possible diagnoses, it's more useful and relevant to appreciate the one or two most likely threats to life and use them to direct questions and the physical examination. This process ensures that the most life-threatening possibility in each clinical scenario is considered and sought in the initial evaluation of the patient.

BEDSIDE

The protocols for what to do on arrival at the patient's bedside are divided into the following parts:

- Quick-look test
- Airway and vital signs
- Selective history
- Selective physical examination
- Selective chart review
- Management

The bedside assessment begins with the quick-look test, which is a rapid visual assessment that helps the physician categorize the patient's condition in terms of severity: well (comfortable), sick (uncomfortable or distressed), or critical (about to die). Next is an assessment of the airway and vital signs, which is important in the evaluation of any potentially sick patient. Because of the variety of problems that must be assessed by the on-call physician, the order of the remaining components of evaluation is not uniform. For example, the selective physical examination may either precede or follow the selective history and chart review, and either of these may be superseded by management if the clinical situation dictates.

Occasionally, the "Selective Physical Examination" and "Management" sections are subdivided, allowing the reader to focus on life-threatening problems and leaving less urgent problems to be reviewed later.

It is hoped that the principles and protocols offered will provide a logical, efficient system for the assessment and management of common on-call problems.

Documentation of On-Call Problems

Accurate and concise documentation of on-call problems is essential for the continuity of care of hospitalized patients. In many instances you will not know the patient you are asked to see, and you may not be involved in their continued care after your night on call. Some problems can be handled safely over the phone, but most situations require a selective history and physical examination to correctly diagnose and treat the problem. Documentation is recommended for every patient you examine. If the problem is straightforward, a brief note is sufficient; if the problem is complicated, however, your note should be concise but complete.

Begin by recording the date, time, and who you are. For example:

April 10, 2023, 0200H. "Medical student on-call note" or "Resident on-call note."

State who called you and what time you were called. For example:

Called to see patient by RN at 0130H because the patient "fell out of bed."

If your assessment was delayed by more urgent problems, say so. A brief one- or two-sentence summary of the patient's admission diagnosis and major medical problems should follow. For example:

This 74-year-old woman with a history of chronic renal failure, type 2 diabetes mellitus, and rheumatoid arthritis was admitted 10 days ago with increasing joint pain.

Next, describe the history of present illness (HPI)—the "fall out of bed"—from the viewpoint of both the patient and any witnesses. This HPI is no different from the HPI you would document in an admission history. For example:

HPI. The patient was on the way to the bathroom to void, tripped on her bathrobe, and fell to the floor, landing on her left side. She denied palpitations, chest pain, lightheadedness, nausea, and hip pain. The fall was not witnessed. The RN found the patient lying on the floor. Vital signs were normal. There was no difficulty walking unaided and no pain afterward.

If your chart review has relevant findings, include these in the HPI. For example:

Three previous "falls out of bed" on this admission. Patient has no recall of these events.

Documentation of your examination should be selective. For example a call regarding a fall out of bed requires an assessment of the vital signs, the head and neck, and the cardiovascular, musculoskeletal, and neurologic systems. It is not necessary to examine the respiratory system or the abdomen unless there is a second, separate problem (e.g., you arrive at the bedside and find the patient febrile).

For on-call problems, a complete history and complete physical examination are not required; these were done when the patient was admitted. Your history taking, physical examination, and chart documentation should be directed (i.e., problem oriented). It may be useful to underline the abnormal physical findings both for yourself (it aids your summary) and for the house staff who will be reviewing the patient in the morning. For example:

Vital signs	Blood pressure (BP): 140/85 mmHg
	Heart rate (HR): <u>104</u>/min
	Respiratory rate (RR): <u>36</u>/min;
	Oxygen saturation 97%
	Temperature (Temp): <u>38.9</u>°C PO
Head, ears, eyes, nose, and throat (HEENT)	No tongue or cheek lacerations; No hemotympanum
Cardiovascular system (CVS)	Pulse rhythm normal; jugular venous pressure (JVP) 2 cm > sternal angle (SA)
Musculoskeletal system (MSS)	No skull or face lacerations or hematomas
	Spine and ribs normal
	Full, painless range of motion (ROM) of all 4 limbs
	7 × 9 cm hematoma, left thigh

Reflexes	
Motor	} Normal
Sensory	
Neurologic system	Alert; oriented to time, place, and person

Relevant laboratory, electrocardiographic, or radiographic data should be documented. Again, it is useful to underline abnormal findings. For example:

Glucose	6.1 mmol/L
Sodium	141 mmol/L
Potassium	3.9 mmol/L
Calcium	Not available
Urea	12 mmol/L
Creatinine	180 mmol/L

Your diagnostic conclusion regarding the problem for which you were called must be clearly stated. It is not enough to write "Patient fell out of bed"; any caregiver could have written that without consulting you. The information gathered must be synthesized to achieve the highest level of diagnostic integration possible. This provisional diagnosis should be followed by a differential diagnosis, listing the most likely alternative explanations in order. For a patient who fell out of bed, your diagnostic conclusion might be as follows:

1. "Fell out of bed" because of difficulty reaching the bathroom to void—diuretic-induced nocturia (?), contribution of sedation (?)
2. Large hematoma (7 × 9 cm), left thigh

Your plan must be clearly stated—both the measures taken during the night and the investigations or treatment you have organized for the morning. Avoid writing "Plan—see orders." It is not always obvious to the staff handling the patient's care the next day why certain measures were taken. If you informed the intern, resident, or attending physician of the problem, document the name of the person with whom you spoke and the recommendations given. Record whether any of the patient's family members were informed and what they were told. Finally, sign or print your name clearly so that the staff knows whom to contact should there be questions about the management of this patient the following day.

Assessment and Management of Volume Status

The assessment of volume status is an integral part of the physical examination. As a medical student and intern, and later as a practicing physician, you will find that this skill plays a key role in choosing the appropriate investigation and management in many clinical situations.

Ideally, this skill is learned at the patient's bedside. However some background knowledge will help you in the accurate assessment and interpretation of a patient's volume status.

First, terminology must be clarified. The human body is composed mostly of water (Fig. 3.1). In fact, total body water (TBW) makes up 60% of the weight of the adult male body. Of this, two-thirds are intracellular fluid and one-third is extracellular fluid (i.e., water that is outside of cells). Of the extracellular fluid, two-thirds are interstitial fluid, such as fluid bathing the cells, cerebrospinal fluid, and intraocular fluid. Only 7% of total body weight is intravascular fluid (plasma). Clinically, it is the extracellular fluid, consisting of intravascular and interstitial fluids, that physicians assess when determining the volume status of a patient.

Assessment of Volume Status

There are only three basic states of volume status that a patient can have:
- Volume depleted
- Normovolemic (euvolemic)
- Volume overloaded

On approaching the patient's bedside, ask yourself whether the patient is volume depleted, normovolemic, or volume overloaded.

QUICK-LOOK TEST

*Does the patient look well (comfortable), sick (uncomfortable or distressed), or **critical** (about to die)?*

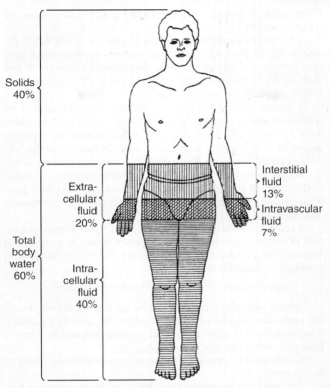

Solids
40%

Extra-
cellular
fluid
20%

Total
body
water
60%

Intra-
cellular
fluid
40%

Interstitial
fluid
13%

Intravascular
fluid
7%

FIG. 3.1 Body fluid compartments.

In most instances when you first enter the room and see the patient, a serious fluid balance abnormality, when present, is apparent. Patients who are seriously volume depleted look wan, drawn, and tired, whereas patients who are volume overloaded look uncomfortable, anxious, and restless. Of course, these are only general guidelines; a more detailed physical examination is required.

VITAL SIGNS

In most cases, simply measuring the patient's vital signs will help you determine whether there is significant volume depletion.

Measure the heart rate (HR) and blood pressure (BP) first with the patient supine and then after the patient stands for 1 minute. If the patient is unable to stand alone, ask for assistance or have the patient sit up and dangle his or her legs over the side of the bed.

If the patient is hypotensive in the supine position, this maneuver is not necessary.

A fall in systolic BP of more than 15 mm Hg or any fall in diastolic BP signifies the presence of postural hypotension, which may indicate intravascular volume depletion. An increase of HR of more than 15 beats/minute without a fall in BP may indicate a milder degree of volume depletion.

A patient with autonomic dysfunction (e.g., that caused by α-blockers, diabetic neuropathy, Shy-Drager syndrome) may also have a pronounced postural fall in BP but without the expected degree of compensatory tachycardia. Also, in contrast to the volume-depleted condition, there should be no other features of extracellular fluid deficit in a patient with uncomplicated autonomic dysfunction. A patient taking beta-blockers may also have postural hypotension without the expected degree of compensatory tachycardia.

A resting tachycardia may be seen with either volume depletion or volume overload. Volume depletion results in a low stroke volume (SV). The patient must therefore generate a tachycardia to maintain cardiac output:

$$\text{Cardiac output} = \text{Heart rate (HR)} \times \text{Stroke volume (SV)}$$

Volume-overloaded patients also have a low SV, usually due to left ventricular systolic or diastolic dysfunction, and they generate a tachycardia in an effort to increase forward flow and thereby relieve pulmonary vascular congestion.

Normovolemic patients without other complicating features have a normal HR.

Measure the respiratory rate (RR). The most important feature to look for when measuring the RR is tachypnea, which may be present in a volume-overloaded patient in whom pulmonary edema has developed.

SELECTIVE PHYSICAL EXAMINATION

Head, Ears, Eyes, Nose, and Throat
Look at the oral mucous membranes. An adequately hydrated patient has moist mucous membranes. It is normal for a small pool of saliva to collect at the undersurface of the tongue in the area of the frenulum, and this should be looked for.

Respiration
Listen for crackles. Pulmonary edema with bilateral basilar crackles and, occasionally, wheezes or pleural effusions may be a manifestation of volume overload.

Cardiovascular System

Look at the neck veins. Examination of the internal jugular veins is one of the most helpful components of the volume status examination. The jugular venous pressure (JVP) can be assessed with the patient at any inclination from 0 to 90 degrees, but it is easiest to begin looking for the JVP pulsation with the patient at a 45-degree inclination. If you are unable to visualize the neck veins when the patient is positioned at 45 degrees, this usually signifies that the JVP is either very low (in which case you need to lower the head of the bed) or very high (in which case you may need to sit the patient upright to see the top of the column of blood in the internal jugular vein). Once the internal jugular vein pulsation is identified, measure the perpendicular distance from the sternal angle to the top of the column of blood (Fig. 3.2). This distance represents the patient's JVP in centimeters of water above the sternal angle. Its value represents a composite of the volume of venous return to the heart, the central venous pressure, and the efficiency of right atrial and right ventricular emptying. A JVP of 2 to 3 cm H_2O above the sternal angle is normal in adult patients. A significantly volume-depleted patient has flat neck veins, which may fill only when the patient is placed in the Trendelenburg position. A volume-overloaded patient usually has an elevated JVP of >3 cm above the sternal angle.

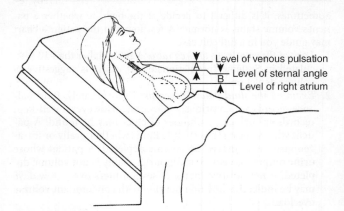

Level of venous pulsation
Level of sternal angle
Level of right atrium

FIG. 3.2 **Measurement of jugular venous pressure.** (A) represents the perpendicular distance from the sternal angle to the top of the column of blood; (B), the distance from the center of the right atrium to the sternal angle is commonly accepted as measuring 5 cm, regardless of inclination.

Listen for an S_3. A third heart sound (S_3) is most often associated with a volume-overloaded state due to left ventricular systolic dysfunction and is best heard with the patient in the left lateral position.

Abdomen

Examine the liver. An enlarged, tender liver and hepatojugular reflux may be manifestations of volume overload due to right ventricular dysfunction or severe tricuspid regurgitation.

Skin

Check the skin turgor. This is best evaluated in an adult by raising a fold of skin from the anterior chest area over the sternal angle. In a normovolemic patient, the skin should return promptly to its usual position. A sluggish return is suggestive of an interstitial fluid deficit. Taut, nonpliable skin that cannot be raised in a fold is suggestive of interstitial fluid excess.

Look at the skin creases and check for edema. Accentuated skin creases from bed sheets pressing against the posterior thorax and sacral or pedal edema are indicative of interstitial fluid excess.

SELECTIVE CHART REVIEW

Sometimes, it is difficult to decide at the bedside whether a patient's volume status is normal. A few items in the patient's chart may guide you in a difficult case.

1. *Look at the creatinine-to-urea ratio.* A ratio higher than 12 (calculated in Système Internationale [SI] units) is suggestive of volume depletion.

2. *Examine the fluid balance records.* Unfortunately, fluid balance records are notoriously inaccurate. However if well-kept records are present, a number of clues may be found. A patient who is taking in very little fluid (whether orally or intravenously) may indeed be volume depleted. A patient whose urine output exceeds 20 mL/hour probably is not volume depleted. A net positive intake of several liters over a few days may be indicative of fluid retention with concomitant volume overload.

3. *Look for a change in weight.* A gain or loss of a kilogram since admission may indicate a significant fluid gain or loss, respectively.

4. *In the volume-depleted patient, look at the chart for contributing causes:*

Gastrointestinal (GI) losses	Vomiting
	Nasogastric suction
	Diarrhea
Urinary losses	Diuretics
	Osmotic diuresis (hyperglycemia, mannitol administration, hypertonic intravenous [IV] contrast material)
	Postobstructive diuresis
	Diabetes insipidus
	Recovery phase of acute tubular necrosis
	Adrenal insufficiency
Surface losses	Skin (increased sweating caused by fever, evaporation in patients with burns)
	Respiratory tract (hyperventilation, nonhumidified inhalation therapy)
Fluid sequestration	Pancreatitis
	Ileus
	Burns
Blood losses	GI tract
	Surgical
	Trauma
	Iatrogenic (laboratory sampling)
Other	Inadequate oral or parenteral intake

Classic States of Volume Status

Only rarely does a patient have every feature of volume depletion or volume overload. Nevertheless, it is useful when examining a patient to carry a mental picture of the three *classic* states of volume status.

CLASSIC VOLUME DEPLETION

Quick-Look Test

The patient looks wan, tired, and drawn.

Vital Signs

HR	Resting tachycardia
	Postural rise in HR of >15 beats/min
BP	Normal or low resting BP
	Postural drop in systolic BP of >15 mm Hg or any drop in diastolic BP
RR	Normal
HEENT	Dry oral mucous membranes

Respiration (Resp)	Clear
Cardiovascular system (CVS)	JVP flat
	No S_3
Abdomen (ABD)	Normal
Skin	Poor turgor
	No edema

CLASSIC VOLUME OVERLOAD

Quick-Look Test

The patient looks sick and is short of breath. Often, they are sitting upright and appear uncomfortable, anxious, and restless.

Vital Signs

HR	Resting tachycardia
	Postural rise in HR of <15 beats/min
BP	May be low, normal, or high
	No postural fall in systolic or diastolic BP
RR	Tachypnea
Resp	Crackles bilaterally at bases
	Wheezing may or may not be present
	Pleural effusions may or may not be present
CVS	JVP >3 cm H_2O above the sternal angle
	S_3 present
ABD	Hepatojugular reflux present
	Liver may or may not be enlarged and tender
Extremities (Ext)	Accentuated skin creases on posterior thorax
	Sacral or pedal edema

CLASSIC NORMAL VOLUME STATUS

Quick-Look Test

The patient looks well!.

Vital Signs

HR	Normal
	Postural rise in HR of <15 beats/min
BP	Normal
	Postural fall of <15 mm Hg in systolic BP and no fall in diastolic BP
RR	Normal
HEENT	Moist oral mucous membranes
Resp	Clear
CVS	JVP 2-3 cm H_2O above the sternal angle No S_3
ABD	Normal
Ext	No edema

Choosing the Correct Intravenous Fluid

Selection of an appropriate IV fluid for a particular clinical situation need not be a guessing game. A basic understanding of physiology will help you make rational and effective decisions about fluid management.

Water is important in the body because it serves as a solvent for a variety of solutes. Solutes can be either electrolytes or nonelectrolytes.

Electrolytes are substances that dissociate into charged components (ions) when placed in water, and they include the following commonly measured substances:

Sodium
Potassium } Cations
Calcium
Magnesium

Chloride } Anions
Bicarbonate

In physiologic solutions, the total number of cations always equals the total number of anions.

Nonelectrolytes are solutes that have no electrical charges, and they include such substances as glucose and urea.

As mentioned previously, intravascular volume is made up mostly of water, which acts as a solvent to dissolve and transport electrolytes and nonelectrolytes. Water is able to move from one body compartment to the next by the process of osmosis. When two solutes are separated by a semipermeable membrane, such as a cell membrane, water tends to flow across the membrane from the solution of lower concentration to that of higher concentration; the net effect is that the solute concentrations on each side of the membrane are equalized (Fig. 3.3).

Suppose you decided to infuse a liter of pure water into a patient without any solutes. What would happen to the patient's red blood cells (RBCs)? By understanding the process of osmosis, you can reason that because the solute concentration inside the RBCs is vastly higher than that in the water infused, water would move across the cell membrane into the RBCs (Fig. 3.4). There is a limit to how much the RBC membrane can stretch, and eventually the RBCs would burst. Similarly, you can see that if a hypertonic solution were infused directly into the patient's vein, the RBCs would shrink (crenate) as water moved out of the RBCs and into the surrounding solution.

For these reasons, most IV solutions that are prepared for hospital use are usually close to isotonic—that is, they have the same solute concentration as blood—to minimize such fluid shifts. Although cell membranes allow water to pass freely by the process

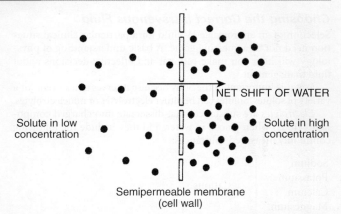

FIG. 3.3 **Osmosis.** Water flows across a semipermeable membrane to equalize solute concentrations on each side of the membrane.

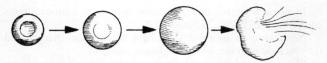

FIG. 3.4 **Osmosis.** Effect of infusion of pure water on red blood cell volume.

of osmosis, they limit the passage of solutes to varying degrees. Some solute molecules cross membranes more readily than others, depending on their size and physical properties.

For hospitalized patients, you need to consider only three solutes in order to effectively diagnose and treat disorders of fluid balance: glucose, which is distributed widely throughout both intracellular and extracellular spaces; sodium, which is limited primarily to the extracellular space; and albumin, which remains largely within the intravascular space. The distribution of these three solutes is a fundamental principle that will be useful in guiding your choices of fluid therapy.

The combination of 50 g of dextrose dissolved in 1 L of water is known as *D5W* (Table 3.1). It has an osmolality of 252 mOsm/L, which prevents the patient's RBCs from shrinking or swelling. Dextrose can be expected to equilibrate rapidly among the intravascular, interstitial, and intracellular spaces, and water follows along quickly by osmosis.

Normal saline is another commonly used IV solution. It has an osmolality of 308 mOsm/L, and although it is slightly hypertonic,

TABLE 3.1   Commonly Used Intravenous Fluids

Fluid	Glucose (g/L)	Sodium (mmol/L)	Chloride (mmol/L)	Potassium (mmol/L)	Calcium (mmol/L)	Lactate (mmol/L)	Approximate Osmolality (mOsm/L)
D5W	50	—	—	—	—	—	252
D10W	100	—	—	—	—	—	505
D20W	200	—	—	—	—	—	1010
D50W	500	—	—	—	—	—	2525
0.45% NaCl (1/2; NS)	—	77	77	—	—	—	151
0.9% NaCl (NS)	—	154	154	—	—	—	308
D5NS	50	154	154	—	—	—	560
D5/0.5% NS	50	77	77	—	—	—	432
D5/0.2% NS	50	34	34	—	—	—	321
Ringer's lactate	—	130	109	4	3	28	272
Albumin[a]	—	145	145	—	—	—	—
Fresh-frozen plasma[b]	—	—	—	—	—	—	—
Stored plasma[c]	—	—	—	—	—	—	—

D5W, 50 g of dextrose in 1 L of water; *D10W*, 100 g of dextrose in 1 L of water; *D20W*, 200 g of dextrose in 1 L of water; *D50W*, 500 g of dextrose in 1 L of water; *NS*, normal saline.
[a]Available in 5% concentrations (50, 250, or 500 mL) or 25% concentrations (20, 50, or 100 mL).
[b]200-250 mL of plasma that has been separated from whole blood and frozen within 8 hours of collection; it contains all coagulation factors.
[c]200-250 mL of plasma that has been separated from whole blood and frozen 8-72 hours after collection; it contains all coagulation factors but has reduced levels of factors V and VIII.

it is not sufficiently different from blood tonicity to cause cell shrinkage. Normal saline stays predominantly in the extracellular space longer than a glucose infusion does because sodium does not readily move intracellularly.

Albumin and *plasma* stay in the intravascular space for many hours because albumin is a large molecule that does not easily traverse the endothelial pores of the blood vessels. The half-life of albumin within the intravascular space is 17 to 20 hours.

With this knowledge of solutes and their membrane permeability, you can make logical choices regarding fluid management.

In patients with intravascular volume depletion, the goal of treatment is to correct and maintain adequate intravascular volume and tissue perfusion. Hence, a volume-depleted patient could be treated with IV normal saline, albumin, or plasma. Because normal saline is more readily available and much less expensive, it is the treatment of choice for the initial resuscitation of a volume-depleted patient. Infusion of D5W would be of little benefit because the glucose and water would be distributed rapidly throughout the intravascular, interstitial, and extravascular spaces.

In patients with intravascular volume excess, the goal of treatment is to improve and maintain adequate cardiac function and tissue perfusion. This usually necessitates the use of preload-reducing measures, as outlined in Chapter 24. However, because these patients are often critically ill, medication must be administered intravenously. The best fluid to give, usually at a rate to keep the vein open, is D5W, which quickly leaves the intravascular space. Infusion of normal saline or albumin could worsen the patient's condition by further increasing intravascular volume. This is why patients with cardiac disease, who are at risk for volume overload, are usually given an IV infusion of D5W when medication must be administered intravenously. An alternative is to use a heparin lock flush-injection (Hep-Lock) at the IV site.

Another IV solution, ⅔ to ⅓, contains 33 g/L of glucose and 51 mmol/L each of sodium and chloride and is isotonic at approximately 269 mOsm/L.

REMEMBER

Volume status abnormalities should be corrected at a rate similar to that at which they developed. Biologic systems are more responsive to rates of change than to absolute amounts of change. It is safest to correct half the deficit and then reevaluate the patient's condition. There is no substitute for frequent repeated examination of the patient when you are trying to effect changes in volume status.

On occasion, you will be faced with a patient in whom there is a discrepancy between the two compartments of the extracellular fluid, such as a decrease in intravascular volume and an excess of interstitial fluid (i.e., edema). This discrepancy is most commonly observed in states of marked hypoalbuminemia.

Fluid transfer from the intravascular space to the interstitial space depends on the permeability of the capillary bed, how much hydrostatic pressure is being exerted to force fluid out of the intravascular space, and the difference in oncotic pressure between the intravascular and interstitial spaces (Fig. 3.5).

Oncotic pressure is exerted by plasma protein (i.e., albumin). There is little, if any, protein in the interstitium; hence the intravascular oncotic pressure exerted by albumin tends to draw water out of the interstitium and into the intravascular space. This knowledge is important for treating the occasional

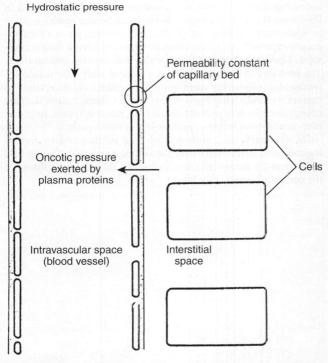

FIG. 3.5 **Factors influencing fluid transfer between the intravascular and extravascular spaces.**

patient with both intravascular volume depletion (as assessed by your clinical examination) and interstitial fluid excess (i.e., edema). To help shift fluid from the interstitium to the intravascular space in such a patient, a logical choice is to administer IV albumin. Artificial plasma expanders (e.g., gelofusine, polygeline, dextran, hetastarch) also may be used. These are glucose polymers of high molecular weight that remain in the intravascular space because of their large size. Although they are useful in shifting fluid from the interstitium to the intravascular space, each has specific contraindications and should only be used by physicians familiar with their properties and with the specific patient for whom they are being considered.

Remember that oncotic pull comes from albumin. It does not come from sodium, and so normal saline is not an appropriate fluid to give in this situation. It does not come from RBCs, and so a blood transfusion is an equally inappropriate choice. Note that albumin is available in two concentrations: 5% and 25%. The 25% concentration is preferred when you are trying to effect a shift in fluid from the interstitial space to the intravascular space.

Unfortunately, albumin, plasma, and artificial plasma expanders are expensive, and their effect in removing edema fluid is transient. Thus their continued use for this indication is controversial. The best way to correct edema in a patient with a decreased intravascular volume but an excess of interstitial fluid is certainly to correct the underlying cause of interstitial volume excess. In most cases, the cause is hypoproteinemia (e.g., malabsorption, liver disease, nephrotic syndrome, protein-losing enteropathy).

In summary, most disorders of fluid balance can be treated logically and successfully with the simple principles of water and solute transfer across cell membranes. See Table 3.1 for a listing of the commonly used IV fluids.

Viruses and the House Officer

The 21st century has seen an emergence of transmissible viruses that have challenged healthcare worldwide—SARS-CoV (serious acute respiratory syndrome) in 2003, MERS (Middle East respiratory syndrome) in 2012, Ebola in 2013, and SARS-CoV-2 (COVID-19) in 2019.

As a house officer, you may be the first person in a position to recognize that a patient has a transmissible disease and is a risk to other patients, healthcare workers, and yourself. As a conscientious house officer, you will have taken advantage of the best preventive measures for yourself by being fully vaccinated. Others may not be so fortunate.

If an infectious disease is a possibility, you should ascertain the patient's vaccination status against viruses—seasonal influenza, coronavirus, hepatitis A and B, measles, as well as the bacteria—pneumococcus, Haemophilus influenzae, and meningococcus.

Predominantly Respiratory Aerosol-Transmitted Viruses

With patients suspected of having an infectious illness transmitted by respiratory aerosols, you should wear a fit-tested N95 or higher respirator in addition to gloves, gown, and face–eye protection—so-called PPE or personal protective equipment. Strict adherence to standard precautions minimizes the risk of transmission (Table 4.1).

CORONAVIRUS

The risk of transmission of the coronavirus is high. The most frequent symptoms are low-grade fever, cough, wheezing, shortness of breath, anorexia, ageusia (loss of taste), and anosmia (loss of smell). Such symptoms are similar to those of other respiratory viruses such as rhinovirus and seasonal influenza. Ageusia and anosmia may be distinguishing features. About 5% of patients presenting to

TABLE 4.1   **Recommendations for Application of Standard Precautions for the Care of All in All Healthcare Settings**

Standard precautions are recommended for the care of all patients in hospitals, regardless of their diagnosis or presumed infection status. Standard precautions apply to the following:

1. Blood
2. All body fluids, secretions, and excretions except sweat, regardless of whether they contain visible blood
3. Nonintact skin
4. Mucous membranes

Standard precautions are designed to reduce the risk of transmission of microorganisms from both recognized and unrecognized sources of infection in hospitals. Standard precautions include the following:

Component	Recommendations
Hand hygiene	Wash hands in soap and water for 30 to 45 seconds before and immediately after patient contact and after touching blood, body fluids, secretions, excretions, contaminated items; and after removing gloves
Gloves	Use for touching blood, body fluids, secretions, excretions, contaminated items; for touching mucous membranes and nonintact skin
Gown	Use during procedures and patient-care activities when contact is anticipated between clothing/exposed skin and blood/body fluids, secretions, and excretions
Mask, eye protection (goggles), face shields	During aerosol-generating procedures on patients with suspected or proven infections transmitted by respiratory aerosols (e.g., coronavirus infection: wear a fit-tested N95 or higher respirator)
Needles and other sharps	Do not recap, bend, break, or hand-manipulate used needles; if recapping is required, use a one-sided scoop technique only; use safety features when available; place used sharps in puncture-resistant container
Patient resuscitation	Use mouthpiece, resuscitation bag, other ventilation devices to prevent contact with mouth and oral secretions

TABLE 4.1	Recommendations for Application of Standard Precautions for the Care of All in All Healthcare Settings—cont'd
Component	**Recommendations**
Patient placement	Prioritize for single-patient room if patient is at increased risk of transmission, is likely to contaminate the environment, does not maintain appropriate hygiene, or is at increased risk of acquiring infection or developing adverse outcome after infection
Respiratory hygiene/cough etiquette	Instruct symptomatic persons to cover mouth/nose when coughing/sneezing; use tissues and dispose in no-touch receptacle; perform hand hygiene after soiling of hands with respiratory secretions; wear surgical mask if tolerated or maintain spatial separation, >3 feet if possible

hospital become critically ill with respiratory failure, septic shock, and multiple organ failure. However, patients may be asymptomatic or can transmit the virus before developing symptoms.

Confirmation of the diagnosis should be immediately initiated so that decisions can be made regarding appropriate preventive measures. NAATs (nucleic acid amplification tests) on nasopharyngeal secretions can provide immediate results.

There is currently no specific treatment for the asymptomatic healthcare worker who has contracted coronavirus at work. Your institution should have specific policies regarding quarantine or isolation following exposure. The potential treatments for coronavirus do not rely solely on test positivity but take into account the stage and severity of disease, with antivirals being most effective in the early stages, antibody therapy being more effective in mild/moderate illness, and anti-inflammatories playing a greater role in severe or critical illness.

Among the original antiviral agents are nirmatrevir-ritonavir, which inhibits coronavirus protease, and molnupiravir that inhibits viral DNA polymerase. The initial long-acting monoclonal antibodies are combined in the products tixagevimab/cilgavimab and bebtelovimab. Glucocorticoids (e.g., dexamethasone), Janus kinase inhibitors (e.g., baricitinib), and interleukin-6 pathway inhibitors (e.g., tocilizumab) have been used in severe illness for their immunomodulatory effects.

INFLUENZA

Influenza (flu) affects between 5% and 29% of the population of the United States every year; more than 200,000 people are hospitalized with complications of flu. Patients with diabetes, asthma, and heart disease are particularly susceptible to serious flu complications. Influenza is usually seasonal. However, in 2009, a subtype of influenza A virus, H1N1, caused a pandemic that did not respect seasons.

The symptoms suggestive of a diagnosis of flu include fever (usually high), extreme fatigue, headache, muscle aches, dry cough, sore throat, runny or stuffy nose, and—particularly in children—nausea, vomiting, and diarrhea.

If you suspect that a patient has flu, you should inform staff responsible for infection control, who will have developed protocols to control the spread of flu in the institution. This includes vaccination of healthcare workers and perhaps susceptible patients, particularly those who are elderly or infirm.

Vaccination results in a rise in antibodies after about 2 weeks. Antiviral agents provide more rapid prevention. They may also diminish the severity of the illness in a patient if given within 24 to 48 hours of onset, although they are less effective in ill, hospitalized patients. Unfortunately, the flu virus rapidly develops resistance; thus the selection of an antiviral drug may change from year to year.

Antiviral treatment is recommended for patients who are severely ill or at increased risk of complications. Neuroamidase inhibitors (oral oseltamivir, IV peramivir, and inhaled zanamivir) and the oral cap-dependent endonuclease inhibitor, baloxavir, can slightly shorten the duration of symptoms (by 1 day). To be effective the drugs must be initiated without delay. The drug of choice is oseltavir (Tamiflu) 75 mg PO bid.

Postexposure prophylaxis should be considered in healthcare personnel or patients at very high risk for influenza complications.

RESPIRATORY SYNCYTIAL VIRUS (RSV) AND HUMAN METAPNEUMOVIRUS (HMPV)

RSV and HMPV infections are seasonal illnesses like flu. They are very contagious. Frequent in children, RSV and HMPV can also infect adults. Most infected children are under 2 years of age. Most healthy children and adults have mild symptoms like those of a common cold lasting about a week. In adults over age 65 and individuals with a compromised immune system, chronic lung disease or congenital heart condition RSV and HMPV infections can lead to pneumonia and bronchiolitis.

A vaccine (AREXVY) against RSV became available in 2023.

Predominantly Blood/Body Fluid–Transmitted Viruses

Despite attention to safe practices, you may, in the course of your training, be accidentally exposed to potentially infectious blood or body fluids. The hospital should have an established policy for helping you, and you should contact the appropriate individual if you have been exposed.

Exposures that might place you at risk for HBV, HCV, HIV, or monkeypox infection include a needlestick injury, a cut from a sharp object, or contact of your mucous membranes or nonintact (cut, scraped, chapped, or inflamed) skin with blood, tissue, or other potentially infectious secretions from an individual infected with one of these viruses.

The following general guidelines are recommended if you have been exposed to blood or body fluids.

First Aid

1. Seek assistance from a more senior staff member.
2. Immediately cleanse the contaminated site.
   a. Needlestick
      i. Allow the puncture site to bleed.
      ii. Thoroughly wash the site for 2 to 4 minutes with soap and water.
   b. Skin contamination
      i. Open wound: flush the area with water or saline.
   c. Mucous membrane or eye contact
      i. Mouth: rinse with water; repeat several times.
      ii. Eyes: rinse well with water for 3 to 5 minutes.
3. Save the instrument, without washing, in a sharps container.
4. Report immediately to the designated officer responsible for helping you.

Immediate Management

Treatment of parenteral exposure (i.e., nonintact skin, mucous membrane, or skin puncture) may include the following:

1. Tetanus prophylaxis: **tetanus toxoid 0.5 mL**, if indicated
2. HBV prophylaxis after exposure (Table 4.2)
3. HIV prophylaxis after exposure
4. HCV prophylaxis after exposure

MONKEYPOX

In 2022, there were several outbreaks of Mpox (monkeypox), predominantly affecting men who have had sex with men. This febrile illness is characterized by a macular rash beginning on the face then spreading and becoming pustular. The monkeypox virus is related to the smallpox virus and can be prevented with smallpox vaccination.

| TABLE 4.2 | Prophylaxis After Parenteral Exposure to Hepatitis B Virus |

Postexposure management of healthcare personnel after occupational percutaneous or mucosal exposure to blood or body fluids, by healthcare personnel HepB vaccination and response status

	Postexposure Testing		Postexposure Prophylaxis		
HCP Status	Source Patient (HBsAg)	HCP Testing (anti-HBs)	HBIG	Vaccination	Postvaccination Serologic Testing
Documented responder after complete series	No action needed				
Documented nonresponder after two complete series	Positive/unknown	—*	HBIG × 2 separated by 1 month	—	N/A
	Negative	No action needed			
Response unknown after complete series	Positive/unknown	<10 mIU/mL	HBIG × 1	Initiate revaccination	Yes
	Negative	<10 mIU/mL	None		
	Any result	<10 mIU/mL	None	Initiate revaccination	Yes
			No action needed		
Unvaccinated/incompletely vaccinated or vaccine refusers	Positive/unknown	—	HBIG × 1	Complete vaccination	Yes
	Negative	—	None	Complete vaccination	Yes

Abbreviations: *anti-HBs* = antibody to hepatitis B surface antigen; *HBIG* = hepatitis B immune globulin; *HBsAg* = hepatitis B surface antigen; *HCP* = healthcare personnel

N/A = not applicable

*A seroprotective (adequate) level of anti-HBs after completion of a vaccination series is defined as anti-HBs ≥10 mIU/mL; a response <10 mIU/mL is inadequate and is not a reliable indicator of protection.

Adapted from: CDC Prevention of Hepatitis B Virus Infection in the United States. (2018). Recommendations of the Advisory Committee on Immunization Practices. *MMWR Recomm Rep, 67*(1).

HEPATITIS B VIRUS (HBV) EXPOSURE

The risk of transmission of the hepatitis B virus (HBV) is many times that of HIV. In the United States, hundreds of healthcare workers become infected with HBV each year. Hepatitis B vaccination is strongly recommended for all staff. A variety of antiviral drugs are available to treat hepatitis B including the antiretroviral agents entecavir (Baraclude) and tenofavir (Viread). In the event of a suspected exposure to HBV, see Table 4.2.

HUMAN IMMUNODEFICIENCY VIRUS EXPOSURE (HIV) EXPOSURE

The risk of transmission of the human immunodeficiency virus (HIV) from patient to healthcare worker is extremely low. The rate of transmission is less than 0.5% after direct inoculation of infected blood through a needlestick puncture and even lower after other types of exposures. Circumstances that may increase the risk of seroconversion include procedures involving a needle placed directly in a vein or artery, a deep injury, the presence of visible blood on the device, or a high viral load in the source patient (e.g., at the time of seroconversion or in the terminal stages of acquired immunodeficiency syndrome [AIDS]).

Infection with the human immunodeficiency virus induces an acquired immunodeficiency syndrome (HIV/AIDS). HIV/AIDS is one of the deadliest pandemics with 79 million people infected and 36 million deaths by 2022. Over 1 million people continue to be infected annually.

Initially the patient may be asymptomatic or have a flu-like illness. This is followed by a long incubation period until a variety of opportunistic infections and malignancies develop as part of the acquired immunodeficiency syndrome (AIDS). After 3 to 8 years or longer patients begin to suffer fever, weight loss, muscle pains, diarrhea, and generalized lymphadenopathy. The most common conditions that should alert you to the presence of AIDS include pneumocystis pneumonia, Kaposi's sarcoma, lymphoma, esophageal carcinoma, cachexia due to the HIV wasting syndrome, and respiratory tract infections.

A variety of antiretroviral drugs are available for treatment as well as for post- and pre-exposure prophylaxis. Procedures for assessing the source person vary among institutions. Current recommendations differ slightly, depending on whether the exposure involves a percutaneous injury, mucous membranes, or nonintact skin. Therapy should be initiated as soon as possible, preferably within 1 to 2 hours after exposure, and should involve three or more antiretroviral drugs. Choosing a drug regimen based on the severity of exposure is no longer recommended. The choice of agents to use is empirically based. Resistance of the source virus (suspected in a source patient if there has been progression of disease, increasing viral load, or a fall in CD4+ T-cell count despite therapy) to specific antiretroviral drugs may influence the choice of agents for postexposure prophylaxis. If it is unclear which agents to choose, then it is best to begin with a three-drug regimen immediately, obtain consultation, and modify the regimen later as more information becomes available. Postexposure prophylaxis should be started as soon as possible after exposure when indicated. The preferred three-drug regimen is *emtricitabine (Emtriva) 200 mg daily plus tenofovir (Viread) 300 mg daily (the two are available as a combination tablet, Truvada), plus raltegravir (Isentress) 400 mg twice a day (BID) or Dolutegravir (Tivicay) 50 mg once daily*. Other antiretrovirals are available but should be used only after consulting an expert in this field. One month of therapy is recommended. Raltegravir can cause headaches, nausea, fatigue, diarrhea, itching, and rash. The tenofovir/emtricitabine combination can produce nausea, diarrhea, and headache.

In the absence of a postexposure prophylaxis policy or of knowledge among senior staff at your hospital, a good resource is the National Clinicians' Post-Exposure Prophylaxis Hotline (PEPline) 1-888-448-4911.

HEPATITIS C VIRUS (HCV) EXPOSURE

The risk of seroconversion after percutaneous exposure to hepatitis C virus (HCV) is very low, in the range of 1.8%.

Current guidelines do not support the use of antiviral agents in the postexposure prophylaxis of HCV. After a potential exposure, the source patient should be tested for the presence of hepatitis C antibody (anti-HCV), and if positive, additional testing for HCV RNA should be performed. If the source patient is anti-HCV negative or is anti-HCV positive but has undetectable levels of HCV RNA, then no further evaluation of the healthcare worker is necessary. If the source patient has active hepatitis C, then the healthcare worker should consult a physician knowledgeable in the risk of transmission of HCV for further advice.

Hepatitis C infection is often asymptomatic; however, it can lead to the development of cirrhosis and hepatocellular carcinoma. A variety of antivirals, direct-acting agents (DAAs) that target viral proteins, are available for treatment (see Formulary Anti-hepatitis C agents).

EBOLA VIRUS

The Ebola virus (named after the river site where it originated) differs from the coronavirus in being spread by contact with body fluids, thus being less easily transmitted.

The first symptoms are fever, sore throat, muscle pain, and headache. These are usually followed by vomiting, diarrhea, rash, and hepatic and renal failure. Finally, some patients suffer internal and external hemorrhages. Mortality rates vary from 25% to 90%, ushered in by shock from fluid loss that occurs between 6 and 16 days after the first symptoms. The largest outbreak was in Africa in 2016; however, sporadic cases have appeared elsewhere on the Congo. Currently the disease is limited to subtropical Africa. At the time of this writing, there is no approved form of postexposure prophylaxis. Experimental therapies are in development, and in the event of a known exposure, advice should be sought from a filovirus expert. Although current treatment consists of supportive measures, early detection is important to minimize intravascular volume depletion, correct electrolyte disorders, and provide nutritional support.

MPOX (MONKEYPOX)

Endemic in the Congo and Nigeria, an outbreak due to the Mpox virus began in Western Europe and North America in 2022. After a febrile period with constitutional symptoms, a diffuse and sometimes painful rash develops that progresses through stages to become bullous then pustular with scab formation. The disease is largely spread through sexual contact between homosexual men but may be contracted by contact with the rash in infected individuals. Imvamune vaccine (a modified small pox vaccine) is effective in postexposure administration in individuals at high risk (Table 4.3 and Table 4.4).

TABLE 4.3	Vaccinations Recommended for Healthcare Workers

Hepatitis B
If you don't have documented evidence of a complete hepB vaccine series, or if you don't have a blood test that shows you are immune to hepatitis B (i.e., no serologic evidence of immunity or prior vaccination), then you should
- Get a three-dose series of Recombivax HB or Engerix-B (dose #1 now, #2 in 1 month, #3 approximately 5 months after #2) or a two-dose series of Heplisav-B, with the doses separated by at least 4 weeks.
- Get an anti-HBs serologic test 1-2 months after the final dose.

Influenza virus
Get one dose of influenza vaccine annually.
If you were born in 1957 or later and have not had the MMR vaccine, or if you don't have a blood test that shows you are immune to measles or mumps (i.e., no serologic evidence of immunity or prior vaccination), get two doses of MMR (one dose now and the second dose at least 28 days later).

Mumps, measles, and rubella
If you were born in 1957 or later and have not had the MMR vaccine, or if you don't have a blood test that shows you are immune to rubella, only one dose of MMR is recommended.

Continued

TABLE 4.3	Vaccinations Recommended for Healthcare Workers—cont'd

Varicella (Chickenpox)
If you have not had chickenpox (varicella), if you haven't had varicella vaccine, or if you don't have a blood test that shows you are immune to varicella (i.e., no serologic evidence of immunity or prior vaccination), get two doses of varicella vaccine, 4 weeks apart.

Tetanus, diphtheria, pertussis
Get a one-time dose of Tdap as soon as possible if you have not received Tdap previously.
Get either a Td or Tdap booster shot every 10 years thereafter.

Neisseria meningitidis
If you are in an environment where meningitis is endemic (e.g., college dorms), you should get meningococcal conjugate vaccine and serogroup B meningococcal vaccine.

TABLE 4.4	Vaccines	

Vaccine		Duration of Immunity
Viruses		
COVID-19		Variable, months rather than years
MERS-CoV		Under development
Diphtheria, Tetanus, Pertussis	DTP	10 years
Dengue fever	CYD-TDV	Lifelong
Hepatitis A	HepA	At least 30 years
Hepatitis B	HepB	At least 30 years
Herpes Zoster (Shingles)	RZV	Declines after 5-10 years
Human Papilloma Virus	HPV	At least 30 years
Influenza (Flu)	LAIV	3-6 months
Measles, Mumps, Rubella	MMR	Lifelong
Monkey pox	Imvamune	? 2 years
Polio		Lifelong
RSV	AREXVY	not known
Smallpox		30-40 years
Varicella (Chickenpox)	V VAP	10-20 years
Yellow fever		Lifelong
Bacteria		
Hemophilus influenzae Type Bacteria	Hib	Years
Meningococcus	MenACWY	3-5 years
Pneumococcus	PPSV223	10 years

Useful URLs
Coronavirus treatment www.fda/gov/drugs
Infection control guidelines https://ipac-canada.org/evidence-based-guidelines
www.cdc.gov/infection-control

Patient-Related Problems: The Common Calls

Abdominal Pain

Many patients complain of abdominal pain during their hospital stays. It is essential to distinguish the acute abdominal emergency from the recurrent nonemergency. The former necessitates urgent medical or surgical intervention, whereas the latter necessitates thorough but less urgent investigation. Avoid ordering analgesic agents until a preliminary diagnosis has been made. Narcotic analgesic agents may mask the physical findings of an acute abdomen and thereby delay recognition and treatment of a serious intra-abdominal disorder.

PHONE CALL

Questions

1. How severe is the patient's pain?
2. Is the pain localized or generalized?
3. What are the patient's vital signs?

   Fever and abdominal pain are suggestive of intra-abdominal infection or inflammation.

   Hypotension or tachycardia, in association with abdominal pain, suggests intra-abdominal or retroperitoneal hemorrhage, necrosis of a viscus, or intra-abdominal sepsis.
4. Is this pain a new problem?
5. Why was the patient admitted?
6. Is the patient taking steroids or other antiinflammatory drugs?

   Steroids may mask the pain and fever of an inflammatory process, which may lead you to underestimate the nature or severity of a patient's abdominal pain. If the patient is taking steroids, even mild abdominal pain should be assessed soon.

Orders

If the abdominal pain is mild and the vital signs are normal, ask the registered nurse (RN) to call you immediately if the pain becomes worse before you are able to assess the patient.

Informing the Registered Nurse

Tell the RN, "I will arrive at the bedside in … minutes."

If the abdominal pain has an acute onset, is severe, or is associated with fever or hypotension, you must see the patient immediately. Mild recurrent abdominal pain is a less urgent problem and may be assessed in an hour or two if you have other patients with higher-priority problems.

ELEVATOR THOUGHTS

What causes abdominal pain?

The causes of *localized abdominal pain* are numerous. A useful system for approaching the problem is *diagnosis by location.* Fig. 5.1 illustrates a differential diagnosis by location.

The causes of *generalized abdominal pain* are fewer. These are listed in the key to Fig. 5.1. Disorders producing either localized or generalized pain are indicated in the key to Fig. 5.1 by an asterisk.

MAJOR THREAT TO LIFE

- Perforated or ruptured viscus
- Ascending cholangitis
- Necrosis of a viscus
- Exsanguinating hemorrhage
- Myocardial infarction
- Aortic dissection

A perforated or ruptured viscus may result in hypovolemic shock (from third-space losses), septic shock (from bacterial peritonitis), or both. Progression of infection from an initial localized site (e.g. ascending cholangitis) to septic shock may occur rapidly (i.e., within hours of the patient's first presenting symptom). Necrosis of a viscus, as in severe pancreatitis, intussusception, volvulus, strangulated hernia, or ischemic colitis, may cause hypovolemic or septic shock and electrolyte and acid-base disturbances. Exsanguinating hemorrhage with hypovolemic shock may result from a leaking abdominal aortic aneurysm, a ruptured ectopic pregnancy, or a splenic rupture; the cause is occasionally iatrogenic, such as a liver or renal biopsy or a misdirected thoracentesis.

Patients with myocardial infarction and aortic dissection occasionally present with abdominal pain. These cardiovascular diagnoses should be considered, especially if no local abdominal signs can be identified.

BEDSIDE

Quick-Look Test

Does the patient look well (comfortable), sick (uncomfortable or distressed), or critical (about to die)?

Appearances are often deceptive in acute abdominal disease. If the patient has recently received narcotic analgesics or high-dose steroids, they may appear well despite a serious underlying problem.

Patients with severe colic are often restless; those with peritonitis, in contrast, lie immobile, avoiding movement that exacerbates the pain. With peritonitis, patients may have their knees drawn up to reduce abdominal tension.

Airway and Vital Signs

What is the blood pressure?

Hypotension associated with abdominal pain is an ominous sign suggestive of impending hypovolemic, hemorrhagic, or septic shock.

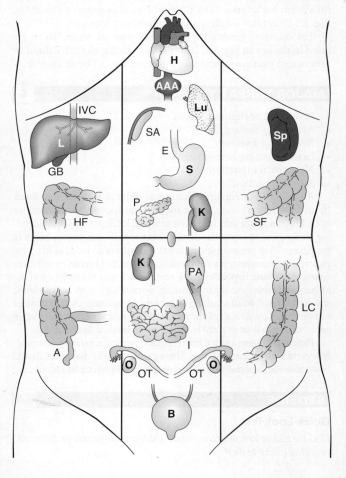

FIG. 5.1 **Differential diagnosis by abdominal quadrant.** Key: Right upper quadrant: *GB*, gallbladder (cholecystitis, steatosis, cholangitis, choledocholithiasis); *HF*, hepatic flexure [obstruction]; venous obstruction (*IVC*, inferior vena cava (Budd-Chiari syndrome), portal vein thrombosis); *HZ,* herpes zoster; *L*, liver (hepatitis, abscess, perihepatitis). Right lower quadrant: *A*, appendix (appendicitis,* abscess); *O*, ovary (torsion, ruptured cyst, carcinoma); *HZ,* herpes zoster. Left upper quadrant: *Sp,* spleen (rupture, infarct, abscess), *SF*, splenic flexure (obstruction); *HZ,* herpes zoster. Left lower quadrant: *LC*, left colon (diverticulitis, ischemic colitis); *O*, ovary (torsion, ruptured cyst, carcinoma); *HZ,* herpes zoster. Epigastrium: *AAA*, abdominal aortic aneurysm; *E,* esophagus (gastroesophageal reflux disease); *H*, heart (myocardial infarction, pericarditis, aortic dissection); *K*, kidney (pyelonephritis, renal colic); *Lu*, lung (pneumonia, pleurisy); *P*, pancreas (pancreatitis); *S*, stomach and duodenum (peptic ulcer, gastroparesis); *SA*, subphrenic abscess. Hypogastrium: *B,* bladder (cystitis, urinary retention); *I*, intestine (infection,* obstruction,* inflammatory bowel disease*); *K*, kidney (renal colic); *O*, ovary (torsion, ruptured cyst, carcinoma); *OT*, ovarian tube (ectopic pregnancy, salpingitis, endometriosis); *PA*, psoas abscess. Generalized abdominal pain: (1) See conditions marked with an asterisk (*), (2) peritonitis (any cause), (3) diabetic ketoacidosis, (4) sickle cell crisis, (5) acute intermittent porphyria, and (6) acute adrenocortical insufficiency resulting from steroid withdrawal.

Does the patient have postural changes (lying and standing) in the blood pressure and heart rate?

If the supine blood pressure is normal, recheck the blood pressure and heart rate with the patient standing.

📖 A drop in blood pressure that is associated with an increased heart rate (>15 beats/minute) is suggestive of volume depletion.

What is the temperature?

Fever associated with abdominal pain is suggestive of intra-abdominal infection or inflammation. However, lack of fever in an elderly patient or in a patient receiving an antipyretic or immuno-suppressive drug does not rule out infection.

Selective History and Chart Review

Diagnosis is often dependent on a careful history that addresses the following issues:

1. The pain at onset and its subsequent progression
2. Any associated symptoms
3. The past medical history

Pain

Is the pain localized?

The location of the pain's maximum intensity can provide a clue to the site of origin (see Fig. 5.1). Remember that a patient may complain of diffuse abdominal pain, but on careful examination the pain may be found to be localized.

Does the patient characterize the pain as severe or mild, burning or knifelike, or constant or waxing-and-waning, as in colic?

Pain associated with certain diseases has characteristic descriptions. The pain of a peptic ulcer tends to be burning, whereas that of a perforated ulcer is sudden, constant, and severe. The pain of biliary colic is sharp and constricting ("taking one's breath away"); that of acute pancreatitis is deep and agonizing; and that of obstructed bowel is gripping, with intermittent worsening.

Did the pain develop gradually or suddenly?

The severe pain of colic (renal, biliary, or intestinal) develops within hours. An acute onset with fainting is suggestive of perforation of a viscus, ruptured ectopic pregnancy, torsion of an ovarian cyst, or a leaking abdominal aortic aneurysm.

Has the pain changed since its onset?

A ruptured viscus may be initially associated with localized pain that subsequently shifts or becomes generalized, with the development of chemical or bacterial peritonitis.

Does the pain radiate?

Pain radiates to the dermatome or cutaneous areas that are supplied by the same sensory cortical cells that supply the deep-seated structure (Fig. 5.2). For example, the diaphragm is supplied by cervical roots C3, C4, and C5. Many upper abdominal or lower

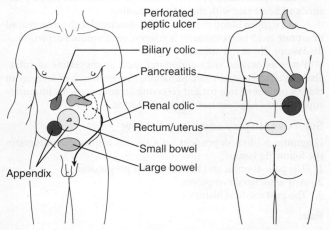

FIG. 5.2 **Common sites of referred pain.**

thoracic conditions that cause irritation of the diaphragm refer pain to the cutaneous supply of C3, C4, and C5 (i.e., the shoulder and neck). The liver and gallbladder are derived from the right seventh and eighth thoracic segments. Thus in biliary colic, pain is frequently referred to the inferior angle of the right scapula. The pain of pancreatitis may radiate to the midback or scapula.

Does the patient have any aggravating or alleviating factors?

Pain that increases with meals, decreases with passage of bowel movements, or does both is suggestive of a hollow viscera origin. An exception is pain from a duodenal ulcer, which is often relieved by the ingestion of food. The pain of pancreatitis is often worse after eating and may be relieved by sitting up or leaning forward. Pain that increases with inspiration is suggestive of pleuritis or peritonitis, and pain that is aggravated by micturition is suggestive of a urogenital cause.

Associated Symptoms

Does the patient have nausea or vomiting?

Vomiting that occurs with the onset of pain frequently accompanies both acute peritoneal irritation and perforation of a viscus. It is also commonly associated with acute pancreatitis and with obstruction of any muscular hollow viscus. Pain relieved by vomiting suggests a hollow viscera origin (e.g., bowel obstruction). Vomiting many hours after the onset of abdominal pain may be a clue to intestinal obstruction or ileus.

What is the nature of emesis?

Brown, feculent emesis is pathognomonic of bowel obstruction, either paralytic or mechanical. Frank blood is suggestive of upper gastrointestinal bleeding, either from peptic ulcer disease or esophageal varices and portal hypertensive gastropathy as may be seen in Budd-Chiari syndrome. Vomiting food after fasting is consistent with gastric stasis or gastric outlet obstruction.

Does the patient have diarrhea?

Diarrhea and abdominal pain are observed in infectious gastroenteritis, ischemic colitis, appendicitis, and partial small bowel obstruction. Acute portal vein thrombosis sometimes involves the superior mesenteric vein, and these patients may have diarrhea. Diarrhea alternating with constipation is a common symptom of diverticular disease.

Does the patient have fever or chills?

Fever and chills that accompany abdominal pain are suggestive of an intra-abdominal infection. Check the record of temperature since admission. Also check the medication sheet for antipyretic or

steroid use; remember that fever may be masked by the administration of these medications.

Past History and Chart Review

*Does the patient have a history of peptic ulcer disease or antacid
ingestion?*

Peptic ulcer disease is a chronic, recurring disease. If the
patient has a history of peptic ulcer, check for the presence of
a new one.

*Does the patient have a history of blunt or penetrating trauma to
the abdomen? Has there been a liver or kidney biopsy or has thoracentesis been performed since admission?*

A subcapsular hemorrhage of the spleen, liver, or kidney may
result in hemorrhagic shock 1 to 3 days later.

Does the patient have a history of alcohol abuse and ascites?

Spontaneous bacterial peritonitis must always be considered in
an alcoholic patient with ascites and fever.

*Does the patient have a history of coronary or peripheral vascular
disease?*

Atherosclerosis is a diffuse process and may affect the vascular
supply to several body systems. In addition to the possibility of a
myocardial infarction that manifests with abdominal pain, you
should consider a leaking abdominal aortic aneurysm, aortic dissection, and ischemic colitis caused by atherosclerosis of the mesenteric
arteries.

*If the patient is a premenopausal woman, what was the date of
her last normal menstrual period?*

Abdominal pain associated with a missed period raises the possibility of an ectopic pregnancy. Hypotension in this situation is
suggestive of a ruptured fallopian tube as the result of an ectopic
pregnancy, which is a life-threatening situation.

*Does the patient have a history of previous abdominal
surgery?*

Adhesions are responsible for 70% of bowel obstructions.

Has the patient received drugs that affect blood clotting?

Intra-abdominal hemorrhage may occur in the anticoagulated patient, especially if the patient has a history of peptic ulcer
disease.

*Does the patient have a history of use of aspirin or nonsteroidal
antiinflammatory drugs, alcohol, or other ulcerogenic drug?*

Peptic ulcer should be a consideration in a patient who has
been taking one or more of these agents.

Does the patient have a prothrombotic disorder?

Recent abdominal surgery, malignancy, cirrhosis, pregnancy, oral
contraceptive use, inflammatory disorders (e.g., collagen vascular

disease, inflammatory bowel disease), and inherited thrombophilic disorders are risks for hepatic or portal vein thrombosis.

Selective Physical Examination

Vitals	Repeat measurements now
Head, ears, eyes, nose, and throat (HEENT)	Icterus (cholangitis, choledocholithiasis)
	Spider nevi (risk of spontaneous bacterial peritonitis if ascites is present)
Respiratory system	Generalized or localized restriction of abdominal wall movement in respiration (localized or generalized peritoneal inflammation)
	Stony dullness to percussion, decreased breath sounds, decreased tactile fremitus (pleural effusion)
	Dullness to percussion, diminished or bronchial breath sounds, crackles (consolidation and pneumonia)
Cardiovascular system (CVS)	Decreased jugulovenous pressure (JVP) (volume depletion)
	New onset of dysrhythmia or mitral insufficiency murmur (myocardial infarction)
ABD	Before examining the abdomen, make sure that your hands are warm and the head of the bed is flat. It may be helpful to flex the patient's hips to relax the abdominal wall. When examining for tenderness, begin in a nonpainful region. Watch the patient's face as you examine for the following:

- Visible peristalsis (bowel obstruction)
- Bulging flanks (ascites)
- Hepatomegaly (Budd-Chiari syndrome)
- Loss of liver dullness (perforated viscus)
- Localized tenderness, masses (see Fig. 5.1)
- Rigid abdomen, guarding, rebound tenderness (peritonitis)
- Shifting dullness, fluid wave (ascites)
- Absent bowel sounds (paralytic ileus or late bowel obstruction)
- All hernia orifices (strangulated hernia) (Fig. 5.3)
- Murphy's sign (cholecystitis) (Fig. 5.4)
- Psoas sign (appendicitis) (Fig. 5.5)
- Obturator sign (appendicitis) (Fig. 5.6)
- Skin unilateral maculopapular rash or vesicles in a dermatomal pattern (herpes zoster)

Rectal   Tenderness (retrocecal appendicitis,
                      prostatitis)
                   Mass (rectal carcinoma)
                   Rectal fissure (Crohn's disease)
                   Stool positive for occult blood (ischemic
                      colitis, peptic ulcer)

Pelvic   Tenderness (ectopic pregnancy, ovarian
                      cyst, pelvic inflammatory disease)
                   Mass (ovarian cyst or tumor)

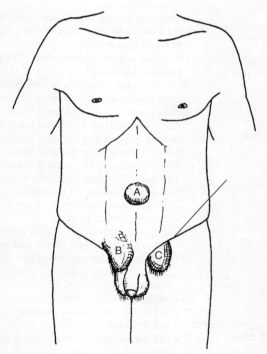

FIG. 5.3 Hernial orifices. *A,* Umbilical hernia; *B,* inguinal hernia; *C,* femoral hernia. Note that the bulge of the inguinal hernia begins superiorly to the inguinal ligament, whereas the bulge of the femoral hernia originates inferiorly to the inguinal ligament.

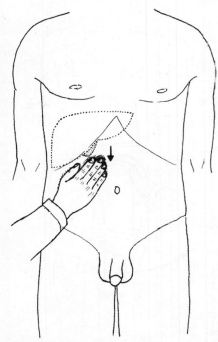

FIG. 5.4 Examination for Murphy's sign. Murphy's sign is manifested by pain and inspiratory arrest when the patient takes a deep breath while the examiner applies pressure against the abdominal wall in the region of the gallbladder. Murphy's sign is often observed in the presence of cholecystitis.

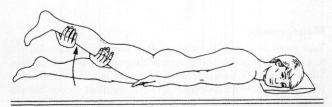

FIG. 5.5 Examination for psoas sign. A psoas sign is manifested by abdominal pain in response to passive hip extension. (This test may also be performed with the patient lying on the side.) This sign is often observed in patients with appendicitis or a psoas abscess.

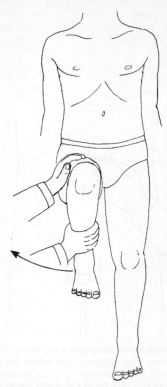

FIG. 5.6 Examination for obturator sign. An obturator sign is manifested by abdominal pain in response to passive internal rotation of the right hip from the 90-degree hip-knee flexion position when the patient is supine. This sign is often observed in patients with appendicitis.

Management

Your assessment and investigation thus far may not have led you to a specific diagnosis of the cause of the patient's abdominal pain. You will, however, have determined from the physical examination whether the patient has developed shock, the most serious complication from disorders that cause abdominal pain.

Shock

For either hypovolemic or septic shock, the initial treatment is the same and is aimed at immediate expansion of the intravascular volume:

1. Rapid volume repletion can be achieved with the use of 500 to 1000 mL of normal saline, Ringer's lactate, or other crystalloid intravenously as rapidly as possible, followed by an intravenous (IV) rate titrated to the JVP and vital signs. In this situation, IV fluids should be given through a large-bore peripheral IV or central line.

2. Blood should be drawn for a "stat" crossmatch for 4 to 6 U of packed red blood cells (RBCs), for a platelet count, and to measure hemoglobin, prothrombin time, and activated partial thromboplastin time. Baseline values of electrolytes, urea, creatinine, blood glucose, and amylase; a white blood cell (WBC) count; and manual differential are also useful. Two sets of blood cultures should be drawn if septic shock is suspected.

3. If hemorrhagic shock is suspected, packed RBCs should be given in place of, or in addition to, the crystalloid, normal saline, or Ringer's lactate as soon as the crossmatch has been completed. In extreme circumstances, O-negative blood may be used during the wait for the crossmatched supply.

4. When shock occurs in the setting of a disorder causing abdominal pain, urgent surgical consultation is almost always required. Ensure that the patient has nothing by mouth (NPO status). Consider inserting a nasogastric tube if the patient is vomiting.

5. As resuscitation measures are being initiated, additional investigations can be arranged, as follows:

   a. Order an ultrasound of the abdomen. An ultrasound is the initial imaging test of choice for patients with upper right quadrant pain. Computed tomography (CT) is recommended for right or left lower quadrant pain.

   b. Conventional radiography has limited value in the diagnosis of abdominal pain. However, if more advanced imaging is not available, order three radiographic views of the abdomen (anteroposterior abdomen in supine and either erect or lateral decubitus positions and posteroanterior chest in erect position). If the patient looks unwell or critical, these radiographs must be obtained on a stat portable basis. Examine the radiographs for the following conditions:

      i. Toxic megacolon is manifested by an increase in diameter of the midtransverse colon (>7 cm) and a mucosal pattern of thumbprinting or thickening. This condition is a medical or surgical emergency.

      ii. Air that is visible under the diaphragm in the chest film or between the viscera and subcutaneous tissue in the lateral decubitus film is indicative of a perforated viscus.

      iii. Air-fluid levels are suggestive of bowel obstruction or ileus.

    iv. Calcified gallstones could be a cause of cholecystitis or pancreatitis.

    v. Pancreatic calcifications, if present, may be a clue that the patient is having a recurrent attack of chronic pancreatitis.

  c. If septic shock is suspected, specimens for Gram stain, culture, and sensitivity testing should be obtained immediately from sputum, if available; from urine, for which catheterization may be required; and from wounds. If ascites is present, an immediate diagnostic paracentesis should be performed.

In a case of suspected septic shock, once culture specimens have been obtained, therapy with empirical broad-spectrum antibiotics should be started immediately to treat infection with coliforms and gut anaerobes. Commonly used broad-spectrum regimens include one of the following: a third- or fourth-generation cephalosporin plus metronidazole or vancomycin; a betalactam/betalactamase inhibitor (e.g., ticarcillin-clavulanate or piperacillin-tazobactam); or a carbapenem (e.g., imipenem or meropenem).

Acute Surgical Abdomen

If the patient is not in shock or has been successfully resuscitated from shock, you must consider the possible underlying conditions responsible for the complaint of abdominal pain. Of utmost importance at this point is to determine whether the patient has an acute *surgical* abdomen (i.e., necessitating surgery). Look for the following:

- *Perforated or ruptured viscus.* The presence of air under the diaphragm on the upright chest radiograph or between the viscera and subcutaneous tissue on the lateral decubitus film is indicative of a perforated or ruptured viscus. Immediate surgical consultation is required. Ensure that the patient's status is NPO.
- *Intra-Abdominal hemorrhage.* An intra-abdominal hemorrhage almost always necessitates immediate surgical consultation. Ensure that the patient is kept on NPO status and that blood has been sent for a stat crossmatch for 4 to 6 U of packed RBCs.
- *Ruptured intra-abdominal abscess.* An intra-abdominal abscess that has ruptured often results in acute peritonitis and, if left untreated, may lead to septic shock. Urgent surgical consultation for proper drainage is required. Ensure that the patient is kept on NPO status.
- *Necrosis of a viscus.* Necrosis of an intra-abdominal viscus as a result of intussusception, volvulus, strangulated hernia, or ischemic colitis necessitates urgent surgical consultation. Ensure that the patient is kept on NPO status.

Other Conditions

Other conditions that may not cause an acute surgical abdomen are common and should be considered if none of the previously mentioned conditions is present. Each condition has features that mandate specific attention from the physician on call.

- *Pancreatitis* should be suspected in any patient with abdominal pain but no evidence of upper gastrointestinal bleeding or ascites. The abdominal x-ray films may reveal a sentinel loop, colonic distention, left pleural effusion, or calcification within the pancreas (Fig. 5.7). An elevated level of serum amylase or lipase supports the diagnosis, but normal levels do not exclude the possibility of pancreatitis. Abdominal imaging with a computed tomographic (CT) scan, magnetic resonance imaging (MRI), or ultrasonography is helpful in confirming the diagnosis and is especially important in the patient with severe abdominal pain, fever, or marked leukocytosis, in whom necrotizing pancreatitis or a pancreatic abscess should be suspected. The patient's status should be NPO. IV fluids with normal saline should be ordered to replace any losses. Narcotic analgesic agents are usually required. **Meperidine (Demerol), 50 to 150 mg intramuscularly (IM) or subcutaneously (SC) every 3 to 4 hours (as needed)**, is the drug of choice. In cases of severe pancreatitis with sepsis, abscess formation, or generalized

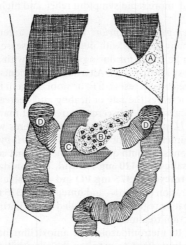

FIG. 5.7 Locations of radiographic features of pancreatitis. *A,* Left pleural effusion; *B,* calcification within the pancreas; *C,* sentinel loop; *D,* colonic distention.

peritonitis, broad-spectrum antibiotics directed against bowel flora are appropriate, and surgical consultation is indicated.

- *Contained intra-abdominal abscess* requires delineation by ultrasonography, CT scan, or MRI. This can be arranged in the morning, if the patient is otherwise stable. Abscesses may be treated with ultrasonographically guided percutaneous drainage, surgical drainage, or antibiotics alone, depending on the circumstance.

- *Peptic ulcer disease or gastroesophageal reflux disease* (GERD). Cases of suspected peptic ulcer disease or GERD should be considered for endoscopy, particularly if the patient has so-called alarm features such as bleeding, anemia, dysphagia, odynophagia, persistent vomiting, or weight loss. Antisecretory agents may be initiated on call, even before the patient has undergone endoscopy. Proton pump inhibitors (PPIs) are common initial therapy for both conditions, and once-daily dosing before breakfast is effective. The six generally available PPIs are similar in effectiveness: **omeprazole (Losec and generic preparations), 20 mg orally (PO); esomeprazole (Nexium), 20 mg; lansoprazole (Zoton), 15 mg; pantoprazole (Protium), 40 mg; dexlansoprazole (Kapidex, Dexilant) 30 mg; and rabeprazole (Pariet and generic preparations), 20 mg.** These drugs are expensive; costs can be reduced by using generic formulations. PPIs are preferable to H2-receptor antagonists in treatment of peptic ulcer disease because of their greater acid suppression, more rapid symptom relief, and higher ulcer healing rates.

- *Helicobacter pylori.* H. pylori infection is a remediable risk factor in many patients with peptic ulcer disease. *H. pylori* infection can be tested for during endoscopy with a urea biopsy test or biopsy for histology. Alternatively, patients can be tested with the urea breath test (UBT) or stool antigen. Eradication of *H. pylori* increases the rate of healing and decreases the likelihood of recurrence. Antisecretory treatment may suppress the growth of *H. pylori* to a degree that interferes with the UBT. Several regimens exist for the treatment of *H. pylori.* The preferred option is bismuth quadruple therapy that consists of **bismuth subsalicylate 420 mg PO qid, metronidazole 375 mg PO qid, tetracycline 375 mg PO qid**—available as a prepackaged preparation (Pylera)—and **omeprazole 375 mg PO bid or qid.** Alternative regimens are detailed in the Formulary (see *H. pylori* infection treatments).

Resistance to metronidazole and amoxicillin has developed; therefore it is important to monitor the sensitivities of *H. pylori* locally. When you encounter a patient in whom peptic ulcer disease is suspected, empirical triple therapy of *H. pylori* is not recommended; this should be reserved for patients in whom peptic ulcer disease is confirmed by endoscopy or in whom *H. pylori* infection is confirmed.

- *Pyelonephritis.* Pyelonephritis associated with severe systemic symptoms such as high fever, chills, and impending shock necessitates immediate blood and urine cultures and empirical IV antibiotics such as a carbapenem (e.g., imipenem or meropenem) and vancomycin until the specific organism has been identified.

- *Renal colic.* Patients with severe pain from renal stones may be managed in the acute phase with IV hydration to increase urine output and with morphine, 3 mg IV, repeated (usually once or twice) as needed. Diclofenac, 75 mg IM or 100 mg rectally, may be a useful adjunctive measure. Surgical removal, basket extraction, or lithotripsy may be required if the stone has not passed within a few days or if an associated infection persists.

- *Infectious gastroenteritis.* Patients with infectious gastroenteritis may require specific antibiotics if the results of the stool culture reveal a bacterial cause. Viral gastroenteritis is treated supportively with IV fluids and antiemetics. *Clostridium difficile* infection should be suspected in any patient who develops diarrhea during or after a course of antibiotics. Sigmoidoscopy may reveal a characteristic pseudomembrane, in which case the inciting antibiotic should be stopped. Metronidazole (Flagyl), 250 to 500 mg PO tid or qid, vancomycin (Vancocin), 125 PO qid, or fidaxomicin (Dificid), 200 mg PO bid, may be instituted before confirmation by *C. difficile* culture or toxin assay.

- *Hepatic venous outflow tract obstruction (Budd-Chiari syndrome).* Treatment for Budd-Chiari syndrome is aimed at restoring hepatic venous flow. If the obstruction is due to thrombosis, therapies may include thrombolysis, anticoagulation, angioplasty and stenting, transjugular intrahepatic portosystemic shunt (TIPS), or surgical shunting. When on call, if you suspect Budd-Chiari syndrome in a patient with abdominal pain, provide analgesia and organize appropriate bloodwork (CBC, transaminases, PT, albumin), an abdominal ultrasound, and referral to a gastroenterologist or surgeon.

- *Acute portal vein thrombosis.* In patients suspected of acute portal vein thrombosis, an abdominal ultrasound, abdominal CT, or MRI scan is usually diagnostic. Referral to a gastroenterologist or surgeon experienced in management of this condition is important. Thrombolysis and surgical thrombectomy are sometimes required, but the usual treatment is anticoagulation. Some patients with acute portal vein thrombosis also have cirrhosis, and UGI endoscopy to exclude esophageal varices is often done before initiating anticoagulation.

- *Ovarian cyst, tumor, or salpingitis.* These conditions are best managed by referral to a gynecologist.

Abdominal Pain in the Immunocompromised Patient

Symptoms such as chronic abdominal pain, nausea, and vomiting are common in the critically ill immunocompromised patients including those with malignancy, HIV-AIDS, an organ or bone marrow transplant, as well as patients on immunosuppressive drugs.

The following special features are pertinent in the evaluation of abdominal pain in a patient with immune suppression:

1. Fever is a sensitive sign of infection in a patient with immune suppression. Unfortunately, it is a nonspecific finding and may be due to nonabdominal occult infections. In patients who are immunocompromised who have temperatures of 38.5°C or higher, blood cultures should be drawn twice, although frequently no causative agent is isolated.
2. Enteric infections are common causes of abdominal pain (usually cramping in quality and associated with diarrhea); they include enteritis caused by *Cryptosporidium, Shigella, Salmonella, Cytomegalovirus,* and *Campylobacter* organisms.
3. Patients with immune suppression commonly have leukopenia. Thus even a normal WBC level, especially if accompanied by an increase in band cells ("left shift"), should be interpreted as a sign of possible infection in a patient with immune suppression who has fever and abdominal pain. Neutropenic enterocolitis (typhlitis), consisting of transmural inflammation and submucosal hemorrhage in the cecum or ascending colon, is associated with severe abdominal pain in immunocompromised patients.
4. Acalculous cholecystitis is relatively common. However, gallbladder disease may also be caused by infections with *Cryptosporidium* organisms, *Cytomegalovirus* organisms, or *Mycobacterium avium–intracellulare.*

Abdominal Pain in Elderly Patients

Abdominal pain in an elderly patient should be investigated and managed as in other patients. Of note in elderly patients is that abdominal pain may be very mild despite the presence of an acute abdomen. You should not underestimate the seriousness of mild abdominal pain in an elderly patient, especially if it is associated with acute confusion, fever, elevated WBC level, or metabolic acidosis.

Two conditions causing abdominal pain that are usually confined to elderly persons are colonic perforation as a result of diverticular disease and mesenteric ischemia as a result of atherosclerosis.

Chest Pain

In developed countries, where coronary artery disease is the leading cause of death, it is logical that when a patient complains of chest pain, you wonder whether he or she has an *acute coronary syndrome*. This term refers to a range of acute myocardial ischemic states and encompasses unstable angina, non-ST-segment elevation myocardial infarction (NSTEMI), and ST-segment elevation myocardial infarction (STEMI). There are also several other, equally serious causes of chest pain that may go undiagnosed if you do not specifically look for them. In the assessment of chest pain, history taking is your most powerful tool.

PHONE CALL

Questions

1. How severe is the patient's pain?
2. What are the patient's vital signs?
3. Why was the patient admitted?
4. Does the patient have a history of angina or myocardial infarction (MI)? If so, is the pain similar to that of his or her usual angina or the previous MI?

Orders

If acute coronary syndrome is suspected, order the following:
1. Electrocardiogram (ECG) stat
2. Pulse oximetry reading

   If pulse oximetry is available, and the oxygen saturation level is 93% or less, supplemental oxygen should be given to maintain a saturation of 94% or more. If pulse oximetry is unavailable, **oxygen by face mask or nasal prongs at 4 L/minute** can be initiated until you are able to assess the patient at the bedside. If the patient is a carbon dioxide (CO_2) retainer, you must be cautious when giving oxygen; in this case it is best to limit the initial **fraction of inspired oxygen [FiO_2] to 0.28 by mask or 2 L/minute by nasal prongs**.

3. Insert an IV. Intravenous access may be needed to deliver medications and fluids.

   Nitroglycerin, 0.3 to 0.6 mg sublingually every 5 minutes, provided there is no contraindication. Contraindications include recent (within 24 to 48 hours) ingestion of a phosphodiesterase-5 enzyme inhibitor, a systolic blood pressure less than 90 mm Hg, a heart rate less than 50/minute or greater than 100/minute, hypertrophic cardiomyopathy, severe aortic stenosis, and suspected right ventricular infarct. In most cases you will not be able to determine whether the patient has a right ventricular infarct until he or she can be assessed at the bedside and a right-sided ECG performed. If you can determine, with minimal delay, that the patient has a right ventricular infarct, nitroglycerin can be withheld for a few minutes. Ask the RN to take the patient's chart to the bedside.

Informing the Registered Nurse

Tell the RN, "I will arrive at the bedside in . . . minutes."

   Most causes of chest pain are diagnosed according to information from the history. It is impossible to obtain an accurate and relevant history by speaking to the RN over the telephone; the history must be obtained firsthand from the patient. Because some causes of chest pain represent medical emergencies, the patient should be assessed immediately.

ELEVATOR THOUGHTS

What causes chest pain?

Cardiac	Acute coronary syndrome
	Aortic dissection
	Pericarditis
Respiratory	Pulmonary embolism or infarction
	Pneumothorax
	Pleuritis (with or without pneumonia)
Gastrointestinal (GI)	Esophageal spasm, dysmotility; esophagitis (reflux, pill, eosinophilic, infectious)
	Peptic ulcer disease
Musculoskeletal system (MSS)	Costochondritis
	Arthropathies
	Xiphodynia
	Rib fracture
Skin	Herpes zoster
Psychiatric	Panic disorder
	Anxiety disorder

MAJOR THREAT TO LIFE

- Acute coronary syndrome
- Aortic dissection
- Pneumothorax
- Pulmonary embolus

Cardiogenic shock or fatal dysrhythmias may occur as a result of an acute coronary syndrome. Aortic dissection may result in death from cardiac tamponade, aortic rupture, acute aortic insufficiency, or MI and may damage other organ systems by compromising vascular supply. A pneumothorax may cause hypoxia by compressing the ipsilateral lung. A tension pneumothorax may also lead to hypotension as a result of positive intrathoracic pressure that decreases venous return to the heart. Pulmonary embolism may cause hypoxia and, in more severe cases, may result in acute right ventricular failure.

BEDSIDE

Quick-Look Test

Does the patient look well (comfortable), sick (uncomfortable or distressed), or critical (about to die)?

Most patients with chest pain from an acute coronary syndrome look pale and anxious. Patients with pericarditis, pneumothorax, or pulmonary embolism involving the pleural surface look apprehensive and breathe with shallow, painful respirations. If the patient looks well, suspect esophagitis or a musculoskeletal problem such as costochondritis.

Airway and Vital Signs

What is the blood pressure?

Most patients with chest pain have normal blood pressure. Hypotension may be seen with MI, massive pulmonary embolism, aortic dissection that results in cardiac tamponade, or tension pneumothorax. Hypertension, occurring in association with myocardial ischemia or aortic dissection, should be treated urgently (see Chapter 16).

A wide pulse pressure should raise the suspicion of aortic insufficiency, which may be observed as a complication of a proximal aortic dissection.

A pulsus paradoxus (see page 284) may be a clue to the presence of a pericardial effusion, which may be present with an aortic dissection or pericarditis.

What is the heart rate?

Does the patient have tachycardia?

Severe chest pain of any cause may result in sinus tachycardia. Heart rates of more than 100 beats/minute should also alert you to the possibility of a tachydysrhythmia, such as atrial fibrillation, other supraventricular tachycardias, or ventricular tachycardia. The presence of these conditions, depending on the specific dysrhythmia, may necessitate IV drug therapy to slow or convert the dysrhythmia, or electrical cardioversion to restore hemodynamic stability.

Does the patient have bradycardia?

Bradycardia in a patient with chest pain may represent sinus or atrioventricular nodal ischemia (as may occur with MI), β-blockade, or calcium channel blockade caused by drugs. Immediate treatment of bradycardia is not required unless the rate is extremely slow (<40 beats/minute) or the patient is hypotensive (see Chapter 18).

What is the breathing pattern?

Tachypnea may accompany any type of chest pain. Shallow, painful breathing is suggestive of a pleural cause (pleuritis, pneumothorax, pericarditis, pulmonary embolism) or a musculoskeletal cause.

What does the ECG show?

The ECG should be reviewed immediately after the vital signs are measured, to avoid delays in administering reperfusion therapy if the patient is having an acute ST-segment elevation MI.

There are five main ECG patterns that are important to recognize when considering a patient for emergency reperfusion therapy. Typical anterior and inferior STEMI patterns are shown in Figures 6.1 and 6.2, respectively. In the context of ischemic chest pain, other STEMI-equivalent ECG patterns that warrant immediate reperfusion include new-onset left bundle branch block (Figure 6.3), ST depression and peaked T waves in the precordial leads (De Winter's sign – Figure 6.4), and deeply inverted or biphasic T waves in the precordial leads (Wellen's syndrome – Figure 6.5). A second ECG performed with right-sided chest leads may help diagnose a right ventricular infarct, which is often associated with inferior myocardial infarctions.

Variations on these typical ECG patterns are common. If you are uncertain whether the patient's ECG qualifies them for immediate reperfusion therapy, call your resident or attending physician for help.

Remember that a normal ECG does not rule out the possibility of an acute coronary syndrome.

📖 The ECG in a case of aortic dissection may look perfectly normal. The presence of left ventricular hypertrophy may be evidence of long-standing hypertension, which is a risk factor for a dissection.

📖 In a patient with pulmonary embolism, the most common finding on an ECG is sinus tachycardia, but you should also look for a rightward axis.

📖 The ECG in a patient with pericarditis may show diffuse, usually mild ST elevations and sometimes PR depression.

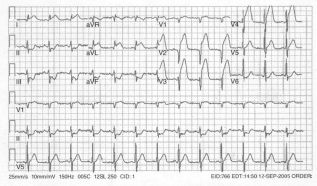

FIG. 6.1 **Typical anterior STEMI ECG pattern.**

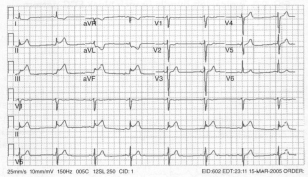

FIG. 6.2 **Typical inferior STEMI ECG pattern.**

Management I: Acute Coronary Syndrome: ST-segment Elevation Myocardial Infarction (STEMI)

If the ECG shows an acute ST-segment elevation MI or its equivalent, call your resident and a cardiologist immediately to assess the patient for emergency reperfusion therapy. Percutaneous intervention (angioplasty/stenting) is the preferred treatment. If unavailable in your hospital, then fibrinolysis with alteplase, reteplase, tenecteplase, or streptokinase should be considered; this is most effective when performed within the first 4 hours of symptoms. While reperfusion therapy is being organized, ask yourself the following questions:

Could the patient's STEMI be due to an aortic dissection?

An aortic dissection that involves a coronary ostium (usually the right coronary artery) may cause an acute STEMI, and this is treated differently than other STEMIs. Urgent surgical referral is

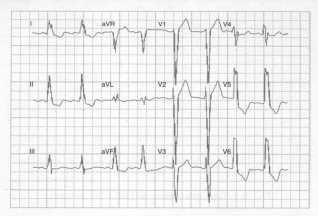

FIG. 6.3 **Typical left bundle branch block ECG pattern.**

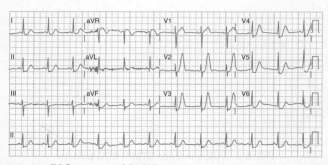

FIG. 6.4 **ECG pattern of De Winter suggesting acute left anterior descending coronary artery occlusion.**

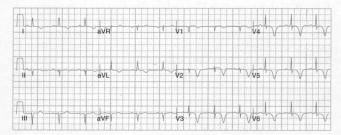

FIG. 6.5 **ECG pattern of Wellens syndrome suggesting acute left anterior descending coronary artery occlusion.**

necessary. Severe tearing chest or back pain, widening of the mediastinum on chest radiograph (CXR), and differential limb pulses may be clues that the STEMI is secondary to an aortic dissection. If a dissection-related STEMI is a consideration, call your resident or attending immediately for guidance.

Has the patient received aspirin?

If the patient has not taken aspirin and has no aspirin allergy, give aspirin, 160 to 325 mg, to chew.

Is the patient receiving oxygen?

Ensure that the patient is receiving oxygen at an appropriate concentration. Attach a pulse oximeter, and keep the oxygen saturation level at 94% or above.

Does the patient have chest pain now?

If chest pain is still present, there are no contraindications to nitroglycerin, and the last dose was administered more than 5 minutes ago, administer another dose immediately. If, after an additional 5 minutes, the pain is still present, administer a third nitroglycerin dose.

If the pain continues despite three doses of nitroglycerin, or there are contraindications to administering nitroglycerin, ask the RN to draw 10 mg (1 mL) of morphine into a syringe diluted with 9 mL of normal saline. Give the morphine in 2- to 4-mg aliquots intravenously (IV) over 1 to 5 minutes until the pain is relieved, provided that the systolic blood pressure is more than 90 mm Hg.

Morphine sulfate may cause hypotension or respiratory depression. Measure the patient's blood pressure and respiratory rate before each dose is given. If necessary, naloxone hydrochloride (Narcan), 0.2 to 2 mg IV, intramuscularly (IM) or subcutaneously (SC) may be given every 5 minutes, up to a total of 10 mg to reverse these side effects. Naloxone can also be given by nasal spray as Narcan 4 mg or Kloxxado 8 mg. Nausea or vomiting may also occur and can usually be controlled with dimenhydrinate, 25 mg IV or 50 mg by mouth (PO), every 4 to 6 hours as needed.

In addition to these measures, the patient should be transferred to the ICU/CCU as soon as possible, where ongoing myocardial ischemia can be treated with intravenous nitroglycerin, anticoagulants, $P2Y_{12}$ inhibitors, and β-blockers if required.

Selective History and Chart Review

How does the patient describe the pain?

Crushing, squeezing, viselike pain or pressure is characteristic of MI. Severe tearing or ripping pain is characteristic of an aortic dissection.

Is the pain the same as that of the patient's usual angina?

If the patient recognizes the current discomfort as his or her usual angina, the patient is probably correct.

Is the chest pain worse with deep breathing or coughing?

Pleuritic chest pain is suggestive of pleuritis, pneumothorax, rib fracture, pericarditis, pulmonary embolism, pneumonia, or costochondritis.

Does the pain radiate?

Radiation of the pain to the jaw, shoulders, or arms is suggestive of myocardial ischemia or MI. Radiation of pain to the back is suggestive of myocardial ischemia, MI, or aortic dissection distal to the left subclavian artery. Dissection proximal to the left subclavian artery characteristically causes nonradiating anterior chest pain. A burning sensation that radiates to the neck and is accompanied by an acid taste in the mouth is suggestive of esophageal reflux.

Does the patient also have nausea, vomiting, diaphoresis, or light-headedness?

Cardiogenic nausea and vomiting are associated with larger MIs.

Is the chest pain worse with swallowing?

Chest pain that is made worse by swallowing is suggestive of an esophageal disorder or pericarditis.

Selective Physical Examination

Vitals	Repeat measurements now
Body habitus	Does the patient look marfanoid? (A tall, thin patient with long limbs and arachnodactyly may have a connective tissue disorder, predisposing them to aortic dissection.)
Head, eyes, ears, nose, throat (HEENT)	White exudate in oral cavity or pharynx (thrush with possible concomitant esophageal candidiasis)
Respiratory system	Asymmetric expansion of the chest (pneumothorax)
	Deviation of the trachea to one side (large pneumothorax on the side opposite the deviation)
	Hyperresonance to percussion (on the side of a pneumothorax)
	Diminished breath sounds (on the side of a pneumothorax)
	Crackles (congestive heart failure [CHF] secondary to acute myocardial infarction [MI], pneumonia)
	Consolidation (pulmonary infarction, pneumonia)
	Pleural rub (pulmonary embolism, pneumonia)
	Pleural effusion (pulmonary embolism, pneumonia, ruptured aortic dissection)

Chest wall	Tender costal cartilage (costochondritis)
	Erythema, swelling of costal cartilage (costochondritis, arthritis)
	Tender xiphoid process (xiphodynia)
	Localized rib pain (rib fracture)
Cardiovascular system (CVS)	Unequal carotid pulses (aortic dissection)
	Unequal upper limb blood pressure or diminished femoral pulses (aortic dissection)
	Elevated jugulovenous pressure (JVP) (right ventricular failure secondary to MI or pulmonary embolism; tension pneumothorax)
	Right ventricular heave (acute right ventricular failure secondary to pulmonary embolism)
	Left ventricular heave (CHF)
	Displaced apical impulse (away from the side of a pneumothorax)
	Loud P_2 (acute cor pulmonale), S_3 (CHF)
	Mitral insufficiency murmur (papillary muscle dysfunction resulting from ischemia or MI)
	Aortic stenosis murmur (angina)
	Aortic insufficiency murmur (proximal aortic dissection)
	Pericardial rub (pericarditis; pericardial rubs are biphasic or triphasic scratching sounds that vary with position)
Abdomen (ABD)	Guarding, rebound tenderness (perforated ulcer)
	Epigastric tenderness (peptic ulcer disease)
	Generalized abdominal pain (mesenteric infarction from aortic dissection)
Central nervous system (CNS)	Hemiplegia (aortic dissection involving a carotid artery)
Skin	Unilateral maculopapular rash or vesicles in a dermatomal pattern (herpes zoster)

LOOK AT THE CHEST RADIOGRAPH

Review the CXR as soon as possible.

If a pneumothorax is suspected, upright inspiratory and expiratory films should be ordered. A pneumothorax is identified by a peripheral hyperlucent area, which represents free air in the pleural space and partial or complete collapse of the affected lung

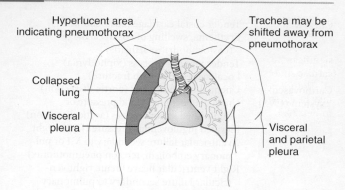

Hyperlucent area indicating pneumothorax

Trachea may be shifted away from pneumothorax

Collapsed lung

Visceral pleura

Visceral and parietal pleura

FIG. 6.6 Pneumothorax.

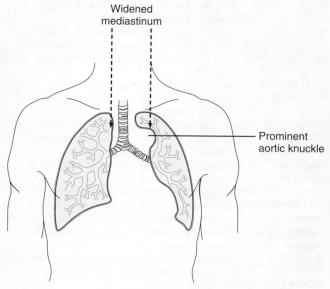

Widened mediastinum

Prominent aortic knuckle

FIG. 6.7 Aortic dissection.

(Fig. 6.6). A tension pneumothorax is a medical emergency and should be treated urgently, as outlined in Chapter 20.

The CXR may be normal in a patient with angina or an MI. Sometimes pulmonary venous congestion is seen if significant left ventricular dysfunction is associated.

If an aortic dissection is suspected, look specifically for a widened mediastinum or prominent aortic knuckle (Fig. 6.7). If aortic dissection is suspected, you must proceed urgently with the appropriate investigation and management (see page 59).

The CXR may be normal in a patient with pericarditis unless significant pericardial fluid has accumulated, in which case the cardiac silhouette may be enlarged.

The CXR of a patient with suspected pulmonary embolism may be entirely normal or may show any of the features illustrated in Fig. 24.3.

Management II (conditions other than ST-segment elevation MI)

1. Acute Coronary Syndrome: Non-ST-segment Elevation Myocardial Infarction (NSTEMI) or Unstable Angina

If angina has been relieved with one to three nitroglycerin tablets, review the precipitating cause. An adjustment in the antianginal medication may be required and should be made in consultation with the resident and the attending physician. However if the angina occurred at rest or this is the first episode of angina, the patient should be assessed by the intensive care unit/critical care unit (ICU/CCU) staff, regardless of whether the pain was relieved with three or fewer nitroglycerin tablets.

If the angina necessitated more than three doses of nitroglycerin or intravenous morphine, serial measurements of cardiac enzymes and ECGs should be ordered. Cardiac troponin is the cardiac enzyme marker of choice. It is elevated relatively early proportional to the size of the infarction. Negative troponin levels after 6 hours rule out infarction in most patients. If the clinical impression is of possible MI, the patient should be transferred to a unit with telemetry capabilities or the ICU/CCU. A patient with an acute coronary syndrome should be treated in a similar way to the patient with acute STEMI, with two exceptions: (1) Unless contraindicated, the patient with ACS should, in addition to aspirin, receive a platelet $P2Y_{12}$ receptor blocker such as **ticagrelor 180 mg oral load followed by 90 mg PO bid, prasugrel 60 mg oral load followed by 10 mg PO daily, or clopidogrel 600 mg oral load followed by 75 mg PO daily.** (2) Patients with ACS should not receive fibrinolysis. Emergency cardiac catheterization and percutaneous intervention is warranted in high-risk patients with ACS, including those with hemodynamic instability or shock, significant left ventricular dysfunction or heart failure, persistent angina despite maximal medical therapy, sustained ventricular arrhythmias, significant mitral regurgitation, or new ventricular septal defect.

2. Aortic Dissection

If aortic dissection is suspected, investigation and management as follows is urgent:

1. Arrange for an urgent computed tomographic scan of the thorax or transesophageal echocardiography. If neither can be performed within an hour, transthoracic echocardiography may reveal a dilated aortic root, aortic valvular insufficiency, or a pericardial effusion, any of which may be a clue to the presence of a dissection. On occasion, an aortic dissection flap is visualized directly with this test.
2. Draw blood for a stat crossmatch for 6 to 8 U of packed red blood cells and for CBC, electrolytes, urea, creatinine, and glucose, as well as measurements of prothrombin time and activated partial thromboplastin time.
3. Review the ECG for evidence of an acute MI. This finding suggests that the aortic dissection involves the coronary ostia.
4. The patient should be transferred to the ICU/CCU as soon as possible for careful control of blood pressure (see Chapter 16).
5. Surgical consultation should be obtained early if aortic dissection is present.

3. Pericarditis

If pericarditis is suspected, a nonurgent echocardiogram should be obtained to look for pericardial effusions or signs of hemodynamic compromise. Ninety percent of acute pericarditis cases are either viral or idiopathic, and initial therapy is aimed at relief of chest pain and inflammation. **Ibuprofen, 600 to 800 mg PO q8h; indomethacin (Indocin), 25 to 50 mg PO three times a day; and aspirin, 650 to 1000 mg PO q8h,** may be used; ibuprofen is preferable because of a lower incidence of adverse effects. The addition of colchicine to nonsteroidal anti-inflammatory drug (NSAID) therapy reduces symptoms and decreases the rate of recurrence. The dose depends on the patient's weight. **If ≥ 70 kg, give colchicine 1 to 1.2 mg PO q12h on day 1, followed by 0.5 to 0.6 mg PO q12h thereafter; if < 70 kg, give 0.5 to 0.6 mg every 12 hours on day 1 followed by 0.5 to 0.6 mg once daily thereafter.**

NSAIDs are contraindicated in a patient with NSAID or salicylate (aspirin) hypersensitivity, nasal polyps, and bronchospasm; in a patient who is taking anticoagulants; and in a patient who has active peptic ulcer disease. Because of the sodium-retaining properties of NSAIDs, caution should be used in giving these drugs to patients with CHF. Caution should also be used in giving NSAIDs to patients with renal insufficiency, because these drugs may inhibit renal prostaglandins, which are responsible for maintaining renal perfusion in patients with prerenal conditions.

4. Pulmonary Embolus

The management of pulmonary embolus is discussed in Chapter 24.

5. Pneumothorax

A pneumothorax may necessitate chest tube drainage, depending on its size. If the patient develops a tension pneumothorax, immediate treatment is necessary to relieve the pressure; a 16-gauge intravenous catheter as described on page 224 is used.

6. Pneumonia

Suggested antibiotics for pneumonia are discussed in Chapter 24 and should be chosen according to the results of the Gram stain and the patient's characteristics.

7. Esophagitis

The pain of esophagitis may be treated temporarily with antacids. Choose carefully: Magnesium-containing antacids (Gelusil, Maalox) may cause diarrhea, whereas antacids containing solely aluminum (Amphojel, Basaljel) may cause constipation. In treating gastrointestinal complaints, do not substitute one complaint for another. **The combination of aluminum, magnesium, and simethicone (Gelusil), 30 to 60 mL every 1 to 2 hours during the acute phase and 30 to 60 mL PO every 1 to 4 hours after meals and at bedtime,** is a standard antacid order. More frequent doses may be required if the pain is severe. An alginate such as the mixture of buffering agents with **sodium alginate and magnesium alginate (Gaviscon), 10 to 20 mL PO or 2 to 4 tablets (chewed) after meals and at bedtime,** followed by a glass of water, may also be used. Elevation of the head of the bed and avoidance of nighttime snacks are also helpful.

Treatment with a proton pump inhibitor—such as omeprazole (Losec and generic preparations), 20 mg PO daily; esomeprazole (Nexium), 20 to 40 mg PO daily; lansoprazole (Prevacid, Zoton), 15 to 30 mg PO daily; pantoprazole (Protonix, Protium), 40 mg PO daily; dexlansoprazole (Kapidex, Dexilant), 30 to 60 mg PO daily; and rabeprazole (Aciphex, Pariet, and generic preparations), 20 mg PO daily—should be started to aid in the long-term treatment of this disease. H2 antagonists are less costly but also less effective and can be used when cost is an issue.

Esophageal candidiasis does not respond to antacids. Immunocompromised patients may experience severe chest pain from this condition. Diagnosis should be confirmed by endoscopy. Nystatin (Mycostatin), although useful in the treatment of thrush, is not effective against esophageal candidiasis. In patients with acquired immunodeficiency syndrome (AIDS) or who are immunocompromised, **fluconazole (Diflucan), 200 to 400 mg PO daily,** has been shown to be more effective than ketoconazole (Nizoral) in eradicating *Candida* organisms from the esophagus; fluconazole also has a more rapid onset of action and produces faster resolution of symptoms. It may be given parenterally when necessary. An alternative is itraconazole (Sporanox) oral solution, 200 mg PO daily, voriconazole (Vfend) 200 mg PO daily, or posaconazole (Posanol) 200 m PO bid. Caspofungin (Cancidas) injectable, 70 mg IV over 1 hour, then 50 mg IV daily, is useful against candidiasis resistant to other agents. Resistant cases may also be treated with amphotericin (Fungazone) 0.3 to 0.7 mg/kg by slow IV infusion od, but its use should be restricted because of serious side effects.

8. Peptic Ulcer

The pain of peptic ulcer disease may be treated temporarily with antacids. Gelusil, 30 to 60 mL every 1 to 2 hours during the acute phase and 30 to 60 mL PO every 1 to 4 hours after meals and at bedtime, is a standard antacid order. More frequent doses may be required if the pain is severe. Proton pump inhibitors such as omeprazole (Losec and generic preparations), 20 to 40 mg PO daily; esomeprazole (Nexium), 20 to 40 mg PO daily; lansoprazole (Prevacid, Zoton), 15 to 30 mg PO daily; pantoprazole (Protonix, Protium), 40 mg PO daily; dexlansoprazole (Kapidex, Dexilant), 30 to 60 mg PO daily; and rabeprazole (Aciphex, Pariet, and generic preparations), 20 mg PO daily, have been shown to be more effective than H2 antagonists in the healing of gastric ulcers. If proton pump inhibitors are unavailable, an H2 antagonist such as cimetidine (Tagamet), 800 to 1200 mg PO daily at bedtime; famotidine (Pepcid), 40 mg PO daily at bedtime; nizatidine (Axid), 300 mg PO daily at bedtime; and ranitidine (Zantac), 300 mg PO daily at bedtime, may be used. When you encounter a patient in whom peptic ulcer disease is suspected but when tests are not available (e.g., at night), empirical triple therapy of *Helicobacter pylori* is not recommended; this should be reserved for patients in whom peptic ulcer disease is confirmed by endoscopy or in whom *H. pylori* infection is confirmed by a urea breath test (UBT) or stool testing. A patient with suspected peptic ulcer disease should be referred for a possible endoscopy and *H. pylori* evaluation when testing is available.

9. Costochondritis

Costochondritis may be treated with an NSAID, such as ibuprofen (Advil, Motrin), 400 mg PO every 4 to 6 hours, or naproxen (Naprosyn), 500 mg, and then 250 mg PO every 6 to 8 hours.

10. Herpes Zoster

Unilateral chest pain in a dermatomal distribution may precede the typical skin lesions of herpes zoster (*shingles*) by 2 or 3 days. The rash begins as a reddened, maculopapular area that rapidly evolves into vesicular lesions. Treatment of acute herpes zoster neuritis may be difficult, and affected patients often require narcotic analgesics, amitriptyline hydrochloride, and, in some cases, steroids. Topical preparations of capsaicin (Zostrix) may also provide temporary relief of neuralgic pain but should not be applied directly to open skin lesions. Antiviral agents such as **valacyclovir 1000 mg three times daily for 7 days; famciclovir 500 mg three times daily for 7 days; or acyclovir 800 mg five times daily for 7 days,** may reduce the severity and duration of localized flares of herpes zoster. Immunocompromised patients may initially require intravenous **acyclovir 10 mg/kg IV every 8 hours.**

11. Panic and Anxiety Disorders

Panic attacks are defined as *discrete periods of discomfort or fear* and are often associated with chest pain, dyspnea, diaphoresis, and dizziness. These symptoms may also be accompanied by feelings of depersonalization and a fear of dying, of "going crazy," or of "losing control." Chest pain may also be a feature of an anxiety disorder. Because of the possibility of a life-threatening cause of chest pain, panic and anxiety disorders should be diagnoses of exclusion. Short-acting benzodiazepines such as **midazolam (Versed) 2–5 mg IM clonazepam (Klonopin) 0.25 to 0.5 mg PO, or lorazepam (Ativan) 0.5 to 2 mg PO, SL, IM or IV** as needed, may be helpful in the short-term treatment of these disorders. IM midazolam is rapidly absorbed with a maximum effect in 10 minutes and a duration of effect up to 2 hours.

Combativeness: The Out-of-Control Patient

Every once in a while you will be paged by an exasperated nurse who has been trying to reason with a patient who is out of control. "Out of control" does not refer to moody or uncooperative; it refers to hostility in individuals whose temporary behavior poses a real physical threat to themselves, other patients, or hospital staff. Your job is not to act as the strong arm of the hospital law. Your role is to determine the medical reasons, if any, that are responsible for the patient's behavior and to administer appropriate treatment. In general, restraints, whether chemical or physical, should be used only as a last resort. In deciding whether a patient should be restrained, you must be sure that the restraints are medically necessary and that other interventions (usually calm reasoning) have been ineffective.

PHONE CALL

Questions

1. Is the patient delirious, highly agitated, and dangerous to self and/or staff (so-called excited delirium)?

    If so, ask the RN to call a code blue or code white alert and/or call security. You are going to need help.
2. Why was the patient admitted?
3. What measures have been used so far to calm or reason with the patient?
4. What medications is the patient taking now and what calming medicines have already been given? Is there an obvious reason for the patient's combative behavior?
5. What additional hospital personnel are available to help you now?

Orders

1. Ask the registered nurse (RN) to call the hospital's security personnel now, if this has not already been done. Your job is not to hurry to the ward to help hold down the patient. Your role is

to determine the cause of the patient's behavior and to institute appropriate treatment.

2. In general, patients can be given lorazepam 1 to 2 mg SL, midazolam 2 to 5 mg IM, or the antipsychotic that has previously been effective in this patient.

   Midazolam is rapidly absorbed with a maximum effect within 10 minutes lasting up to 2 hours. IM diazepam is poorly absorbed, and IM lorazepam is slowly and erratically absorbed.

3. If the code white or blue team has arrived, they may choose to use ketamine 5 mg/kg IV or a combination of haloperidol 5 to 10 mg IM or IV with lorazepam 1 to 2 mg IV or IM.

   Ketamine should not be used in the absence of resuscitation equipment and experienced staff.

Informing the Registered Nurse

Tell the RN, "I will arrive at the bedside in . . . minutes."

The out-of-control patient requires your immediate attention.

ELEVATOR THOUGHTS

What causes dangerously combative behavior?

Any confusional state resulting from an acute or chronic medical or psychiatric condition can result in temporary hostile or combative behavior. How an individual reacts in a given situation is often a reflection of his or her premorbid personality. The out-of-control patient is most commonly a young individual who feels frustrated, confined, and overwhelmed by the illness and the hospital environment. A second common type of out-of-control patient is an elderly person who becomes disoriented and combative, particularly at night (the sundown phenomenon).

Numerous other medical conditions may set off this behavior in a hospitalized patient, including intracranial disease, systemic disorders (drugs, organ failure, metabolic and endocrine disorders, infection, inflammation), and psychiatric disorders. Once the patient is safely approachable, you should carefully assess for the presence of these conditions (see Chapter 8, pages 70–71).

MAJOR THREAT TO LIFE

Physical Injury

Patients who are acutely agitated and hostile are not reasoning properly and may appear to be *looking for a fight*. The typical out-of-control patient has pulled out an intravenous line, a nasogastric tube, or a Foley catheter and is cursing, threatening, and pummeling any hospital personnel within striking distance. The patient loses regard for his or her own safety and risks both new injury and worsening of the underlying medical condition that necessitated the hospitalization.

BEDSIDE

Quick-Look Test

Does the patient look well (comfortable), sick (uncomfortable or distressed), or critical (about to die)?

Determine the severity of the condition:

Mild	agitated but cooperative
Moderate	disruptive but without danger
Severe	excited delirium—dangerous to self and/or staff

The combative patient looks very much alive, agitated, and (often) ready for a fight.

Stand back from the situation for a moment and observe the patient. You must judge from a distance how dangerous the patient is and what immediate measures are needed to calm him or her and regain control. Look for any obvious signs or conditions that may necessitate specific treatment:

- Is the patient cyanotic or having difficulty breathing (as a result of hypoxia)?
- Does the patient appear to be hallucinating (as a result of drug intoxication or withdrawal)?
- Is the patient in pain?

Management

The first priority is to calm the patient and regain control of the situation. In performing this task, the first rule is to remain calm yourself. It is not necessary to jump into the brawl, and you will be far more effective if you can think clearly in this situation. Be calm and supportive and acknowledge that the patient is suffering. Your tone of voice and body language should transmit this.

1. Some patients become calm simply because *the doctor* has arrived, and they feel less helpless and more in control of themselves with a physician there to address their immediate concerns. You will be able to judge within the first 30 seconds whether this is the case.
2. Some patients are so completely out of control that calm reasoning is ineffective. You may try to explain that you are going to give the patient a *shot* to calm him or her down and make him or her feel better. If the patient does not allow you to approach because of aggressive behavior, the patient may need to be held down while medication is administered. Should you need to

physically restrain a violent individual, the general rule is to have at least one person per limb plus one.

If the patient has already been given the antipsychotic you ordered over the telephone, allow adequate time for the medication to take effect. If the patient remains agitated 30 minutes after the initial dose, you may give an additional dose of midazolam 2 to 5 mg IM. The dose may be repeated every 2 to 4 hours. Always use the lowest effective dosage.

📖 Inform the patient's family, explain what has happened, and see whether the family can shed any light on the patient's behavior.

3. Patients with schizophrenia or bipolar disorder can be treated with **sublingual dexmedetomidine (Igalmi), an alpha-adrenergic receptor agonist, 120 or 180 ug SL.**

Restraints should be avoided or only used as a last resort.

If physical restraints (wrist and ankle restraints or a Posey restraint) are required, inform the family immediately and reassure them that the restraints are probably needed only temporarily. Emphasize that these measures are intended to protect the patient from injuring himself or herself. Nothing is more upsetting than for uninformed and unsuspecting family members to walk into their loved one's room the next day and find the patient tied down to the bed.

4. Delirium is a cardinal presentation not a diagnosis. There is an underlying cause that should be determined. Once the acute crisis is over, underlying causes of confusion (any of which may lead to combative behavior) should be thoroughly evaluated (see Chapter 8). Once the patient is safely approachable, you should perform a directed physical examination, in which you look for life-threatening or correctable (see pages 72–75) causes of confusion. You will have to use your judgment, because sometimes these patients are best left alone to sleep for a while. Just as often, however, a patient who was recently out of control will be grateful for the additional attention received from a concerned medical student or physician.

Confusion/Decreased Level of Consciousness

Confusion is a common problem in hospitalized patients, especially among the elderly. Unfortunately, the terms *delirium, toxic psychosis, acute brain syndrome,* and *acute confusional state* are often used interchangeably to refer to any cause of confusion. The term *metabolic encephalopathy* implies that the condition does not arise from psychiatric disorders or structural intracranial lesions.

The two recommended terms are *delirium* and *dementia*. Delirium is characterized by restlessness, agitation, clouding of consciousness, and, in some patients, bizarre behavior, hallucinations, delusions, and illusions. Dementia is a state of usually irreversible loss of memory and a global cognitive deficit. The level of consciousness is an important distinguishing feature between delirium and dementia. Delirium is characterized by a clouding of consciousness (a decreased clarity of awareness of the environment), whereas dementia is associated with a normal level of consciousness. Also, delirium usually develops over a short period of time (hours to days), and the signs fluctuate during the day, whereas the confusion seen with dementia is generally more constant.

Drowsiness, stupor, and *coma* refer to various degrees of unresponsiveness or diminished levels of consciousness.

PHONE CALL

Questions

1. Clarify the situation: In what way is the patient confused?
2. What are the patient's vital signs, including pulse oximetry?
3. Has the patient's level of consciousness changed?
4. Has the patient had previous episodes of confusion?
5. Why was the patient admitted?

6. Is the patient diabetic?

Confusion can be caused by too much or too little glucose in the blood. Hypoglycemia (resulting from excess insulin or excess oral hypoglycemic agents) and marked hyperglycemia (resulting from inadequate insulin or inadequate oral hypoglycemic agents) are prime considerations when confusion occurs in a diabetic patient.

7. How old is the patient?

Confusion in a 30-year-old patient is much more likely to have a serious yet reversible cause than is confusion in an 80-year-old patient receiving multiple medications.

Orders

Blood glucose and finger-prick blood glucose should be measured; hypoglycemia is a rapidly reversible cause of confusion.

Informing the Registered Nurse

Tell the registered nurse (RN), "I will arrive at the bedside in . . . minutes."

Confusion in association with hypotension, hypoxia, fever, decreased level of consciousness, or acute agitation (see Chapter 7) mandates that you evaluate the patient immediately.

ELEVATOR THOUGHTS

What causes confusion or a decreased level of consciousness?

Many disorders that begin with confusion may progress to a diminished level of consciousness and, ultimately, coma (in the following list, such items are marked with an asterisk). For the level of consciousness to be diminished, both cerebral hemispheres must be affected (e.g., by drugs or toxins), or the reticular activating system of the brain stem must be suppressed.

CENTRAL NERVOUS SYSTEM (INTRACRANIAL) CAUSES

1. Dementia
    *   Alzheimer disease
    *   Multi-infarct dementia
    *   Parkinson disease
    *   Normal-pressure hydrocephalus
2. Malignancy (primary central nervous system [CNS] tumor, CNS metastasis, paraneoplastic syndrome)
3. Head trauma (subdural and epidural hematoma, concussion, cerebral contusion)
4. Postictal state
5. Transient ischemic attack (TIA) or stroke

6. Hypertensive encephalopathy
7. Wernicke encephalopathy (thiamine deficiency)
8. Vitamin B_{12} deficiency

SYSTEMIC CAUSES

Drugs

1. Alcohol: in an alcoholic patient, confusion may occur when the patient is intoxicated, during early withdrawal, or later as part of delirium tremens.
2. Narcotic and sedative drug excess or withdrawal: even *normal* doses of these drugs frequently cause confusion in elderly patients.
3. Nonsteroidal anti-inflammatory drugs (NSAIDs), including aspirin
4. Antihypertensive agents (methyldopa, β-blockers)
5. Psychotropic medications or withdrawal: even *normal* doses of these drugs frequently cause confusion in elderly patients (tricyclic antidepressants, lithium, phenothiazines, monoamine oxidase [MAO] inhibitors, benzodiazepines, selective serotonin reuptake inhibitors [SSRIs])
6. Miscellaneous (steroids, cimetidine, antihistamines, anticholinergics)
7. Herbal remedies (St. John's wort, jimson weed)
8. Illicit drugs such as cocaine, amphetamines

Organ Failure

1. Respiratory failure (hypoxia, hypercapnia)
2. Renal failure (uremic encephalopathy)
3. Liver failure (hepatic encephalopathy)
4. Congestive heart failure (CHF) (hypoxia), hypertensive encephalopathy

Metabolic Disorders

1. Hyperglycemia, hypoglycemia
2. Hypernatremia, hyponatremia
3. Hypercalcemia

Endocrine Disorders

1. Hyperthyroidism or hypothyroidism
2. Hyperadrenocorticism or hypoadrenocorticism

Infection or Inflammation

1. Meningitis, encephalitis, brain abscess
2. Lyme disease
3. Cerebral vasculitis (systemic lupus erythematosus [SLE], polyarteritis nodosa)

Psychiatric Disorders

1. Mania, depression
2. Schizophrenia

COINCIDENTAL CAUSES

1. Confusion may be precipitated by environmental factors such as multiple room changes, lack of a clock or window, or lack of glasses or a hearing aid. A distended bladder or the insertion of a bladder catheter can lead to confusion, particularly in an elderly patient.

MAJOR THREAT TO LIFE

- Hypotension
- Hypoxia
- Delirium tremens
- Meningitis
- Intracranial mass

In some patients confusion will be due to hypotension or hypoxia, both of which may be life-threatening. Among patients with untreated delirium tremens, the mortality rate can be as high as 15%. Meningitis must be recognized early if antibiotic medication is to be effective. An intracranial mass (e.g., subdural or epidural hematoma, brain abscess, tumor) may initially manifest with confusion.

BEDSIDE

Quick-Look Test

Does the patient look well (comfortable), sick (uncomfortable or distressed), or critical (about to die)?

Most patients with delirium look sick, whereas most otherwise healthy patients with dementia look well.

Airway, Vital Signs, and Finger-Prick Glucose Results

Is the patient receiving oxygen?

A fraction of inspired oxygen (FiO_2) of more than 0.28 in a patient with chronic obstructive pulmonary disease (COPD) may depress the respiratory center, resulting in hypercapnia and then confusion.

What is the blood pressure?

Hypotension may sometimes present as confusion, especially in the elderly.

Hypertensive encephalopathy is rare; diastolic blood pressure is usually higher than 120 mm Hg. Confusion in association with a systolic blood pressure of less than 90 mm Hg may result from impairment of cerebral perfusion secondary to shock. Drug overdose, adrenal insufficiency, and hyponatremia are metabolic causes that should be considered in a hypotensive, confused patient.

What is the heart rate?

Tachycardia is suggestive of sepsis, delirium tremens, hyperthyroidism, or hypoglycemia, but it may also occur in any agitated, anxious patient.

What is the temperature?

Fever is suggestive of infection, delirium tremens, or cerebral vasculitis.

What is the respiratory rate?

The presence of confusion in association with tachypnea should alert you to the possibility of hypoxia. Tachypnea with confusion and petechiae in a young patient with a femoral fracture is a classic manifestation of fat embolism syndrome.

What is the blood glucose result?

Hypoglycemia is most commonly seen in a patient with diabetes mellitus who has received the usual insulin dose but has not eaten. In rare cases, an incorrect dose of insulin, surreptitious insulin use, or an insulinoma is the cause (see Chapter 33, page 401 for the management of hypoglycemia and pages 394–400 for the management of hyperglycemia).

Selective Physical Examination I

Is there evidence on physical examination of one of the other major threats to life?

Head, eyes, ears, nose, throat (HEENT)	Nuchal rigidity (meningitis)
	Papilledema (hypertensive encephalopathy, intracranial mass)
	Pupil size and symmetry
	📖 Dilated pupils suggest increased sympathetic outflow, such as may be seen in delirium tremens or cocaine ingestion, whereas pinpoint pupils suggest narcotic excess or recent application of constricting eye drops
	Palpate the skull for fractures, hematomas, and lacerations (subdural or epidural hematoma, concussion)
	Hemotympanum or blood in the ear canal (basal skull fracture)

Neurologic system	General appearance: behavior and attitude
	Level of consciousness: alert, drowsy
	Mood, affect: depressed, agitated, restless
	Form of thought: flight of ideas, circumstantiality, loosening of associations, perseveration
	Thought content: delusions, concrete thinking
	Perceptions: illusions, hallucinations (auditory, visual)
	Mental status: a detailed mental status examination is required in the assessment of a confused patient; however, if the patient has a decreased level of consciousness or is agitated or uncooperative, not all the categories listed as follows will be appropriate.
	Orientation: check whether the patient is aware of the correct time, place, and person.
	Registration: name three objects (e.g., *apple, pencil, car*) and have the patient repeat them.
	Attention and calculation: have the patient count by serial 7s.
	Recall: ask the patient to name the three aforementioned objects (*apple, pencil, car*).
	Language: ask the patient to point to and identify objects, follow a three-stage command, and write a sentence.
	Long-term memory: ask the patient his or her birth date and the name of his or her hometown.
	Judgment: test hypothetical situations.
	A full neurologic examination is required (within the limits posed by the mental status examination).
	Does the patient have any tremor (indicative of delirium tremens, Parkinson disease, or hyperthyroidism)?
	Is any asymmetry present in the pupils, visual fields, eye movement, limbs, tone, reflexes, or plantar flexors?
	📖 Any such asymmetry is suggestive of structural brain disease.

Management I

Hypotension

For the investigation and management of hypotension, see Chapter 18, page 189.

Hypoxia

For the investigation and management of hypoxia, see Chapter 24, page 281.

Bacterial Meningitis

If you suspect bacterial meningitis, refer immediately to Chapter 12, page 108, for further information on investigation and management.

Delirium Tremens

Delirium tremens (confusion, fever, tachycardia, dilated pupils, diaphoresis) and alcohol withdrawal must be treated urgently with sedation. Benzodiazepines are of proven benefit. Administer **midazolam 2 to 5 mg IM**. Midazolam is rapidly absorbed with a maximum effect within 10 minutes lasting up to 2 hours. **Lorazepam 0.5 to 2 mg SL** is an alternative benzodiazepine but may be difficult to administer to an uncooperative patient. IM diazepam is poorly absorbed, and IM lorazepam is slowly and erratically absorbed. **Thiamine, 100 mg IV (given slowly over 5 minutes), IM or PO daily for up to 3 days**, if not already administered during this hospitalization, should be given to prevent the development of Wernicke encephalopathy in an alcoholic or malnourished patient. If necessary, 5% dextrose in normal saline (D5NS) IV may be given to correct volume depletion after the initial dose of thiamine. Barbiturates may be useful in patients with refractory delirium tremens. However, respiratory depression is common with the higher doses that are required. Call your resident or attending physician for help before instituting higher doses.

Intracranial Lesion

A structural intracranial lesion (e.g., stroke, tumor, subdural hematoma, epidural hematoma) should be suspected in a patient with new findings of asymmetry on neurologic examination. Urgent computed tomography (CT) of the head helps define the intracranial lesion. A CT scan is the preferable imaging technique when speed is important, as in stroke and trauma. An MRI (magnetic resonance imaging) or PET (positive emission tomography) is the imaging technique of choice where details are important, as in cancer, dementia, and neurological disease. Prompt referral to a neurosurgeon is required for a subdural or epidural hematoma and for a cerebellar hemorrhage.

Selective Physical Examination II

Are there other correctable causes of confusion?

Vitals	Hypertension and bradycardia may signify rising intracranial pressure.
	Hypothermia is suggestive of myxedema or alcohol, barbiturate, or phenothiazine intoxication
HEENT	Subhyaloid hemorrhage (subarachnoid hemorrhage)
	Conjunctival and fundal petechiae (fat embolism syndrome) (Fig. 8.1)
	Lacerated tongue or cheek (postictal)
	Goiter (hyperthyroidism or hypothyroidism)
Respiratory system	Cyanosis (hypoxia)
	Barrel chest (COPD with hypoxia or hypercapnia)
	Bibasilar crackles (CHF with hypoxia)
Cardiovascular system	CHF
	Elevated jugular venous pressure (JVP)
	S_3
	Pitting edema
Abdomen (ABD)	Costovertebral angle tenderness (pyelonephritis)
	Liver, spleen, or kidney tenderness (infection)
	Guarding, rebound tenderness (intraabdominal infection)
	Shifting dullness, dilated superficial veins, caput medusae (liver failure), bladder distention
Neurologic system	Argyll Robertson pupils accommodate but do not react to light (neurosyphilis, neurosarcoidosis, multiple sclerosis) (Fig. 8.2).
	Cranial nerve palsies (Lyme disease)
	Asterixis, constructional apraxia (liver failure) (Fig. 8.3)
Skin	Axillary fold, neck, upper chest petechiae (fat embolism syndrome)

Selective History and Chart Review

What drugs is the patient receiving?

Even the usual doses of some drugs can cause confusion in elderly patients because of alterations in drug clearance.

Does the patient have a history of alcohol abuse?

It is important to establish when alcohol was last ingested, because withdrawal symptoms are unlikely after 1 week of abstinence.

Has the patient recently undergone surgery?

During the postoperative period, patients are predisposed to confusion because of CNS effects of anesthetic and analgesic medications, nutritional deficiencies (e.g., thiamine), and fluid and electrolyte disturbances. These physiologic abnormalities may be exacerbated in an elderly patient because of sensory impairment

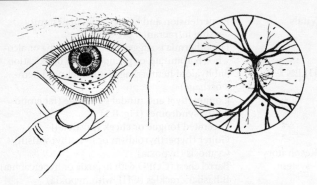

FIG. 8.1 Conjunctival and fundal petechiae observed in fat embolism syndrome.

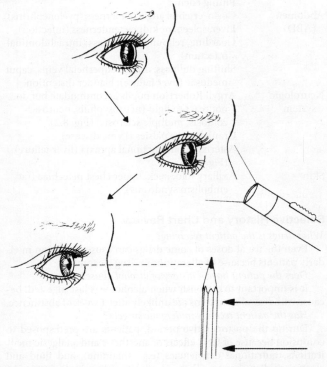

FIG. 8.2 Argyll Robertson pupils. Pupils do not react to light, but they do accommodate.

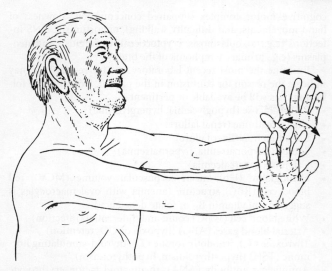

Tests of constructional apraxia
a. Copy the following:

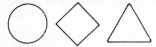

b. Draw a house or a clock face
c. Write signature

FIG. 8.3 *Top,* asterixis. Wrist flapping occurs when the arms are outstretched. *Bottom,* tests of constructional apraxia.

(reduced visual or auditory acuity), psychological factors, and cultural expectations.

If the level of consciousness is decreased, was the change gradual or sudden?

A sudden decrease in the level of consciousness is usually caused by drug ingestion or an acute intracranial catastrophe (hemorrhage, trauma). Unresponsiveness that develops gradually (over days or weeks) is usually caused by a preceding systemic medical disorder (e.g., metabolic or endocrine disorders, hepatic failure, or renal failure).

Does the patient have human immunodeficiency virus (HIV) disease?

HIV infection may result in cognitive impairment in an otherwise asymptomatic patient with AIDS. Patients in the more advanced stages of AIDS may suffer a wide variety of neurologic problems associated with confusion, including HIV-1-associated cognitive–motor complex (impaired concentration, slowness of hand movements, and difficulty walking), opportunistic CNS infections (e.g., toxoplasmosis, cryptococcal meningitis), and neoplasms (e.g., primary lymphoma of the brain).

Examine the most recent laboratory test for results that may indicate the reason for confusion in the patient. Not all of the following tests will be available or pertinent.

- Blood glucose (hypoglycemia, hyperglycemia)
- Urea, creatinine (renal failure)
- Liver function (liver failure)
- Sodium (hyponatremia, hypernatremia)
- Calcium (hypercalcemia)
- Hemoglobin (Hb), mean corpuscular volume (MCV), red blood cell (RBC) structure (anemia with oval macrocytes is suggestive of vitamin B_{12} or folate deficiency)
- White blood cell (WBC) count and differential (infection)
- Arterial blood gases (ABG) (hypoxia or CO_2 retention)
- Thyroxine (T_4), triiodothyronine (T_3), thyroid-stimulating hormone (TSH) (hyperthyroidism, hypothyroidism)
- Antinuclear antibody (ANA), rheumatoid factor, erythrocyte sedimentation rate (ESR), C3, C4 (vasculitis)
- Drug levels (lithium, aspirin, antiepileptic drugs)

Management II

Drugs

If the confusion is secondary to drugs, stop the medication.

If reversal of postoperative narcotic depression is indicated, give naloxone (Narcan), 0.2 to 2 mg IV, IM, or subcutaneously every 5 minutes (maximum total dose, 10 mg), until the desired improved level of consciousness is achieved. Maintenance doses every 1 to 2 hours may be necessary to maintain reversal of the CNS depression. Naloxone should be used with caution in patients known to be physically dependent on opiates.

Reversal of the benzodiazepine effect can be achieved by administering flumazenil (Romazicon), 0.2 mg IV over 30 seconds. Wait 1 minute. If this dose is ineffective, it may be followed by additional doses of 0.2 to 0.5 mg IV every 60 seconds up to the maximum cumulative dose of 5 mg. If there is no response to the maximum dose, the CNS depression is not due to benzodiazepines and another cause should be sought. The effect of flumazenil on respiratory depression caused by benzodiazepines is inconsistent. Also, reversal of the benzodiazepine effect may be associated with seizures. Flumazenil is contraindicated in cases of cyclic antidepressant overdose because of an increased risk of seizures. Its duration of action is relatively short; therefore overdose cases must be monitored for resedation.

Dementia

Dementia is a diagnosis of exclusion. The following investigations are required to rule out a treatable cause of dementia:

- Complete blood cell count (CBC) and electrolyte, urea, and creatinine
- Calcium and phosphorus
- Serum bilirubin (liver disease)
- Serum vitamin B_{12} and folate
- T_4, T_3, and TSH
- Serologic test for syphilis
- CT or MRI of the head

Renal and Hepatic Failure

In endstage kidney and liver failure, ensure that the problem has not been compounded by hepatotoxic or nephrotoxic medications. Aggressive treatment of the kidney failure (dialysis, if necessary) or liver failure (lactulose, neomycin) should be undertaken when indicated.

Hyponatremia or Hypernatremia

For the management of hyponatremia or hypernatremia, refer to Chapter 35.

Hypercalcemia

For the management of hypercalcemia, see Chapter 31.

Vitamin B_{12} Deficiency

Suspected vitamin B_{12} deficiency should be confirmed with a measurement of serum vitamin B_{12} level.

Mania, Depression, or Schizophrenia

For suspected mania, depression, or schizophrenia, psychiatric consultation is necessary for confirmation of diagnosis. Agitation in a confused patient may necessitate **midazolam 2 to 5 mg IM or lorazepam 0.5 to 2 mg SL**.

Cerebral Vasculitis

Cerebral vasculitis is rare. High-dose steroid therapy is the accepted initial treatment.

Fat Embolism

The rate of mortality from fat embolism syndrome can be as high as 8%. The mainstay of treatment is oxygen therapy. If the patient requires an FiO_2 of more than 0.5, he or she should be transferred to the intensive care unit or the cardiac care unit for possible intubation and mechanical ventilation with positive end-expiratory pressure (PEEP).

Decreased Urine Output

Decreased urine output is a problem frequently seen in both medical and surgical services. Proper management of affected patients depends on your skills in assessing volume status.

PHONE CALL

Questions

1. How much urine has the patient passed in the past 24 hours? Urine output of less than 400 mL/day (<20 mL/hour) is oliguria. Absence of urine (anuria) is suggestive of a mechanical obstruction of the bladder outlet or a blocked Foley catheter.
2. What are the patient's vital signs?
3. Why was the patient admitted?
4. Is the patient complaining of abdominal pain? Abdominal pain is a clue to the possible presence of a distended bladder, as may be seen with bladder outlet obstruction.
5. Does the patient have a Foley catheter? If the patient has a Foley catheter in place, the assessment of urine output can usually be assumed to be accurate. If not, you must ensure that the total volume of voided urine has been collected and measured.
6. What is the patient's most recent serum potassium level?

Orders

1. If a Foley catheter is in place and the patient is anuric, ask the nurse to flush the catheter with 20 to 30 mL of normal saline to ensure patency. Clogging of Foley catheters with sediment is a common problem, and it is solved easily before a more detailed investigation for decreased urine output is necessary.
2. Obtain measurements of serum electrolytes, urea, and creatinine. A serum potassium level of more than 5.5 mmol/L is indicative of potentially serious hyperkalemia. This is the most immediate life-threatening complication of renal insufficiency.

A serum bicarbonate (HCO_3) measurement of less than 20 mmol/L is suggestive of metabolic acidosis as a result of renal insufficiency. A serum HCO_3 level lower than 15 mmol/L should prompt you to determine the arterial pH. Elevations in serum urea and creatinine levels can be used as guidelines to assess the degree of renal insufficiency present.

Informing the Registered Nurse

Tell the registered nurse (RN), "I will arrive at the bedside in . . . minutes."

If the patient is not in pain and if a recently measured serum potassium level is not elevated, an assessment of decreased urine output can wait 1 or 2 hours if other problems of higher priority exist.

ELEVATOR THOUGHTS

Causes of Decreases in Urine Output

Prerenal Causes (Underperfusion of Kidneys)

1. Volume depletion
2. Reduced cardiac output (congestive heart failure [CHF], constrictive pericarditis, cardiac tamponade)
3. Drugs that reduce effective glomerular perfusion (diuretics, angiotensin-converting enzyme inhibitors, nonsteroidal anti-inflammatory drugs [NSAIDs], cyclosporine).
4. Hepatorenal syndrome

Renal Causes

1. Glomerulonephritic syndromes (acute glomerulonephritis, subacute bacterial endocarditis [SBE], systemic lupus erythematosus [SLE], other vasculitides)
2. Tubulointerstitial problems
   a. Acute tubular necrosis caused by one of the following:
      i. Hypotension
      ii. Nephrotoxins
         • Exogenous (aminoglycosides, amphotericin B, intravenous [IV] contrast materials, chemotherapy)
         • Endogenous (myoglobin, uric acid, oxalate, amyloid, Bence Jones protein)
   b. Acute interstitial nephritis resulting from drugs (penicillin, other β-lactam antibiotics, NSAIDs, diuretics, allopurinol, cimetidine, sulfonamides), autoimmune disease (e.g., SLE), infiltrative disease, infection
3. Vascular problems
   a. Emboli (from aortic atheroma, SBE, left-sided heart thrombi)
   b. Renal artery thrombosis

Postrenal Causes

1. Bilateral ureteric obstruction (e.g., stones, clots, sloughed papillae, retroperitoneal fibrosis, retroperitoneal tumor)
2. Bladder outlet obstruction (e.g., prostatic hypertrophy, carcinoma of the cervix, stones, clots, urethral strictures)
3. Blocked Foley catheter

MAJOR THREAT TO LIFE

- Hyperkalemia
- Renal failure

A decrease in urine output from any cause may result in or be a manifestation of progressive renal insufficiency, leading to renal failure. Of the complications of renal failure, hyperkalemia is the most immediately life-threatening because it can lead to potentially fatal cardiac dysrhythmias.

BEDSIDE

Quick-Look Test

Does the patient look well (comfortable), sick (uncomfortable or distressed), or critical (about to die)?

A patient who is sick or looks critically ill may have advanced renal insufficiency. Restlessness in a patient is suggestive of pain from a distended bladder. However, both these conditions can be present in a patient who deceptively appears well.

Airway and Vital Signs

Check for postural changes.

A postural rise in heart rate of more than 15 beats/minute, a fall in systolic blood pressure of more than 15 mm Hg, or any fall in diastolic blood pressure is suggestive of significant hypovolemia. *Caution:* A resting tachycardia alone may be indicative of decreased intravascular volume. Fever is suggestive of concomitant urinary tract infection.

Selective Physical Examination

Examine for *prerenal* (volume status), *renal,* or *postrenal* (obstructive) causes of decreased urine output. *Caution:* More than one cause may be present.

Head, eyes, ears, nose, throat (HEENT)	Jaundice (hepatorenal syndrome)
	Facial purpura } Amyloidosis
	Enlarged tongue

Respiratory system	Crackles, pleural effusions (CHF)
Cardiovascular system (CVS)	Pulse volume, jugular venous pressure (JVP)
	Skin temperature and color
Abdomen (ABD)	Enlarged kidneys (hydronephrosis secondary to obstruction, polycystic kidney disease)
	Enlarged bladder (bladder outlet obstruction, neurogenic bladder, blocked Foley catheter)
Rectal	Enlarged prostate gland (bladder outlet obstruction)
Pelvic	Cervical or adnexal masses (ureteric obstruction secondary to cervical or ovarian cancer)
Skin	Morbilliform rash (acute interstitial nephritis)
	Livedo reticularis on lower extremities (atheromatous embolic renal failure)

Selective Chart Review

- Review the patient's history and hospital course; look specifically for possible prerenal, renal, or postrenal causes of decreased urine output (see the Elevator Thoughts section).
- Look for recent blood urea and creatinine values. If the condition is due to prerenal causes, urea reabsorption will be increased, whereas if the condition is due to a renal cause, there will be a reduced reabsorption of urea. Thus the relationship between urea and creatinine levels provides a clue to the cause (Table 9.1)

  📖 A urea-to-creatinine ratio of greater than 110:1 (standard international units) or a BUN-to-creatinine ratio of greater than 20:1 (Imperial units) is suggestive of a prerenal cause. A urine specific gravity higher than 1.020 or a urine sodium concentration lower than 20 mmol/L is also suggestive of a prerenal cause.

- Look for specific combinations of factors that may predispose to renal failure, such as a patient receiving angiotensin-converting enzyme inhibitors, diuretics, and NSAIDs in combination, a septic patient receiving aminoglycosides, a patient receiving an angiotensin-converting enzyme inhibitor and IV contrast material, or a patient with CHF who was given an NSAID.

Management I

Your job becomes simpler when you can find a prerenal or postrenal cause for decreased urine output.

TABLE 9.1	Urea and BUN Creatinine Ratios		
Urea:Cr (SI Units) Ratio	BUN:Cr (Imperial Units) Ratio	Condition	Mechanism
>110:1	>20:1	Prerenal	Urea reabsorption is **increased**. Urea is disproportionately elevated relative to creatinine in serum.
40-110:1	12-20:1	Normal or postrenal	Normal range. Urea reabsorption is within normal limits.
<40:1	<12:1	Renal	Renal damage causes **reduced reabsorption** and increased loss of urea, therefore lowering the Urea:Cr ratio.

Prerenal Cause

First ensure that the intravascular volume is normal. If the patient has CHF, initiate diuresis, as discussed in Chapter 24, pages 290–293. If the patient has volume depletion, replenish the intravascular volume with normal saline. Do not add a potassium supplement to the IV solution until the patient passes urine. Do not administer Ringer's lactate because it contains potassium.

Postrenal Cause

Obstruction in the lower urinary tract can be adequately ruled out by passage of a Foley catheter into the bladder.

1. If the bladder outlet has been obstructed, the initial urine volume on catheterization is usually more than 400 mL, and the patient experiences immediate relief. After catheterization, watch for the development of postobstructive diuresis by monitoring urine volume status carefully for the next few days.
2. If a Foley catheter is already in place, ensure that flushing the catheter with 20 to 30 mL of normal saline allows free flow of fluid from the bladder. This maneuver helps rule out an intraluminal blockage of the Foley catheter as a cause of postrenal obstruction.
3. The presence of a Foley catheter in the bladder rules out obstruction of only the lower urinary tract. If the preceding two steps fail to restore urine output, a renal ultrasound examination should be ordered in the morning to search for upper urinary tract obstruction. Although bilateral ureteric obstruction

TABLE 9.2	Urea, BUN, and Creatinine Values			
Normal values	Units	Urea	BUN	Creatinine
Standard International units	mmol/L	3.0–6.5	2.1–3.8	50–110
Imperial units (USA)	mg/dL	8–18	6–24	0.6–1.2

is rare, additional useful information, such as documentation of the presence of both kidneys and an estimate of renal size, may be obtained.

Renal Cause

If prerenal and postrenal factors are not responsible for the decrease in urine output, you must investigate renal causes. A search for the renal causes of decreased urine output, however, can wait until some additional important questions are answered (see Management II section below).

Management II

Regardless of the cause of decrease in urine output (prerenal, renal, or postrenal), you must now answer the following four questions:
1. Are any of the following five life-threatening complications of decreased urine output present?
   a. Hyperkalemia (the most immediately serious problem):
      i. Order a stat measurement of serum potassium level, if this has not already been done.
      ii. Review the patient's chart for a recent measurement of serum potassium level.
      iii. Order a stat electrocardiogram (ECG) if suspicion of hyperkalemia exists.

      📖 Peaked T waves are early signs of hyperkalemia (Fig. 9.1). More advanced manifestations on the ECG include depressed ST segments, prolonged PR intervals, loss of P waves, and wide QRS complexes.

      iv. Discontinue any potassium supplements and potassium-sparing diuretics.
      v. Treat as outlined in Chapter 34, pages 405–406.
   b. CHF: suggested by tachypnea, elevated JVP, crackles on pulmonary auscultation, an S3, and sacral or pedal edema. Refer to Chapter 24, pages 289–293, for management of CHF.
   c. Severe metabolic acidemia (pH < 7.2): suggested by the presence of (compensatory) hyperventilation and confirmed by arterial blood gas measurement. Investigation should proceed as outlined in Chapter 29, pages 361–362.

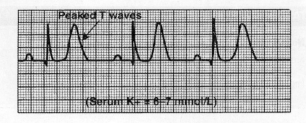

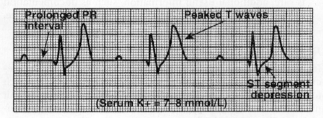

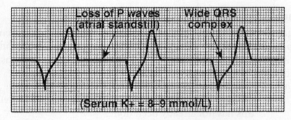

FIG. 9.1 **Progressive electrocardiographic features of hyperkalemia.**

    d. Uremic encephalopathy: manifested by confusion, stupor, or seizures and managed by dialysis. If seizures occur, they should be managed as outlined in Chapter 23 until dialysis can be initiated.

    e. Uremic pericarditis: suggested by the presence of pleuritic chest pain, pericardial friction rub, or diffuse ST-segment elevation on the ECG. It is managed best with dialysis.

2. Is the patient receiving any drugs that may worsen the situation?

    a. Potassium supplements

    b. Potassium-sparing diuretics (eplerenone, spironolactone, triamterene, amiloride)

    c. Nephrotoxic drugs (NSAIDs, aminoglycosides)

       Review the need for these agents and discontinue them immediately, if possible. If aminoglycosides are required, doses will need to be adjusted on the basis of serum levels.

3. Is the patient in oliguric renal failure? If the patient's urine production is less than 480 mL/day (<20 mL/hour), the patient has oliguric renal failure. Although the mortality rate in this condition is higher than that in nonoliguric renal failure, there is little evidence to support efforts to convert oliguric to nonoliguric renal failure through the aggressive use of diuretics. In fact, diuretics may worsen the situation if the renal failure has been caused by IV contrast agents. In general, loop diuretics should be used in this situation only if the patient has coexisting CHF.

4. Does the patient need dialysis?

   a. If the patient does not pass urine despite high doses of diuretics, the indications for urgent dialysis are as follows:

      i. Hyperkalemia
      ii. CHF
      iii. Metabolic acidemia (pH < 7.2)
      iv. Severe uremia (urea level > 35 mmol/L; creatinine level > 800 mmol/L), with or without uremic seizures
      v. Uremic pericarditis

   b. If the patient is in renal failure and if one or more of these conditions are present, request an urgent nephrology consultation about dialysis for the patient. While you await the nephrologist's arrival, all of the problems just listed can be treated temporarily with nondialysis measures:

      i. Hyperkalemia: administer glucose with insulin infusion, sodium bicarbonate (NaHCO$_3$), calcium, sodium polystyene sulfonate or other potassium binder (refer to Chapter 34).
      ii. CHF: preload measures (have the patient sit up; administer morphine, nitroglycerin ointment); give O$_2$ (refer to Chapter 24, pages 289–293).
      iii. Metabolic acidemia: NaHCO$_3$ (refer to Chapter 29, page 360, for assessment of metabolic acidosis).
      iv. Uremic encephalopathy: keep the patient calm and on bed rest until dialysis can be initiated.
      v. Uremic pericarditis: treat symptomatically for pain with an NSAID until dialysis can be initiated.

Once the questions have been addressed, you can consider possible renal causes of decreased urine output. The majority of renal causes are diagnosed from the history, physical examination, and laboratory findings. On occasion, a renal biopsy is required. A simple urinalysis can often provide valuable clues to the diagnosis.

Urine Dipstick Test for Blood and Protein

Urine dipsticks are a rapid and relatively sensitive (>80%) method for detecting hematuria. However, as well as intact red blood cells (RBCs), urine dipsticks may also detect hemoglobin from lysed

RBCs caused by hemolytic conditions, or myoglobin from crush injuries, rhabdomyolysis, or myositis. Microscopic examination of the urine will differentiate between hematuria and hemoglobinuria.

Suspect *rhabdomyolysis* if the orthotolidine test result on dipstick is positive but there are few or no RBCs on urine microscopy. (In this case, order tests for serum levels of creatine phosphokinase, calcium, and phosphate [PO_4] and for urine levels of myoglobin.)

If the test result for urinary protein alone is positive, obtain a serum albumin and 24-hour urine collection for protein and creatinine clearance to identify the *nephrotic syndrome,* if present.

Urine Microscopy

RBC casts are diagnostic for glomerulonephritis. White blood cell casts, particularly eosinophil casts, may be observed in cases of acute interstitial nephritis. Pigmented granular casts may be observed with acute tubular necrosis. Oval fat bodies are suggestive of nephrotic syndrome.

Urine for Eosinophils

Ask for this test if acute interstitial nephritis is suspected.

In most cases, beyond these simple tests, no further investigation is required during the night. For any suspected renal cause of decreased urine output, however, ensure that prerenal and postrenal factors are not additional contributors to the poor urine output.

REMEMBER

All medications that the oliguric or anuric patient is receiving should be reviewed, and any potential nephrotoxins should be discontinued. The actions of many drugs depend on renal excretion, and dosage adjustment may be required. If you are uncertain about the route of excretion of a drug that has been ordered for a patient, it may be safest to withhold the drug until you find out.

Diarrhea

Avoid treating diarrhea as a diagnosis. Diarrhea is always a symptom of another underlying disorder and seldom warrants nonspecific *antimotility therapy*. During the night, when testing services are not always available, your job is to determine the likely cause of the diarrhea, whether additional investigations should be performed, and whether complications have arisen that necessitate treatment.

PHONE CALL

Questions

1. What are the patient's vital signs?
2. Why was the patient admitted?
3. Is the diarrhea a new problem? If not, has the cause of the diarrhea been diagnosed?
4. Has the patient had recent surgery?
5. Is blood, pus, or mucus in the stool?

   Bloody stools with pus or mucus are suggestive of inflammation, as may be present with infection, inflammatory bowel disease, or ischemic colitis.
6. Does the patient have abdominal pain?

   Moderate or severe abdominal pain is suggestive of ischemic colitis, diverticulitis, or inflammatory bowel disease.

Orders

No orders are necessary.

Informing the Registered Nurse

Tell the registered nurse (RN), "I will arrive at the bedside in . . . minutes."

A single episode of diarrhea in an otherwise healthy patient does not usually necessitate bedside assessment. If the diarrhea is frequent, severe, or bloody, the patient should be evaluated at the bedside as soon as possible. If the patient is hypotensive, tachycardic, or febrile, they should be assessed immediately.

ELEVATOR THOUGHTS

What causes diarrhea?

Acute Diarrhea (<2 Weeks' Duration)
The Four I's

Infection	Inflammation and toxins (Box 10.1)
Iatrogenic	Drugs (laxatives, stool softeners, magnesium-containing antacids, sorbitol-containing liquid dosage forms, digoxin, quinidine, colchicine, and xanthines)
	Surgery (gastrectomy, vagotomy, cholecystectomy, intestinal resection)
Ischemia	Mesenteric thrombosis, vascular embolus to the mesenteric artery, volvulus
Impaction	Fecal impaction

Chronic Diarrhea (>2 Weeks' Duration)
The Five I's and Two M's

Infection	Amebiasis, giardiasis, *Clostridioides difficile* infection
Inflammatory bowel disease	Ulcerative colitis, Crohn's disease, collagenous colitis, lymphocytic colitis, radiation enteritis or colitis
Infiltrative disorders	Amyloidosis, lymphoma
Irritable bowel syndrome	
Intake	Laxative abuse, caffeine, sweeteners (sorbitol, fructose, xylitol)
Malabsorption	Celiac disease, short bowel syndrome, bacterial overgrowth
Metabolic/ hormonal	Enzyme deficiencies (lactase deficiency, pancreatic insufficiency)
	Hormone production (gastrinoma, carcinoid, VIPoma, villous adenoma, medullary carcinoma of the thyroid)
	Endocrinopathies (diabetic diarrhea, hyperthyroidism, Addison disease)

Any of the causes of acute diarrhea, if left untreated, may cause chronic diarrhea.

| BOX 10.1 | Etiologic Agents in Infectious Diarrhea |

Inflammatory
Bacteria
- *Salmonella* spp.
- *Shigella* spp.
- *Campylobacter* spp.
- *Yersinia enterocolitica*
- *Vibrio parahaemolyticus* (in uncooked shellfish)
- *Plesiomonas shigelloides* (in uncooked shellfish)
- *Aeromonas hydrophila* (in untreated well water, brackish water)
- *Mycobacterium avium–intracellulare*[a]
- *Mycobacterium tuberculosis*
- *Chlamydia* spp.
- *E. coli*[b]

Viruses
- Norovirus
- Rotavirus
- Cytomegalovirus
- Herpes simplex virus
- Epstein-Barr virus
- Human immunodeficiency virus enteropathy
- Coronavirus

Nematode
- *Strongyloides stercoralis*

Protozoa
- *Entamoeba histolytica*
- *Giardia lamblia*
- *Cryptosporidium* spp.
- *Isospora belli*
- *Enterocytozoon bieneusi* (Microsporidia)
- *Cyclospora* spp.

Toxins
Toxins Produced in Vivo
- *Clostridioides difficile* (after antibiotic administration)
- Clostridioides perfringens (in beef, poultry)
- Vibrio cholerae
- *Bacillus cereus* (in fried rice)
- Enterotoxigenic *E. coli* (in hamburger)

Preformed Toxins
- *Staphylococcus aureus* (in potato salad, mayonnaise, pudding)
- *B. cereus* (fried rice)

[a]Prevalent in human immunodeficiency virus–positive patients.
[b]Enteroinvasive, enterohemorrhagic, and enteroaggregative *E. coli* strains produce an inflammatory diarrheal illness. Enteropathogenic *E. coli* produces a noninflammatory diarrheal illness by attachment to the intestinal brush border, resulting in a disaccharidase deficiency and loss of absorptive surface. Enterotoxigenic *E. coli* attaches to the small intestinal mucosa and produces toxins that result in a secretory diarrhea.

MAJOR THREAT TO LIFE

- Intravascular volume depletion; electrolyte imbalance
- Systemic infection

Volume depletion and *electrolyte disturbances* are the reasons that many children in underdeveloped countries die from diarrhea. Death from diarrhea seldom occurs in hospitalized adult patients, but diarrhea, if left untreated, can certainly progress to serious volume depletion and electrolyte imbalance. Some bacterial causes of diarrhea, if left untreated, may become systemic life-threatening disorders.

BEDSIDE

Quick-Look Test

Does the patient look well (comfortable), sick (uncomfortable or distressed), or critical (about to die)?

Most patients with acute diarrhea do not look unwell. However, if the diarrhea is caused by an invasive organism (e.g., *Salmonella, Shigella*), the patient may look sick and complain of headache, diffuse myalgia, chills, and fever.

Airway and Vital Signs

What is the blood pressure?

Resting hypotension is indicative of significant volume depletion. If the resting blood pressure is normal, examine for postural changes. A postural rise in heart rate of more than 15 beats/min, a fall in systolic blood pressure of more than 15 mm Hg, or any fall in diastolic blood pressure is indicative of significant hypovolemia.

What is the heart rate?

Intravascular volume depletion usually results in tachycardia unless the patient has a coexisting disorder (e.g., β-blockade, sick sinus syndrome, or autonomic neuropathy) that prevents the generation of tachycardia. However, in diarrheal diseases, tachycardia may also be caused by anxiety, pain, or fever. A relative bradycardia despite fever raises the suspicion of *Salmonella* infection.

What is the temperature?

Fever in a patient with diarrhea is nonspecific but is suggestive of the presence of inflammation, as may occur with infectious diarrhea, diverticulitis, inflammatory bowel disease, intestinal lymphoma, tuberculosis, and amebiasis. Some organisms (*Shigella* and *Salmonella* species) may cause systemic sepsis. However, sepsis may occur in the absence of fever, especially in elderly patients.

Selective Physical Examination I

Is the patient volume depleted? Is there evidence of systemic sepsis?

Vitals	(See preceding text)
Cardiovascular system	Pulse volume, jugular venous pressure (JVP) (flat neck veins)
	Skin temperature, color

Management I

What measures need to be taken immediately to correct intravascular volume depletion?

1. Normalize the intravascular volume. This can be achieved quickly by administering an intravenous (IV) fluid that remains in the intravascular space at least temporarily, such as normal saline or Ringer's lactate. Give normal saline, 250 to 500 mL intravenously over 1 to 2 hours, titrating the IV fluid to the patient's vital signs and JVP. Reassess the volume status after each bolus of IV fluid, aiming for a JVP of 2 to 3 cm H_2O above the sternal angle and concomitant normalization of heart rate and blood pressure.

2. Check the chart for a recent electrolyte determination. If the patient's electrolytes have not been checked within the past 24 hours, order measurements of serum electrolytes, urea, and creatinine levels now.

3. In a patient with fever (temperature >38.5°C), two sets of blood should be drawn for cultures. If the patient is also hypotensive, volume replacement should be instituted with normal saline, and empirical antibiotic coverage should be considered (see Chapter 12, page 107).

4. A rectal examination should be performed, and stool samples should be tested for occult blood, culture, ova and parasite determination, *C. difficile* toxin by immunoassay or NAAT (nucleic acid amplification test) and white blood cell (WBC) stain. If unusual organisms are suspected (e.g., in a patient with acquired immunodeficiency syndrome [AIDS]), the laboratory should be alerted so that appropriate culture techniques and media can be used.

Selective Chart Review

Are potential causes of diarrhea apparent from the information in the patient's chart? Is the patient taking any medications that may cause diarrhea?

Medications are the most common cause of diarrhea in the hospital. Frequent offenders include laxatives, stool softeners, magnesium-containing antacids, sorbitol-containing liquid formulations, digoxin, quinidine, colchicine, and xanthines. Laxatives and stool softeners should be discontinued. Magnesium-containing antacids may be withheld or replaced by aluminum-containing preparations. Do not discontinue other medications without first asking the resident or attending physician. Remember also that some medications (e.g., Anacin, Dristan, Dyazide) contain gluten, which is harmful to a patient with celiac disease.

Has the patient received antibiotics recently?

Many antibiotics cause transient diarrhea through alteration of the intestinal flora. In addition, pseudomembranous colitis caused by *C. difficile* enterotoxin may result in persistent diarrhea during or after antibiotic use. Diagnosis is usually made by means of an enzyme-linked immunoassay (ELISA), which is 85% sensitive and 100% specific. Treatment includes discontinuing the offending antibiotic and administering **fidaxomicin (Dificid) 200 mg PO bid for 10 days.** Less expensive treatments that are almost as effective, but accompanied by more frequent recurrence, are **metronidazole 500 mg orally (PO) every 8 hours for 10 to 14 days or vancomycin, 125 to 500 mg PO every 6 hours for 10 to 14 days.**

Comparative prices (USA) in 2022 for 10- to 14-day treatment are fidaxomicin $4262.20, vancomycin $200.00, and metronidazole $15.00.

Does the patient have HIV disease?

Immunocompromised patients and patients with AIDS may develop diarrhea for many reasons, including infections from a variety of pathogens, medications (especially protease inhibitors), and AIDS enteropathy. The most common infectious causes include *Cryptosporidium, Microsporidium, Mycobacterium avium–intracellulare, Salmonella, Shigella,* and *Cytomegalovirus* organisms. If this episode of diarrhea is the first one documented, stool samples should be obtained for acid-fast stain, WBC stain, bacterial and mycobacterial culture, and ova and parasite determination. The test with the highest yield is microscopic examination with a search for ova and parasites. The correct transport medium must be used for specific pathogen cultures, and laboratories often require identification of the possible pathogens—such as *Cryptosporidium, Yersinia,* and *Aeromonas* species and *Escherichia coli* O157—to select the most appropriate laboratory techniques. Diagnosis of anorectal infections may necessitate proctoscopy or sigmoidoscopy, with specimens obtained for gonorrhea testing, herpes simplex viral culture, and dark-field examination for syphilis; this can be arranged in the morning.

Has the patient had recent surgery?

Postgastrectomy dumping of hypertonic boluses of stomach contents into the jejunum is associated with vasomotor symptoms of flushing, anxiety, palpitations, sweating, and dizziness, and diarrhea may occur in association. Resections of the ileum and right colon may result in diarrhea because of bile acid malabsorption.

Does the patient have known inflammatory bowel disease, celiac disease, lactase deficiency, or other conditions known to cause chronic diarrhea?

Any of these preexisting conditions may be responsible for diarrhea occurring while hospitalized; providing the patient does not have volume depletion and is otherwise comfortable, no additional measures are required at night.

Has the patient traveled abroad recently?

E. coli enterotoxin is the most common cause of traveler's diarrhea, although *Salmonella* organisms, *Shigella* organisms, and *Campylobacter jejuni* may be responsible for some cases of acute, self-limited traveler's diarrhea. Giardiasis, amebiasis, and tropical sprue may cause a more chronic picture.

Has the patient been admitted for the investigation of diarrhea?

If so, a plan of investigation has probably already been outlined. If the patient does not have volume depletion and is otherwise comfortable, no additional measures are required at night.

Is the patient receiving tube feedings?

Diarrhea often complicates enteral tube feedings, but in many cases it results from factors other than the feeding formula itself, such as medications or underlying illnesses. On occasion, diarrhea may develop because of the formula's composition (e.g., high fat, high osmolarity, presence of lactose), the manner in which it is delivered (bolus vs. continuous infusion), or contamination of the formula. In most cases, decisions regarding a change in formula or in the manner or rate of delivery can wait until morning.

Selective Physical Examination II

Look for clues to specific causes of diarrhea:

Vitals	Repeat measurements now.
Head, eyes, ears, nose, throat (HEENT)	Lymphadenopathy (lymphoma, Whipple disease, AIDS)
Abdomen (ABD)	Surgical scars (gastrectomy, cholecystectomy, intestinal resection)
	Hepatosplenomegaly (*Salmonella* infection)
	Epigastric tenderness (Zollinger-Ellison syndrome)
	Right lower quadrant: mass or tenderness (Crohn disease, ischemic colitis)
	Left lower quadrant: mass or tenderness (diverticulitis, tumor, inflammatory bowel disease, ischemic colitis, fecal impaction)

Rectal	Rectal fissure (Crohn disease)
	Hard mass (fecal impaction, tumor)
	Fresh blood or stool sample with occult blood (inflammatory bowel disease, infection, tumor)
Musculoskeletal system (MSS)	Arthritis (inflammatory bowel disease, Whipple disease)
Skin	Rose spots (*Salmonella* infection)
	Dermatitis herpetiformis (celiac disease)
	Pyoderma gangrenosum (Crohn disease)
	Hyperpigmentation (Whipple, Addison, or celiac disease)
	Flushing (carcinoid)

Management II

It is unusual for a clinician to be able to pinpoint the specific cause of diarrhea when a patient is seen for the first time at night. On occasion, a patient will say, "I'm sure it's my Crohn disease acting up" or "I have lactose intolerance, and the kitchen gave me yogurt for dinner." In these cases, the patient usually turns out to be right. When the diagnosis is not obvious at night, your goals are to ensure that the patient is adequately hydrated, does not have a serious electrolyte imbalance, and does not have a systemic infection. Additional specialized investigations for diarrhea can, in most cases, wait until the morning to be arranged.

Remember that in many cases of infectious diarrhea, frequent loose stools are the body's way of expelling the offending organism or toxin. Do not compound the problem by inhibiting the body's ability to do this. Diarrhea is always best treated by addressing the underlying cause, which may take a few days (and sometimes weeks) to identify. Unless the diarrhea is profuse or disabling, nonspecific antidiarrheal agents are best avoided. Explain this to the patient and to the nurses caring for him or her so that everyone is clear about the treatment approach.

If the patient's diarrhea is severe and disabling, use of one of the following nonspecific antidiarrheal agents is occasionally warranted. However none of these agents should be prescribed before the patient undergoes examination (including a rectal examination and possibly sigmoidoscopy) and before you decide on an appropriate plan of investigation.

- **Loperamide (Imodium), 4 mg PO every 4 hours**, until diarrhea is controlled, up to a maximum dose of 16 mg in 24 hours. The drug is less effective if given on an as-needed basis (PRN). Side effects include dry mouth; abdominal distention and cramping; on occasion, nausea and vomiting; and, in rare instances, toxic megacolon. Other side effects include rash, drowsiness, dizziness, and tiredness.

- **Diphenoxylate hydrochloride (Lomotil), 5 mg PO three or four times a day,** until diarrhea is controlled, up to a maximum dose of 20 mg in 24 hours. It is as effective as loperamide for treating acute nonspecific diarrhea but has a slower onset of antidiarrheal action. Diphenoxylate is contraindicated in patients with hepatic failure or cirrhosis. Respiratory depression may occur when it is used in combination with phenothiazines, tricyclic antidepressants, or barbiturates. Toxic megacolon may result if ulcerative colitis is present.

- **Bismuth subsalicylate (Pepto-Bismol, Kaopectate in the United States), 30 mL or two tablets (262 mg/tablet) PO every 30 minutes,** up to a maximum of eight doses per day. Bismuth is known to cause blackening of the tongue and stools. It may inhibit the absorption of tetracycline. Salicylate overdose may occur, especially if the patient is also receiving aspirin.

Agents such as anticholinergics, kaolin, and pectin do not reduce fecal water loss in diarrheal illnesses and are best avoided.

Fall Out of Bed

Patients always seem to be falling out of bed, but they can fall in other places, too. This chapter applies to any fall that occurs in the patient's room or elsewhere in the hospital.

PHONE CALL

Questions

1. Was the patient's fall witnessed?
2. Does the patient have an obvious injury?
3. What are the patient's vital signs?
4. Has the level of the patient's consciousness changed?
5. Is the patient receiving anticoagulant, antineoplastic, or other drugs affecting coagulation or antiseizure medications?
6. Why was the patient originally admitted?

Orders

Ask the registered nurse (RN) to call you immediately if the level of consciousness changes before you are able to assess the patient.

Informing the Registered Nurse

Tell the RN, "I will arrive at the bedside in . . . minutes."

If a change in the level of consciousness, a suspected fracture, or a coagulation disorder occurs, you must see the patient immediately. However, when other sick patients are in need of assessment, they take priority over a patient who has had an uncomplicated fall.

ELEVATOR THOUGHTS

Why does a patient fall?

Cardiac   Postural hypotension (volume depletion,
                     drug effects, autonomic failure)
                 Vasovagal attack
                 Dysrhythmia
                 Myocardial infarction

Neurologic	Confusion and cognitive impairment (particularly in elderly patients)
	Drug effects (from narcotics, sedatives, antidepressants, tranquilizers, antihypertensive agents)
	Metabolic disorders (electrolyte abnormalities, renal failure, hepatic failure)
	Dementia (from Parkinson disease, Alzheimer disease, multiple infarctions, normal-pressure hydrocephalus) that results in poor awareness of danger
	Gait and balance disorders
	Visual impairment
	Transient ischemic attack, stroke
	Seizure
Environmental/ accidental	Disorientation at night
	Inaccessible call bell
	Restraints
	Improper bed height
	Wet floors
	Unsafe clothing (e.g., long hospital gowns or pajamas, tractionless slippers)
	Obstacles (e.g., bed rails, intravenous [IV] poles, clutter around bed)

The hospital setting contains many potential environmental hazards. Elderly persons are particularly prone to accidental falls because of a combination of environmental hazards, poor vision, diminished muscular strength, and impaired self-righting reflexes.

MAJOR THREAT TO LIFE

Head Injury/Stroke

The most remediable critical situation is an acute epidural or subdural hemorrhage and stroke. Any patient who may have hit his or her head during a fall requires a complete neurologic examination immediately. Even seemingly minor trauma can result in serious intracranial bleeding in an anticoagulated patient. If a new neurologic problem is identified, an immediate computed tomography (CT) scan of the head is critical in identifying brain injury including subdural and epidural hematomas, skull fractures with hemorrhagic contusions, as well as ischemic and hemorrhagic strokes. If you suspect that a stroke was responsible for the fall, call your senior house staff, neurologist, or stroke team for help (for management of stroke see Chapter 26).

Immediate reversal of anticoagulation should be considered and discussed with the resident and a hematologist (see Chapter 32, pages 388–389, for reversal of anticoagulation). If no neurologic deficit is identified at this time, observation with frequent assessment of the neurovital signs is required.

BEDSIDE

Quick-Look Test

Does the patient look well (comfortable), sick (uncomfortable or distressed), or critical (about to die)?

Most patients do not have life-threatening problems as a result of falling. Usually they look well, and the vital signs are normal.

Airway and Vital Signs

What is the heart rate (HR) and rhythm?

Tachycardia, bradycardia, or irregular rhythm may indicate that a dysrhythmia is the cause of the fall.

Does the patient have postural (lying and standing) changes in blood pressure (BP) and HR?

A postural fall in BP, together with a postural rise in HR (>15 beats/min), is suggestive of volume depletion. A drop in BP without a change in HR is suggestive of autonomic dysfunction. An initial drop in BP that is corrected on standing is also suggestive of autonomic dysfunction. Drugs—particularly antihypertensive agents, sedatives, and antidepressants—are common causes of postural hypotension in elderly patients.

Selective History

Does the patient know why he or she fell out of bed? What was the patient doing just before the fall?

Coughing, micturating, or straining are examples of maneuvers that may result in vasovagal syncope. Question any witnesses who observed the fall. Did the patient trip or slip?

Did the patient have any warning symptoms before the fall?

Lightheadedness and visual disturbances on standing may be indicative of postural hypotension. Palpitations are suggestive of a dysrhythmia. A preceding aura would be rare in this situation but, if present, is highly suggestive of a seizure disorder.

Does the patient have a history of falls?

Recurrent falls suggest an underlying disorder that has gone unrecognized. Although your main duty at night is to detect, document, and treat any injuries that have been sustained, a pattern of falling behavior may be an important clue to an unrecognized but treatable disorder.

Is the patient diabetic?

Hyperglycemia or hypoglycemia may cause confusion, which can contribute to a fall. Order a finger-prick blood glucose reading. Check the patient's diabetic record for the past 3 days.

Is the patient aware of any injury sustained during the fall?

Patients may fracture a wrist or hip as a result of falling. Elderly women are at particular risk because of osteoporosis.

Selective Physical Examination

Look for both the cause and the consequences of the fall.

Vitals	Repeat measurements now; only supine BP and HR values are necessary, provided that both supine and standing measurements were already taken.
Head, eyes, ears, nose, throat (HEENT)	Tongue or cheek lacerations (seizure) Hemotympanum (basal skull fracture)
Cardiovascular system (CVS)	Pulse rate and rhythm (dysrhythmia) Decreased jugular venous pressure (JVP) (volume depletion)
Musculoskeletal system (MSS)	Palpate skull and face Palpate spine and ribs Palpate long bones Check passive range of motion of all four limbs } Fractures, hematomas, and laceration
Neurologic system	Complete neurologic examination; pay particular attention to level of consciousness and any asymmetric neurologic findings. New findings of asymmetry are suggestive of structural brain disease.

Selective Chart Review

Search for the cause of the fall.

1. What was the reason for admission?
2. Does the patient have a history of cardiac dysrhythmia, seizure disorder, autonomic neuropathy, disorientation at night, or diabetes mellitus?
3. What drugs is the patient receiving?
   - Antihypertensive agents
   - Diuretics (volume depletion)
   - Antidysrhythmic agents
   - Antiseizure medications

- Narcotics
- Sedatives, tranquilizers
- Antidepressants
- Insulin, oral hypoglycemic agents
4. Check the most recent laboratory measurements:
   - Glucose: increase or decrease may cause confusion
   - Na: increase or decrease may cause confusion
   - K: increase can cause atrioventricular (AV) block; decrease can cause weakness or tachydysrhythmias
   - Ca: increase causes confusion; decrease may cause seizures
   - Urea, creatinine (uremia can result in confusion and seizures)
   - Antiseizure drug levels (subtherapeutic levels may result in seizure breakthrough; toxic levels may be associated with ataxia)

Management

Treat the Cause

Investigate and treat the suspected cause. A fall is a symptom, not a diagnosis. Establish the reason for the fall (provisional diagnosis). The cause is often multifactorial. For example, if an elderly patient with diuretic-induced nocturia is under the influence of a night-time sedative, the patient's trip to the bathroom will be a struggle in an unfamiliar, dimly lit hospital room.

Immediate CT head scanning should be ordered for patients who are thought to have sustained a head injury and have one or more of the following:
- Glasgow Coma Scale score of less than 15
- Suspected skull fracture
- Any sign of basal skull fracture (hemotympanum, cerebrospinal fluid leakage from the ear or nose, panda eyes, or Battle sign)
- Posttraumatic seizure
- Focal neurologic deficit
- Amnesia for events more than 30 minutes before impact
- Coagulopathy
- More than one episode of vomiting

Reversible Factors

Reversible factors, especially volume depletion and inappropriate drug therapy in elderly patients, must be corrected.

Nocturia

The majority of elderly patients who fall out of bed at night are on their way to the bathroom because of nocturia. Make sure that the nocturia is not iatrogenic (e.g., the result of an evening diuretic order or an unnecessary IV infusion).

Elderly Patient

If the patient is disoriented at night, ensure that the call bell is easily accessible, a nightlight is left on, and the evening's fluid intake is limited. The use of physical restraints (Posey restraints and bed rails) may actually contribute to falls and should be discouraged. It is best to leave the side rails down or lower the bed height.

Complications

Have any complications resulted from the fall? If so, investigate, treat, and record these as a second diagnosis. Hip fractures as a result of a fall are common in elderly patients. A patient who has had a stroke may have unknowingly dislocated or subluxated the shoulder on the paralyzed side during a fall. A patient taking anticoagulants may develop a serious, delayed hemorrhage at any site of trauma. Reexamine these patients frequently.

Fever

It is unusual to spend an entire night on call without being called about a febrile patient. The majority of fevers in hospitalized patients are caused by infections. Locating the source of a fever usually requires some detective work. Whether the cause of a fever necessitates specific immediate treatment depends on both the clinical status of the patient and the suspected diagnosis.

PHONE CALL

Questions

1. How high is the patient's temperature, and by what route was it measured? 37°C oral = 37.5°C rectal or 36.5°C axillary.
2. What are the measurements for the patient's other vital signs?
3. Does the patient have any associated symptoms?

    A cough and hoarseness suggest a contagious respiratory viral illness.
4. Pain may help localize a site of infection or inflammation. A headache, neck ache, seizure, or change in sensorium, together with fever, are suggestive of meningitis or encephalitis.
5. Is this fever *new*?
6. Why was the patient admitted?
7. Has the patient recently undergone surgery?

    Postoperative fever is very common and may result from atelectasis, pneumonia, pulmonary embolism, wound infection, infected intravenous (IV) sites, or urinary tract infection from a Foley catheter.

Orders

1. If the patient is febrile and hypotensive, administer **500 mL of normal saline intravenously**, as rapidly as possible.
2. If the patient is febrile with symptoms of meningitis (headache, neck ache, seizure, or change in sensorium), order a lumbar puncture tray to the bedside now.

3. If a contagious respiratory illness is suspected, ensure that all personnel (including yourself) are using appropriate personal protective equipment (PPE).

Arrange for an immediate test for COVID-19, e.g., NAAT (nucleic acid amplification test)

Informing the Registered Nurse

Tell the registered nurse (RN), "I will arrive at the bedside in . . . minutes."

An elevated temperature alone is seldom life-threatening. However when fever is associated with hypotension or symptoms of meningitis, you must see the patient immediately.

ELEVATOR THOUGHTS

What causes fever?

Infection is by far the most common cause of fever in a hospitalized patient. Common sites of infection are the lung, urinary tract, wounds, and IV sites. Less common sites are the central nervous system (CNS), abdomen, and pelvis. An immunocompromised patient is not only predisposed to infection but also more susceptible to serious complications of infection.

Other common causes of fever are as follows:
• Pulmonary embolism and deep vein thrombosis
• Drug effects
• Neoplasm
• Connective tissue diseases
• Postoperative atelectasis

MAJOR THREAT TO LIFE

• Septic shock
• Meningitis

In hospitalized patients, fever is most commonly a manifestation of infection. Most infections can be brought under control by a combination of the body's natural defense mechanisms and judicious antibiotic use. Infection at any site, if progressive, may lead to septicemia with attendant septic shock. *Meningitis,* by virtue of its location, can result in permanent neurologic deficit or death if it goes untreated.

BEDSIDE

Quick-Look Test

Does the patient look well (comfortable), sick (uncomfortable or distressed), or critical (about to die)?

Toxic signs, such as apprehension, agitation, or lethargy, are suggestive of serious infection.

Airway and Vital Signs

What is the patient's heart rate?

Tachycardia, proportionate to the temperature elevation, is an expected finding in a febrile patient. Normally, the heart rate rises by 16 beats/minute for each degree Celsius of temperature rise. The occurrence of a relative bradycardia with fever has been observed in *Legionella* pneumonia, *Mycoplasma pneumoniae* pneumonia, ascending cholangitis, typhoid fever, and *Plasmodium falciparum* malaria with profound hemolysis.

What is the patient's blood pressure?

Fever in association with supine or postural hypotension is indicative of relative hypovolemia and can be the forerunner of septic shock. Ensure that an IV line is in place. Infuse normal saline or Ringer's lactate to correct the intravascular volume deficit.

Selective Physical Examination I

What is the volume status? Is the patient in septic shock? Are there signs of meningitis?

Vitals	Repeat measurements now.
Head, eyes, ears, nose, throat (HEENT)	Photophobia, neck stiffness
Cardiovascular system (CVS)	Pulse volume, jugular venous pressure (JVP) Skin temperature, color
Neurologic system	Change in sensorium
	Special maneuvers
Brudzinski sign: With the patient supine, passively flex the neck forward; flexion of the patient's hips and knees in response to this maneuver constitutes a positive test result (see Fig. 14.3A, page 134)	*Kernig sign*: With the patient supine, flex one hip and knee to 90 degrees, then straighten the knee; pain or resistance in the ipsilateral hamstrings constitutes a positive test result (see Fig. 14.3B, page 134)

Septic shock is a clinical condition consisting of two states. Early in the development of septic shock, the patient may be warm, dry, and flushed because of peripheral vasodilation and increased cardiac output (*warm shock*). As septic shock progresses, the patient becomes hypotensive, and the skin becomes cool and clammy (*cold shock*) as a result of peripheral vasoconstriction. Delays in treatment may result from failure to recognize the first state and can lead to serious complications.

Fever in an elderly patient, regardless of cause, can produce changes in sensorium ranging from lethargy to agitation. If a specific site of infection is not obvious, a lumbar puncture should be performed to check for meningitis (see page 108).

Management I

What immediate measures need to be taken to prevent septic shock or to recognize meningitis?

Septic Shock

If the patient is febrile and hypotensive, determine the volume status; if the patient is hypovolemic, administer IV fluids (normal saline or Ringer's lactate) promptly until it returns to normal.

📖 *Caution:* Aggressive volume repletion in a patient with a history of congestive heart failure (CHF) may compromise cardiac function. Do not overshoot the goal of volume repletion!

While IV fluid resuscitation is taking place, obtain samples for necessary cultures: usually blood from two different sites, urine (for Gram stain and culture), sputum, and any other potentially infected body fluid.

Septic shock is a major threat to life, and once culture samples are taken, antibiotics must be given to cover both gram-positive and gram-negative organisms. The choice of antibiotic also depends on a knowledge of patterns of local antibiotic susceptibility. Many institutions have protocols to guide empirical antibacterial therapy, particularly in neutropenic patients. A common empirical broad-spectrum regimen includes a third- or fourth-generation cephalosporin (ceftriaxone or cefepime) with an aminoglycoside (gentamicin, tobramycin, natamycin, or amikacin). If pseudomonas is a possibility, ceftaroline is a cephalosporin effective against this organism. Alternatives to cephalosporins include piperacillin/tazobactam with aztreonam. If methicillin-resistant staphylococci are suspected, therapy can be started with ceftaroline or vancomycin.

📖 Some patients are allergic to penicillin. Ensure that the patient is not allergic before you order penicillin or cephalosporin. Aminoglycosides are common causes of nephrotoxicity and ototoxicity. Select maintenance dosing intervals according to the patient's calculated creatinine clearance (see Appendix C, page 430). Monitor the serum aminoglycoside concentrations, usually after the third or fourth dose, and the serum creatinine concentration.

If the volume status is normal and the patient is still hypotensive, transfer him or her to the intensive care unit (ICU)/cardiac care unit (CCU) for inotropic or vasopressor support. (Refer to Chapter 18 for further discussion of septic shock.)

In a patient with septic shock, a Foley catheter should be placed to monitor urine output.

Meningitis

Fever accompanied by headache, seizure, stiff neck, or change in sensorium is considered to be meningitis until proved otherwise.

A lumbar puncture should be performed without delay to confirm the diagnosis and guide antimicrobial therapy. This procedure should not be undertaken if the patient has focal neurologic findings or signs of increased intracranial pressure such as papilledema (see Fig. 14.2, page 133), coma, irregular respirations, bradycardia, or decerebrate posture. Other contraindications include a coagulopathy, because of the risk of intrathecal hematoma formation, which may result in cord compression.

In bacterial meningitis, the cerebrospinal fluid (CSF) usually demonstrates pleocytosis (number of cells >109/L), protein levels higher than 0.4 g/L, and glucose levels lower than 2 mmol/L. However, these findings may not be present early in the course. Gram stain yields positive results in 80% of patients not previously treated with antibacterial agents. In patients who have been partially treated, detection of bacterial antigens with latex agglutination is helpful but unreliable in detecting group B meningococcal antigen.

If you are unable to visualize the fundi or if papilledema or focal neurologic signs are evident (suggestive of a mass lesion), administer the first dose of antibiotics and arrange for an urgent computed tomographic (CT) scan of the head to confirm or rule out a space-occupying lesion before the lumbar puncture is performed. In the presence of an intracranial space-occupying lesion, a lumbar puncture can result in uncal herniation and brainstem compression (coning).

If meningococcal meningitis is a possibility institute antibiotic treatment immediately:

Ceftriaxone 2g IV q12h or
Cefotaxime 2g IV or IM q6h

If culture later identifies the organism to be penicillin-sensitive, treatment can be switched to penicillin G.

Arrangements should be made to protect contacts:

- **Ciprofloxacin 500 mg PO once** or
- **Ceftriaxone 250 mg IM once,** or
- **Rifampin 600 mg PO bid for 48 hrs**

Selective Chart Review

If the patient is not in septic shock and does not have symptoms or signs of meningitis, perform a selective chart review, looking for *localizing clues* (Table 12.1). Also check the chart for the following:

- Temperature pattern during hospital stay
- Recent white blood cell (WBC) count and differential
- Evidence of immunodeficiency (e.g., cancer chemotherapy, immunosuppressive agents, hematologic malignancy, human immunodeficiency virus [HIV] infection, [CD4] lymphocyte count)

TABLE 12.1	Selective Chart Review: Looking for Localizing Clues	
Localizing Clue	Diagnostic Considerations	Comments
Recent surgery	Atelectasis	Postoperative fever caused by atelectasis is a diagnosis made only after infection is ruled out.
—	Pneumonia	—
—	Pulmonary embolism	—
—	Infected surgical wound, infected biopsy site, or deeper infection of biopsy organ	Despite modern surgical techniques, any incision or puncture site may serve as a portal for bacteria.
Blood transfusion	Transfusion reaction	See Chapter 28
Headache, seizure, stiff neck, changes in sensorium	Meningitis	Delirium tremens can mimic meningitis in some patients; is the patient withdrawing from alcohol?
—	Intracranial abscess	—
—	Encephalitis	—
Sinus discomfort	Sinusitis	—
Dental caries, toothache	Periodontal abscess	—
Sore throat	Pharyngitis, tonsillitis	—
Dysphagia	Retropharyngeal abscess	
—	Epiglottitis	Either of these diagnoses is a medical emergency; consult otorhinolaryngology or anesthesia department immediately.
Shortness of breath, cough, or chest pain	Pneumonia	—
	Respiratory virus (e.g., COVID)	Do an immediate NAAT (nucleic acid amplification test)

Continued

TABLE 12.1	Selective Chart Review: Looking for Localizing Clues—cont'd	
Localizing Clue	**Diagnostic Considerations**	**Comments**
—	Lung abscess	—
—	Pulmonary embolus	—
Murmur, CHF, or peripheral embolic lesions	Infective endocarditis	—
Pleuritic chest pain	Pneumonia	—
—	Empyema	—
—	Pulmonary embolus	—
—	Pericarditis	—
Costovertebral angle tenderness	Pyelonephritis	—
—	Perinephric abscess	—
Foley catheter, dysuria, hematuria, or pyuria	Cystitis	Condom catheters and Foley catheters predispose patients to urinary tract infections.
—	Pyelonephritis	—
Abdominal pain	—	If there are peritoneal signs, consider surgical consultation.
RUQ	Subphrenic abscess	—
—	Hepatic abscess	—
—	Hepatitis	—
—	RLL pneumonia	—
—	Cholecystitis	—
—	Ascending cholangitis	Does the patient have the Charcot triad (fever, RUQ pain, jaundice)? If so, consider surgical consultation.
RLQ	Appendicitis	—
—	Crohn disease	—
—	Salpingitis	—
LUQ	Splenic abscess	—
—	Subphrenic abscess	—
—	Infected pancreatic pseudo-cyst	—
—	LLL pneumonia	—
LLQ	Diverticular abscess	—
—	Salpingitis	—

TABLE 12.1	Selective Chart Review: Looking for Localizing Clues—cont'd	
Localizing Clue	**Diagnostic Considerations**	**Comments**
Ascites	Peritonitis	Perform abdominal paracentesis to look for spontaneous bacterial peritonitis in any ascitic patient who becomes unwell
Diarrhea	Enteritis	—
—	Colitis	—
Swollen, red, tender joint	Septic arthritis	A monoarticular effusion or a disproportionately inflamed joint in polyarticular disease must be aspirated to look for infection.
—	Gout or pseudogout	—
Prosthetic joint	Infected prosthesis	—
Vaginal discharge	Endometritis	—
—	Salpingitis	—
Red or tender IV site	Septic phlebitis	—
TPN line	Catheter sepsis	Fever may be the only symptom

CHF, Congestive heart failure; *IV*, intravenous; *LLL*, left lower lobe; *LLQ*, left lower quadrant; *LUQ*, left upper quadrant; *RLL*, right lower lobe; *RLQ*, right lower quadrant; *RUQ*, right upper quadrant; *TPN*, total parenteral nutrition.

- Allergies to antibiotics
- Other possible reasons for fever (e.g., connective tissue disease, neoplasm)
- Antipyretics, antibiotics, or steroids that may modify the fever pattern.

Selective Physical Examination II

Confirm localizing symptoms or signs already documented in the chart review.

Vitals	Repeat measurements now.
HEENT	Fundi: papilledema (intracranial abscess), Roth spots (infective endocarditis) (Fig. 12.1)
	Conjunctival or scleral petechiae (infective endocarditis)
	Ears: red tympanic membranes (otitis media, a complication of intubation)
	Sinuses: tenderness, inability to be transilluminated (sinusitis)
	Oral cavity: dental caries, tender tooth on tongue blade percussion (periodontal abscess)
	Pharynx: erythema, pharyngeal exudate (pharyngitis, thrush)
	Neck: stiff (meningitis)
Respiratory	Crackles, friction rub, signs of consolidation (pneumonia, pulmonary embolism)
CVS	New murmurs (infective endocarditis)
Abdomen (ABD)	Localized tenderness (see page 35)
Rectal	Tenderness or mass (rectal abscess)
Musculoskeletal system (MSS)	Joint erythema or effusion (septic arthritis)
Skin	Decubitus ulcers (cellulitis)
	Osler nodes and Janeway lesions, petechiae (infective endocarditis)
	IV sites (phlebitis, cellulitis)
	All surgical wounds (that means taking off the dressings)
Pelvic	A pelvic examination should be done if a pelvic source of fever is possible.

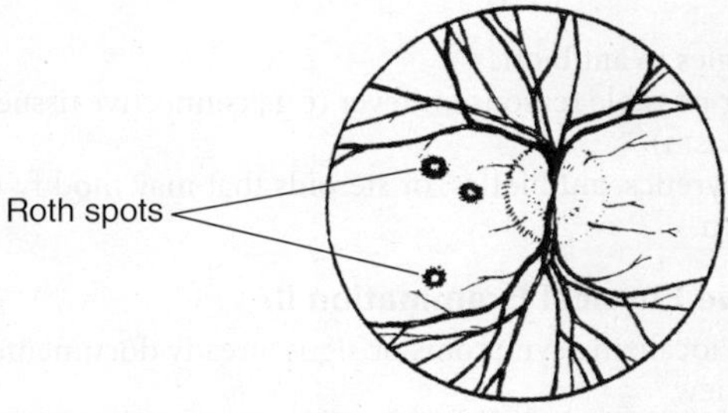

FIG. 12.1 **Roth spots.** Round or oval hemorrhagic retinal lesions with central pallor.

Management II

If an unexplained fever (oral temperature >38.5°C) has developed in the hospital, the following tests should be performed:

- Blood cultures immediately from two different sites
- Urinalysis (routine and microscopic) and urine culture immediately
- WBC count and differential

The performance of other, more selective tests depends on the localizing clues you elicited from your chart review, history, and physical examination. For example:

- Throat swab for Gram stain and culture
- Sputum for Gram stain and culture
- Chest radiography
- Lumbar puncture
- Blood culture for infective endocarditis (refer to your institution's protocol)
- Cervical culture (obtain the specific medium for gonococcal isolation before you perform the pelvic examination)
- Joint aspiration
- Swab of decubitus ulcers or infected or draining wounds for Gram stain and culture
- Fluid from any source for microscopic examination immediately to guide your choice of antibiotics

Remove suspect IV lines and, if necessary, place them at a new site. Central total parenteral nutrition (TPN) lines that may be infected should be replaced in consultation with your resident or TPN service. Catheter tips should be sent to the laboratory for culture.

If a *urinary tract infection* is suspected in a patient with a Foley catheter, remove the catheter. A few days of incontinence is an annoyance for the nursing staff but does not harm the patient if no perineal skin breakdown occurs. An exception to this situation is when a Foley catheter has been placed to treat urinary retention, because urinary stasis predisposes the patient to infection.

Broad-Spectrum Antibiotics

Three types of patients need broad-spectrum antibiotics immediately:

1. A patient with *fever and hypotension*.
2. A patient with *fever and neutropenia* (neutrophil count <500/mm^3 or <1000/mm^3 and falling) in whom a localizing site of infection is not apparent. Anticipate this event in an immunocompromised patient (e.g., one receiving chemotherapy or immunosuppressive agents), and agree on an appropriate broad-spectrum regimen with the hematologist or oncologist well ahead of time.

3. A patient who is febrile, appears toxic and acutely ill, and is suspected of having an infection despite no evidence of a clear-cut source.

  A minimal workup includes the following:

• Blood cultures

  Although the bacterial yield of blood cultures is low for diagnosing bacteremia, they are very valuable when findings are true positive. Optimally, two 20-mL aliquots of blood should be obtained from two venipuncture sites separate from any established venous access sites. This technique helps reduce contamination and the incidence of false-positive results.

• Urinalysis and urine culture
• Sputum for Gram stain and culture
• Chest radiography

  The selection of the initial antibiotics should be based on the most likely source or site of infection, the most likely causative organisms, and their probable antibiotic sensitivities. Your institution should have policies about the availability and appropriateness of specific antibiotics. More than one antibiotic is often required. Common choices include a third-, fourth-, or fifth-generation cephalosporin such as ceftobiprole or extended-spectrum penicillin with an aminoglycoside. However, a gastrointestinal or female pelvic infection may necessitate additional coverage of anaerobic organisms (e.g., metronidazole), and infections in an intravascular device or prosthetic cardiac valve may necessitate an antibiotic effective against methicillin-resistant staphylococci (e.g., vancomycin or another glycopeptide such as teicoplanin or the lipopeptide agent, daptomycin, or a carbapenem such as doripenem, ertapenem, meropenem, or imipenem/cilastatin).

Specific Antibiotics

Two types of patients need specific antibiotics immediately:

1. A patient with *fever and meningitis symptoms* requires antibiotics immediately after the lumbar puncture is performed. However, do not delay initial antibiotic treatment if a CT scan of the head must be performed before the lumbar puncture (see pages 108–109).

2. A patient with *fever and clear localizing clues* should be given specific antibiotics after culture specimens are collected. For diabetic patients, antibiotic therapy should be considered an urgent requirement.

No Antibiotics Until a Specific Microbiologic Diagnosis Is Made

A patient who does not look sick or critical, who is immunologically competent, and in whom the source of fever is not readily apparent (e.g., a patient admitted for workup of fever of unknown origin) should not receive antibiotics until a specific microbiologic diagnosis is made.

Choice of Antibiotics

Unfortunately, infecting organisms can develop resistance to antibiotics, and the widespread use of antibiotics is stimulating the development of these resistant strains. The choice of specific antibiotics depends on knowledge of your institution's local microbial flora and their antibiotic susceptibilities. Most parenteral antibiotics are expensive. Your institution should have guidelines for antibiotic use to diminish the development of resistant organisms and to control costs.

Fever in the Human Immunodeficiency Virus-Positive Patient

In patients with HIV disease, fever is usually caused by infection or lymphoma. In these patients, fever is presumed to be caused by infection until proved otherwise. On occasion, no specific cause of fever is found. In this case, the fever may be caused by the HIV infection itself, but this diagnosis should be considered one of exclusion.

Although HIV-positive patients are susceptible to any of the common infections, a number of opportunistic pathogens should be considered, including pneumocystis carini (pneumonia), Cryptococcus neoformans (meningitis), toxoplasmosis gondii (CNS mass lesion), and candida albicans (esophagitis). In HIV-positive patients, more than in any other patient population, multiple infections are often present.

REMEMBER

1. An immunocompromised patient is especially susceptible to infection and prone to develop complications. You should not hesitate to call for the help of the resident or attending physician.
2. The definition of fever of unknown origin is a temperature higher than 38.3°C for 3 weeks with no cause found despite thorough in-hospital investigation for 1 week.
3. Fever caused by neoplasm, connective tissue disorder, or drug reaction is a diagnosis that should be made only *after* you rule out fever caused by infection.
4. Fever may result from the use of prescription or nonprescription drugs. Even such commonly used drugs as antibiotics can cause a *drug fever,* which usually occurs within 7 days after the patient begins taking the offending drug.

Antipsychotic medications may cause the neuroleptic malignant syndrome, characterized by fever, muscular rigidity, an altered sensorium, tachycardia, and elevations in creatine phosphokinase, WBC count, and liver enzyme levels. The symptoms resolve when the offending drug is discontinued.

Overdoses of some psychostimulants, such as amphetamines and cocaine, may acutely elevate the temperature, resulting in rhabdomyolysis and contributing to fatal cardiac dysrhythmias. Prompt cooling, the use of antipyretics, and the judicious use of tranquilizers may be indicated in this setting.

5. By administering antipyretics for a fever caused by infection, you treat only the symptom. In fact, there is evidence that the ability to mount a febrile response is an adaptive mechanism that inhibits bacterial replication and enhances the ability of macrophages to kill bacteria. It is useful to observe the fever pattern, and if the fever is not very high (>40°C) and the patient is not uncomfortable, it is not necessary to treat with aspirin or acetaminophen.

6. If antipyretics are ordered, ask the RN to mark the bedside temperature chart with an arrow to mark the time of administration. Assessment of the therapeutic response is also made easier by charting the antibiotics given (Fig. 12.2).

7. Steroids may elevate the WBC count and suppress the fever response, regardless of the cause. Defervescence during a regimen with steroids should be interpreted cautiously.

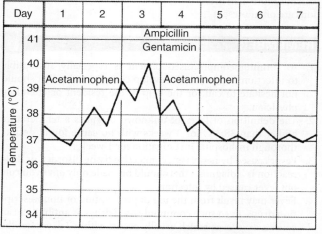

FIG. 12.2 Bedside temperature chart.

8. Microorganisms are attracted to foreign bodies. Look for foreign bodies at sites of infection: IV lines, Foley catheters, ventriculoperitoneal shunts, prosthetic joints, peritoneal dialysis catheters, and bioprosthetic or mechanical heart valves.

9. Fever that occurs while the patient is already on antibiotics may mean the following:
   - You are administering an inappropriate antibiotic.
   - You are administering an inadequate dose.
   - You are not treating the correct organism, or resistance or superinfection has developed.
   - The antibiotic is not reaching the correct place (e.g., thick-walled abscess that must be surgically drained).
   - The fever may not be caused by an infection.

10. Delirium tremens is a serious cause of fever that occurs occasionally in patients withdrawing from alcohol. It is associated with confusion, including delusions and hallucinations; agitation; seizures; and signs of autonomic hyperactivity such as fever, tachycardia, and sweating. This condition is sometimes fatal, and high doses of benzodiazepines are needed to stabilize the patient (see page 74).

Gastrointestinal Bleeding

Gastrointestinal (GI) bleeding is common in hospitalized patients. Whether the bleeding is caused by minor gastric stress ulceration or is part of life-threatening exsanguination of an aortoduodenal fistula, the initial principles of assessment and management are the same.

PHONE CALL

Questions

1. Clarify the situation: Is the bleeding old or new, and from where is it coming? Vomiting of bright red blood or "coffee grounds" and most cases of melena are indicative of upper GI bleeding. Bright red blood passed rectally (hematochezia) is usually indicative of lower GI bleeding but may be seen in upper GI bleeding when blood loss is sudden and massive.

2. How much blood has been lost?

3. What are the patient's vital signs? This information helps determine the urgency of the situation.

4. Why was the patient admitted? Recurrent bleeding from a duodenal ulcer or esophageal varices carries a high mortality rate.

5. Is the patient receiving anticoagulants (heparin, warfarin), direct thrombin inhibitors (dabigatran, fondaparinux, lepirudin, argatroban, bivalirudin), direct factor Xa inhibitors (rivaroxaban, apixaban, edoxaban), fibrinolytic therapy (streptokinase, tissue plasminogen activator, reteplase, tenecteplase), or agents that affect platelet number (chemotherapy) or function (aspirin, clopidogrel, prasugrel, ticagrelor, ticlopidine, glycoprotein IIb/IIIa inhibitors)?

   An actively bleeding patient may require immediate discontinuation of anticoagulants or thrombolytic agents or immediate reversal of their effects.

Orders

1. Do not give the patient anything by mouth.
2. Large-bore intravenous (IV) line (size 16 if possible) immediately, if not already in place. IV access is a priority in a bleeding patient. Two IV sites may be required if the patient is hemodynamically unstable.
3. Hemoglobin stat. *Caution:* The hemoglobin level may be normal during an acute bleeding episode and drops only with correction of the intravascular volume by a shift of fluid from the extravascular space.
4. Crossmatch: Is blood available on hold? If not, order stat crossmatch of 2, 4, or 6 U of packed red blood cells (RBCs), depending on your estimation of blood loss.
5. Ask the registered nurse (RN) to take the patient's chart to the patient's bedside.

Informing the Registered Nurse

Tell the RN, "I will arrive at the bedside in . . . minutes."

If a bleeding patient has hypotension or tachycardia, you must see the patient immediately.

ELEVATOR THOUGHTS

What causes GI bleeding?
1. Upper GI bleeding
   a. Esophagitis
   b. Esophageal varices
   c. Mallory-Weiss syndrome (tear)
   d. Gastric ulcer, gastritis
   e. Duodenal ulcer, duodenitis
   f. Neoplasm (esophageal cancer, gastric cancer)
2. Lower GI bleeding
   a. Angiodysplasia
   b. Diverticulosis
   c. Neoplasm
   d. Colitis (ulcerative, ischemic, infectious)
   e. Mesenteric thrombosis
   f. Meckel diverticulum
   g. Hemorrhoids
3. GI bleeding may also occur in the absence of structural disease in a patient who has recently received a thrombolytic agent, is receiving anticoagulant therapy, or is receiving medications that cause thrombocytopenia or affect platelet function.

   GI bleeding in a patient with human immunodeficiency virus (HIV) may be caused by any of the conditions listed, which are unrelated to the HIV-positive state. However, additional causes should be considered. Upper GI bleeding may result from Kaposi sarcoma, gastric lymphoma, cytomegalovirus (CMV) infection of the esophagus or duodenum, or herpes simplex virus infection of the esophagus. Lower GI bleeding may result from Kaposi sarcoma or from colitis caused by CMV, bacterial pathogens (including atypical mycobacteria), or herpes simplex.

MAJOR THREAT TO LIFE

Hypovolemic Shock

The major concern with GI bleeding is the progressive loss of intra-vascular volume in a patient whose bleeding lesion is not identified and managed correctly. If allowed to progress, even minor intermittent or continuous bleeding may eventually result in hypovolemic shock, with hypoperfusion of vital organs.

Initially, lost blood volume can be corrected by infusion of normal saline or Ringer's lactate, but if bleeding continues, lost RBCs must also be replaced, in the form of packed RBC transfusion. Hence, your initial assessment should be directed at the patient's volume status to determine whether a significant amount of intra-vascular volume has been lost.

BEDSIDE

Quick-Look Test

Does the patient look well (comfortable), sick (uncomfortable or distressed), or critical (about to die)?

A patient in hypovolemic shock resulting from blood loss appears pale and apprehensive and may have other symptoms and signs, including cold and clammy skin, as a result of stimulation of the sympathetic nervous system.

Airway and Vital Signs

Are there any postural changes in blood pressure or heart rate?

First, check for changes with the patient in the lying and sitting (with legs dangling) positions. If there are no changes, the blood pressure and heart rate should then be checked with the patient standing.

A rise in heart rate of more than 15 beats/min, a fall in systolic blood pressure of more than 15 mm Hg, or any fall in diastolic blood pressure is indicative of significant hypovolemia.

Caution: A resting tachycardia alone may indicate decreased intravascular volume. If the resting systolic blood pressure is lower than 90 mm Hg, order placement of a second large-bore IV line immediately.

Selective Physical Examination I

What is the patient's volume status? Is the patient in shock?

Vitals	Repeat measurements now.
Cardiovascular system (CVS)	Pulse volume, jugular venous pressure (JVP)
	Skin temperature and color
Neurologic system	Mental status

📖 Shock is a clinical diagnosis, as follows: systolic blood pressure lower than 90 mm Hg with evidence of inadequate tissue perfusion, such as cold and clammy skin and changes in central nervous system function (manifested by agitation or confusion). In fact, the kidney is a sensitive indicator of shock (when urine output <20 mL/hr). The urine output of a patient who is hypovolemic ordinarily correlates with the renal blood flow, which in turn is dependent on cardiac output; therefore, urine output is an extremely important measurement. However, placement of a Foley catheter should not take priority over resuscitation measures.

Management I

What measures must be taken immediately to correct shock or prevent it from occurring?

Replenish the intravascular volume by administering IV fluids. The best immediate choice is a crystalloid (normal saline or Ringer's lactate), which stays in the intravascular space at least temporarily. Albumin or banked plasma can be administered, but both are expensive, carry a risk of hepatitis, and are not readily available.

Blood has been lost from the intravascular space, and ideally, blood should be replaced (see Box 13.1 for steps to take if the patient refuses a blood transfusion). If no blood is on hold for the patient, a stat crossmatch can be made; this usually takes 50 minutes. If blood is on hold, it should be available at the bedside in 30 minutes. In an emergency, O-negative blood can be administered, although this practice is usually reserved for victims of acute trauma.

The incidence of transfusion-associated hepatitis can be minimized by transfusing only when necessary. *Rule:* Maintain a hemoglobin level of 8 to 9 g/100 ml (80 to 90 g/L). An exception to this is suspected variceal bleeding, in which overtransfusion may precipitate further bleeding; in such patients, goal Hb is approximately 7 to 8 g/100 ml (70 to 80 g/L).

Order the appropriate IV rate, which depends on the patient's volume status. For *shock,* run the IV fluid wide open through at least two large-bore IV sites. Elevating the IV bag, squeezing the IV bag, or using IV pressure cuffs may help increase the rate of delivery of the solution. For severe ongoing bleeding requiring massive blood transfusions (more than 3 units packed RBCs/hour or more

| BOX 13.1 | Patients Who Refuse Blood Transfusions |

📖 There are some patients who, for religious or other reasons, may refuse blood transfusions. This refusal should be respected, and local laws should be followed as appropriate. In this case, call your resident or attending physician for help. In general, the following principles apply:

- Immediate endoscopy, with a view toward therapeutic intervention (e.g., sclerotherapy, heater coagulation, laser therapy), is recommended, as is early surgical consultation.
- Avoid resuscitation with synthetic colloids, which may interfere with coagulation.
- Normal saline may be used; however, avoid overaggressive fluid replacement in this patient group, because attempts to achieve normotension before bleeding is controlled may inhibit spontaneous hemostasis and cause further bleeding. In this situation, aim for a systolic blood pressure of 90 to 100 mm Hg in a previously normotensive patient or 20 to 30 mm Hg below a hypertensive patient's usual systolic readings.
- Agents such as IV desmopressin acetate (to raise factor VIII and von Willebrand factor levels and reduce bleeding time) and antifibrinolytic agents (e.g., tranexamic acid) may help prevent ongoing blood loss, but they should be used only after consultation with a hematologist or the patient's attending physician.
- If the hemorrhage is severe, these patients may benefit from hyperbaric oxygen therapy, if it is available.

than 10 units packed RBCs in 24 hours), plasma and platelet transfusions should also be given to prevent dilutional coagulopathy. For *moderate volume depletion,* you can administer 500 to 1000 mL of normal saline as rapidly as possible, with serial measurements of volume status and assessment of cardiac status. If blood is not at the bedside within 30 minutes, designate someone to find out why there is a delay.

📖 Aggressive volume repletion in a patient with a history of congestive heart failure may compromise cardiac function. Do not overshoot the goal of volume repletion!

What can you do at this time to stop the source of bleeding?

Treat the underlying cause. Treating hypovolemia is merely treating a symptom.

- Upper GI bleeding (hematemesis and most cases of melena)

In patients with bleeding from a peptic ulcer, the use of H2-blocking drugs has not been shown to improve outcomes. Proton pump inhibitors, however, may decrease the risk of ulcer bleeding, the need for urgent surgery, and the risk of death. If the patient is actively bleeding, give **esomeprazole or pantoprazole 80 mg IV.** Lower doses, i.e., **esomeprazole or pantoprazole 40 mg IV** may be given if there is no evidence of active bleeding. **Omeprazole, 20 to 40 mg orally (PO) daily; lansoprazole, 15 to 30 mg PO daily; esomeprazole, 40 mg PO daily; pantoprazole, 40 mg PO daily; dexlansoprazole, 30 to 60 mg PO daily; and rabeprazole, 20 mg**

PO daily, may be given once the patient is no longer NPO (nothing by mouth). Antacids are contraindicated if endoscopy or surgery is anticipated; they obscure the field during endoscopy and increase the risk of aspiration during surgery.

- Lower GI bleeding (usually bright red blood per rectum and, occasionally, melena)

  No other treatment is required until the specific site of bleeding is identified, but continue to monitor the volume status.

- Abnormal coagulation

  If the international normalized ratio (INR) is high or the activated partial thromboplastin time (aPTT) is prolonged, or if the patient is thrombocytopenic, fresh-frozen plasma (2 U) or platelet infusion (6 to 8 U), respectively, may be required. If the patient has recently received fibrinolytic therapy, additional agents, such as aprotinin (Trasylol), may be initiated, but only after consultation with your resident or attending physician. Reversal agents for lepirudin and argatroban are not available, but the half-lives of these agents are 1.5 and 1 hours, respectively, and stopping the agent is the best practice. The monoclonal antibody, idarucizumab, is commercially available for reversal of dabigatran effects, and dabigatran is also dialyzable. Andexanet alfa can reverse the effects of rivaroxaban, apixaban, and edoxaban. Dialysis appears to be ineffective. In the advent of serious GI bleeding, these agents should be stopped in consultation with the patient's attending physician. If the patient is receiving an antiplatelet medication, it should be stopped, although the effect of the agent may persist for days. Bleeding disorders resulting from drug-induced platelet dysfunction may necessitate platelet transfusion or other specialized measures (see page 390).

Selective Chart Review

What was the reason for admission?

Has the cause of this GI hemorrhage already been identified during this admission?

Is the patient taking any medication that may worsen the situation?

Nonsteroidal anti-inflammatory drugs (NSAIDs)	Counteract the protective effect of prostaglandins on gastric mucosa; ingestion may result in gastric erosions or peptic ulcers
Steroids	Increased frequency of ulcer disease in patients who take steroids; most disease processes for which a patient is receiving steroids do not allow their immediate discontinuation
Heparin	Prevents clot formation by enhancing the action of antithrombin III
Warfarin	Prevents activation of vitamin K–dependent clotting factors

Dabigatran	Prevents clot formation by direct inhibition of thrombin
Rivaroxaban ⎫ Apixaban ⎬ Edoxaban ⎭	Prevents clot formation by direct inhibition of factor Xa
Fibrinolytic agents	Convert plasminogen to plasmin, a potent fibrinolytic
Antiplatelet	Aspirin, clopidogrel, prasugrel, ticlopidine, ticagrelor, glycoprotein IIb/IIIa inhibitors (e.g., tirofiban), and thrombin receptor antagonists (e.g., vorapaxar) interfere with platelet activation, adhesion, or aggregation and may result in bleeding

What laboratory data should be obtained?
Obtain the following measurements:
- Most recent hemoglobin value
- INR, aPTT, platelet count. Does the patient have any platelet or coagulation abnormalities that may predispose to bleeding?
- Urea, creatinine levels (uremia prolongs bleeding time)

📖 Remember that in prerenal failure, the urea level may be more markedly elevated than the creatinine level. This difference may be accentuated in the presence of GI bleeding by absorption of urea from the breakdown of blood in the GI tract.

Selective Physical Examination II

Where is the site of bleeding?

Vitals	Repeat measurements now.
Head, ears, eyes, nose, throat (HEENT)	Nosebleed
Abdomen (ABD)	Epigastric tenderness (peptic ulcer disease) Right lower quadrant (RLQ) tenderness or mass (cecal cancer) Left lower quadrant (LLQ) tenderness (sigmoid cancer, diverticulitis, ischemic colitis)
Rectal	Bright red blood, melena, hemorrhoids, or mass (rectal cancer)

Also, look for signs of chronic liver disease (hepatosplenomegaly, ascites, parotid gland hypertrophy, spider angiomata, gynecomastia, palmar erythema, testicular atrophy, dilated abdominal veins), which may be suggestive of the presence of esophageal varices.

Management II

Once hypovolemia is corrected, ongoing management includes maintenance of adequate intravascular volume and attempts to determine the specific site of bleeding.

What procedures are available to determine the site of bleeding?
The following procedures are helpful:
- Esophagogastroduodenoscopy
- Tagged RBC scan
- Angiography
- Sigmoidoscopy
- Colonoscopy

When should endoscopy be performed?
For upper GI tract hemorrhages, endoscopy is the cornerstone of diagnosis and treatment; tagged RBC scans or angiography is thus rarely necessary. A variety of risk stratification tools is available to help identify the need for urgent endoscopy, including the Rockall score (see Box 13.2), the Glasgow Blatchford score, the AIMS65 score, and others. For example a *clinical* Rockall

BOX. 13.2	Rockall Score	

			Points
Complete Rockall score	Clinical Rockall score	**Variable age**	
		<60 years	0
		60–79 years	1
		≥80 years	2
		Shock	
		Heart rate >80 beats/min	1
		Systolic blood pressure <100 mm Hg	2
		Coexisting illness	
		Ischemic heart disease, congestive heart failure, other major illness	2
		Renal failure, hepatic failure, metastatic cancer	3
		Endoscopic diagnosis	
		No lesion observed, Mallory-Weiss tear	0
		Peptic ulcer, erosive disease, esophagitis	1
		Cancer of upper GI tract	2
		Endoscopic stigmata of recent hemorrhage	
		Clean base ulcer, flat pigmented spot	0
		Blood in upper GI tract, active bleeding, visible vessel, clot	2

GI, Gastrointestinal.

score (before endoscopy) of 0 identifies patients at low risk for rebleeding or death. In these patients, elective endoscopy can be performed within the next 24 hours. The *completed* Rockall score (after endoscopy) gives additional information to predict the risk of subsequent rebleeding or death.

Urgent endoscopy should be considered if the patient has a high-risk stratification score, if bleeding continues, or if the patient is hemodynamically unstable. The goals of early endoscopy are to define the cause of bleeding, determine prognosis, and administer endoscopic therapy, if indicated.

Some conditions can be temporarily stabilized at the time of endoscopy. Esophageal varices can be treated with ligation or banding; sclerotherapy is also effective but is used less frequently because the complication rates are higher than for ligation or banding. Gastric or duodenal ulcers with active bleeding or a nonbleeding visible vessel at the base may be treated with thermal therapy (electrocoagulation, heater probe, argon plasma coagulation), injection therapy (vasoconstrictors, sclerosing agents, tissue adhesives, saline), or mechanical therapy (e.g., endoscopic clips).

If *esophageal varices* are diagnosed as the cause of upper GI bleeding, then the somatostatin analogue, octreotide (Sandostatin) (50-mcg bolus, then 25 to 50 mcg/hour via IV infusion) or somatostatin (Zecnil) (250 mcg IV bolus, then 250 to 500 mcg/hour via IV infusion), may also be used. If neither of these agents is available, vasopressin (Pitressin) (0.2 to 0.4 U/min intravenously) can be used, although this may cause coronary artery constriction. Terlipressin (Glypressin) (2 mg intravenously every 4 to 6 hours), a synthetic analogue of vasopressin, is available as an orphan drug in the United States and is somewhat safer. Endoscopic confirmation of the diagnosis should be undertaken as soon as possible. Endoscopic hemostatic therapy (EHT) may be undertaken by banding, transjugular intrahepatic portosystemic shunt (TIPS), or scleral treatment. However, there is no evidence that EHT has any advantage over medical therapy in the emergency management of bleeding esophageal varices. If these interventions cannot be performed, a Minnesota tube can be inserted as a temporizing measure to control life-threatening bleeding that is unresponsive to medical treatment (Fig. 13.1). Further surgical treatment may include distal splenorenal shunt (DSRS), devascularization, liver transplant, or esophageal transection.

Patients with lower GI bleeding who are hemodynamically stable should be scheduled for colonoscopy. For unstable patients, urgent tagged RBC scanning should be arranged, followed by angiography, if possible. Tagged RBC scanning and mesenteric angiography are most sensitive if performed while bleeding is still active, but they should not take priority over resuscitation measures.

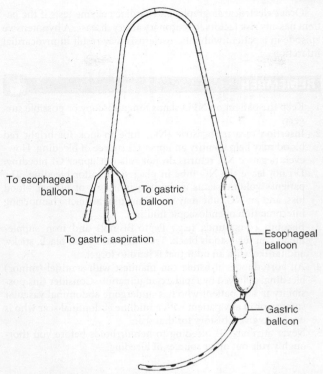

To esophageal balloon

To gastric balloon

To gastric aspiration

Esophageal balloon

Gastric balloon

FIG. 13.1 Sengstaken-Blakemore tube. The Minnesota tube is similar, with an additional port for esophageal aspiration.

As a result of recent improvements in endoscopic therapy, angiographic diagnosis and management of upper GI hemorrhages are rarely necessary. Intra-arterial infusion of vasoconstrictors or selective arterial embolization may be helpful if bleeding is severe or persistent in a patient at high risk for needing surgery or in centers where endoscopic therapy is unavailable. In rare cases, total colectomy is required to treat exsanguinating hemorrhage from an unlocalized colonic source.

When is early surgical consultation appropriate?

Obtain such consultation immediately for the following conditions:

- Exsanguinating hemorrhage
- Continued bleeding with transfusion requirements of more than 5 U/day
- When a patient refuses blood transfusion (see Box 13.1)

Order electrocardiography and cardiac enzyme tests if the patient has any risk factors for coronary artery disease. A hypotensive episode in a patient with atherosclerosis may result in myocardial infarction.

REMEMBER

1. Keep the patient on NPO status for endoscopy or possible surgery.
2. Insertion of a nasogastric (NG) tube to look for bright red blood may help identify an upper GI source of bleeding. However, negative NG returns do not rule out upper GI bleeding. Do not leave the NG tube in place to monitor bleeding. The patient's volume status is the best indicator of further blood loss, and an NG tube may cause mucosal artifacts, hampering interpretation of endoscopic findings.
3. Bismuth compounds (e.g., Pepto-Bismol) and iron supplements can turn stools black. True melena is pitch black, sticky, and tarlike, with an odor that is hard to forget.
4. An aortoduodenal fistula can manifest with sentinel (minor) bleeding, followed by rapid exsanguination. Consider this possibility in any patient who has undergone abdominal vascular surgery or in any patient with a midline abdominal scar who is unable to give a history for that scar.
5. Never attribute GI bleeding to hemorrhoids before you thoroughly rule out other sources of bleeding.

Headache

Patients in the hospital often complain of headache. You must decide whether the headache is chronic and of no urgent concern or a symptom of a more serious problem.

PHONE CALL

Questions

1. How severe is the patient's headache?

    Most headaches are mild and not of major concern unless they are associated with other symptoms.
2. Was the onset of the headache sudden or gradual?

    The sudden onset of a severe headache is suggestive of subarachnoid hemorrhage.
3. What are the patient's vital signs?
4. Has the patient's level of consciousness changed?
5. Does the patient have a history of chronic or recurrent headaches?
6. Why was the patient admitted?

Orders

1. Ask the registered nurse (RN) to take the patient's temperature if it has not been recorded within the past hour.

    Bacterial meningitis may manifest with only fever and headache.
2. If you are confident that the headache represents a chronic or previously diagnosed, recurrent problem, the patient can be given medication that has relieved the headache in the past or a nonnarcotic analgesic agent (e.g., acetaminophen). Ask the RN to call you back in 2 hours if the headache has not been relieved by the medication.

Informing the Registered Nurse

Tell the RN, "I will arrive at the bedside in … minutes."

For headaches associated with fever, vomiting, or a decreased level of consciousness, and for severe headaches with an acute onset, you must see the patient immediately. Chronic, recurrent headaches must be assessed at the bedside if the headache is more severe than usual or if the character of the pain is different.

ELEVATOR THOUGHTS

What causes headaches?

Chronic (Recurrent) Headaches

1. Migraine
2. Tension
3. Cluster
4. Other
   a. Drugs (nitrates, calcium channel blockers, nonsteroidal anti-inflammatory drugs [NSAIDs])
   b. Cervical osteoarthritis
   c. Temporomandibular joint disease

Acute Headaches

1. Infectious causes
   a. Meningitis
   b. Encephalitis
2. Posttraumatic causes
   a. Concussion
   b. Cerebral contusion
   c. Subdural or epidural hematoma
3. Vascular causes
   a. Subarachnoid hemorrhage
   b. Intracerebral hemorrhage
4. Increased intracranial pressure
   a. Space-occupying lesions
   b. Hypertensive encephalopathy
   c. Benign intracranial hypertension
5. Local causes
   a. Temporal arteritis
   b. Acute angle-closure glaucoma

MAJOR THREAT TO LIFE

- Subarachnoid hemorrhage
- Bacterial meningitis
- Herniation (transtentorial, cerebellar, central)

Subarachnoid hemorrhage is associated with a very high mortality rate if it is not recognized and treated to prevent recurrence of bleeding. Bacterial meningitis must be recognized early if antibiotic treatment is to be successful. Any intracranial mass lesion (e.g., tumor, blood, pus) may result in herniation (Fig. 14.1).

BEDSIDE

Quick-Look Test

Does the patient look well (comfortable), sick (uncomfortable or distressed), or critical (about to die)?

Most patients with chronic headaches look well. Those with subarachnoid hemorrhage, meningitis, or severe migraines look sick.

Airway and Vital Signs

What is the patient's temperature?

If fever is associated with a headache, you must make a prompt decision whether a lumbar puncture should be performed.

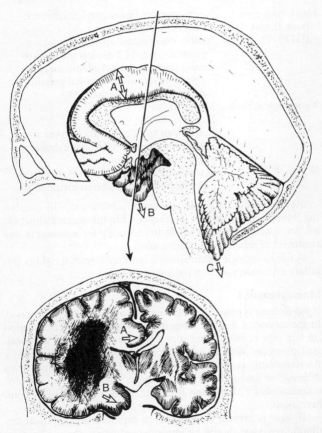

FIG. 14.1 Central nervous system herniation. *A,* Cingulate herniation. *B,* Uncal herniation. *C,* Cerebellar herniation.

What is the blood pressure?

Hypertensive encephalopathy is usually associated with a systolic blood pressure higher than 190 mm Hg and a diastolic pressure higher than 120 mm Hg. Headache is not usually a symptom of hypertension unless blood pressure has increased recently and the diastolic blood pressure is higher than 120 mm Hg.

What is the heart rate?

Hypertension in association with bradycardia may be a manifestation of increasing intracranial pressure.

Selective Physical Examination I

Does the patient have increased intracranial pressure or meningitis?

Head, ears, eyes, nose, throat (HEENT)	Nuchal rigidity (meningitis or subarachnoid hemorrhage)
	Papilledema (increased intracranial pressure): Fig. 14.2 depicts the funduscopic features of papilledema; an early sign of increased intracranial pressure is absence of venous pulsations
Neurologic system	Mental status
	Pupil symmetry
	Kernig sign and Brudzinski sign (meningitis or subarachnoid hemorrhage) (Fig. 14.3)
Skin	Maculopapular rash, petechiae, or purpura may be seen in bacterial meningitis

Asymmetry of the pupils in association with a rapidly decreasing level of consciousness represents a life-threatening situation; ask for a neurosurgical consult immediately for assessment and treatment of probable uncal herniation.

A full neurologic examination is required if nuchal rigidity, pupillary asymmetry, or papilledema is present.

Management I

If *papilledema* is present, intracranial pressure is probably increased. In the context of *headache,* this may be suggestive of a mass lesion (tumor, pus, or blood), but it may also be present with less localized processes such as subarachnoid hemorrhage or meningitis. An immediate computed tomographic (CT) scan of the head helps differentiate among these possibilities. A lumbar puncture is contraindicated if a mass lesion is present, because of the risk of brain herniation.

If *fever* is present in addition to papilledema, empirical antibiotic coverage should be implemented before the CT scan, as follows.

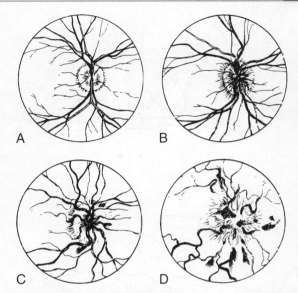

FIG. 14.2 **Disk changes seen in papilledema**. *A,* Normal. *B,* Early papilledema. *C,* Moderate papilledema with early hemorrhage. *D,* Severe papilledema with extensive hemorrhage.

Suspected Bacterial Meningitis

1. In an adult with community-acquired infection (most often *Streptococcus pneumoniae*, Group B streptococci, *Neisseria meningitidis*, *Hemophilus influenzae*, and *Listeria monocytogenes*), pending culture results:
   - **Cefotaxime, 2 g intravenously (IV) every 4 to 6 hours, or ceftriaxone, 2 g IV every 12 hours**, with
   - **Ampicillin, 2 g IV every 4 hours**, for patients over age 50 years to cover the possibility of *Listeria* infection, and
   - **Vancomycin, 15 mg/kg IV every 12 hours, with or without rifampin, 20 mg/kg orally (PO) daily in one or two divided doses**, in cases of serious risk of infection with penicillin-resistant pneumococci
   - **Dexamethasone, 0.15 mg/kg IV every 6 hours**, for 4 days, starting before or with the first dose of antibiotics
2. For patients who are immunosuppressed, alcoholic, or older than 60 years (gram-negative bacilli, staphylococci): **vancomycin, 15 mg/kg IV every 12 hours, plus ampicillin, 2 g every 4 hours**, with either **cefepime, 2 g every 8 hours**, or **meropenem, 2 g every 8 hours**.

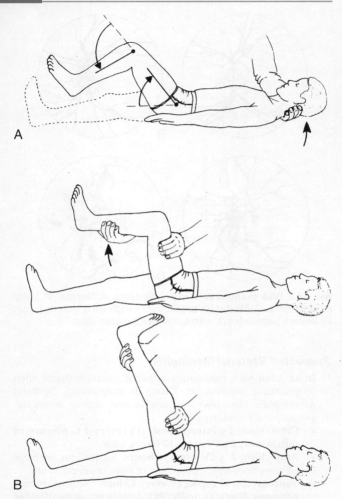

FIG. 14.3 *A,* Brudzinski sign. The test result is positive when the patient actively flexes his or her hips and knees in response to passive neck flexion by the examiner. *B,* Kernig sign. The test result is positive when pain or resistance is elicited by passive knee extension from the 90-degree hip-knee flexion position.

3. For patients after craniotomy, after head trauma, or with cerebrospinal fluid shunt: vancomycin, 15 mg/kg IV every 12 hours, with either ceftazidime, 2 g IV every 4 to 6 hours, or cefepime, 2 g IV every 12 hours, or meropenem, 2 g every 8 hours.

Vancomycin in usual doses may not reach adequate concentrations at the site of infection. Higher doses, up to 4 g/day, may be required in some cases.

Suspected Subdural Empyema or Brain Abscess

1. In patients with headache secondary to frontoethmoid sinusitis, otitis media, mastoiditis, or lung abscess: cloxacillin plus a third-generation cephalosporin plus metronidazole
   Sixty percent to 90% of subdural empyemas are caused by extension of sinusitis or otitis media.
2. In patients after trauma: cloxacillin or nafcillin plus a third-generation cephalosporin

In addition to beginning antibiotics, a patient with a subdural empyema or a brain abscess should be referred for neurosurgical assessment. Steroid treatment, surgery, or both may be necessary to relieve increased intracranial pressure caused by cerebral edema.

If a patient with headache has *fever, nuchal rigidity, and no papilledema,* the likelihood of meningitis is high. In this case, perform a lumbar puncture, followed immediately by intravenous antibiotics, as recommended earlier. If there is a delay of 1 hour or longer in performing the lumbar puncture, antibiotic therapy should be initiated first; the initial dose will have little effect on the evaluation of the cerebrospinal fluid obtained later.

If a patient with headache has *nuchal rigidity, no fever, and no papilledema,* a subarachnoid hemorrhage may be present. In this case, noncontrast CT scanning of the brain should be performed before the lumbar puncture. If a subarachnoid hemorrhage is present, the CT scan shows subarachnoid blood in most cases. If the CT brain scan is normal and a subarachnoid hemorrhage is still suspected, perform a lumbar puncture, looking for xanthochromia. Confirmation of a subarachnoid hemorrhage necessitates immediate neurosurgical consultation.

If a patient with headache has *no papilledema, no fever, and no nuchal rigidity,* obtain a more detailed history and chart review.

Selective History and Chart Review
Was the onset of the headache sudden or insidious?
The abrupt onset of severe headache suggests a vascular cause, the most serious being subarachnoid or intracerebral hemorrhage.

How severe is the headache?

Most muscle contraction headaches are mild and not incapacitating. However, when migraine headaches are associated with severe pain, the patient may look sick.

Is the headache improved or worsened in the supine position?

Most muscle contraction headaches are improved by lying down. Headaches made worse by lying down suggest increasing intracranial pressure, and an intracranial mass should be considered.

Did the patient have any prodromal symptoms?

Nausea and vomiting are associated with increased intracranial pressure but may also occur with migraine or acute angle-closure glaucoma. Photophobia and neck stiffness are associated with meningitis. The classic visual aura (scintillations, migratory scotomata, and blurred vision) that precedes a migraine headache is helpful in making the diagnosis, but the absence of an aura does not rule out migraine.

Does the patient have a history of chronic, recurring headaches?

Migraine and muscle contraction headaches follow a pattern. Ask the patient whether this headache is the same as their *usual* headache. The patient will probably make the diagnosis for you. Migraine is defined as episodic attacks of headache lasting 4 to 72 hours with any two of the following symptoms: unilateral pain, throbbing, aggravation on movement, pain of moderate to severe intensity, and either nausea/vomiting or photophobia/phonophobia.

Does the patient have a history of recent head trauma?

An epidural hematoma may occur after even a relatively minor head injury, particularly in teenagers or young adults. Subdural hematomas can appear insidiously 6 to 8 weeks after seemingly minor trauma and are not uncommon in alcoholic patients.

Does the patient have joint disease in the neck or upper back?

Muscle contraction headaches in elderly patients are often caused by cervical osteoarthritis. These headaches characteristically start in the neck region and radiate to the temple or forehead.

Does the patient have clicking or popping when opening or closing the jaw?

These symptoms are a clue to the presence of temporomandibular joint dysfunction. In addition, the pain may be predominantly in the ear or face.

Has an ophthalmologist or another physician dilated the patient's pupils within the past 24 hours?

Acute angle-closure glaucoma can be precipitated by pupillary dilatation. The patient typically complains of a severe unilateral headache over the brow and may experience nausea, vomiting, and abdominal pain.

Does the patient have any decrease or loss in vision? Does the patient have a history of jaw claudication?

Temporal arteritis is a systemic illness (fever, malaise, weight loss, anorexia, weakness, myalgia) observed in patients older than 50 years. If this condition is suspected, order a stat measurement of the erythrocyte sedimentation rate (ESR). Vision loss in the setting of temporal arteritis is a medical emergency and should be managed in consultation with a neurologist or rheumatologist (for treatment, see page 140).

What drugs is the patient receiving?

Drugs such as nitrates, calcium channel blockers, and NSAIDs can cause headaches. If any head trauma or unusual headache occurs in a patient who is receiving anticoagulants or thrombolytic therapy, suspect an intracranial hemorrhage. In this case, perform a CT scan of the head, and consider reversing the anticoagulant or thrombolytic agent.

Selective Physical Examination II

Vitals	Repeat measurements now.
HEENT	Red eye (acute angle-closure glaucoma)
	Hemotympanum or blood in the ear canal (basal skull fracture)
	Tender, enlarged temporal arteries (temporal arteritis)
	Lid ptosis, dilated pupil, eye deviated downward and outward (posterior communicating cerebral artery aneurysm)
	Tenderness on palpation or failure of transillumination of the frontal and maxillary sinuses (sinusitis or subdural empyema)
	Inability to open the jaw fully (temporomandibular joint dysfunction)
	Cranial bruit (arteriovenous malformation)
Neuro-logic system	Complete neurologic examination
	What is the level of consciousness?
	📖 Drowsiness, yawning, and inattentiveness associated with headache are ominous signs; in a patient with a small subarachnoid hemorrhage, these may be the only signs.
	Does the patient have any asymmetry of pupils, visual fields, eye movements, limbs, tone, reflexes, or plantar responses?
	📖 Asymmetry is suggestive of structural brain disease; if this is a new finding, a CT scan of the head is required.

Musculo-	Palpate skull and face, looking for fractures, hema-
skeletal	tomas, and lacerations.
system	📖 Evidence of recent head trauma is suggestive of the possibility of a subdural or epidural hematoma.

Management II
Muscle Contraction Headache
Chronic muscle contraction headache can be treated temporarily with nonnarcotic analgesics. This is the most common type of headache observed in the hospital. A long-term treatment plan, if not already established, can be discussed in the morning.

Mild Migraine Headache
A mild migraine headache can be treated adequately with analgesics such as **aspirin, 975 to 1300 mg PO every 4 hours, two doses; ibuprofen, 400 to 800 mg PO every 6 hours, two doses; or naproxen sodium, 500 to 1000 mg PO every 4 to 6 hours.** Patients with allergies to these medications may be given **acetaminophen, 1000 mg PO every 4 hours, two doses; or codeine, 30 to 60 mg PO or intramuscularly (IM) every 3 to 4 hours, as needed.**

Severe Migraine Headache
A severe migraine headache is best treated immediately during the prodromal stage, but it is unlikely that you will be called until the headache is well established. Ask the patient what they usually take for migraine headaches; that medication is probably the most effective agent to prescribe immediately.

Serotonin agonists, such as sumatriptan succinate (Imitrex) and many other triptans (almotriptan, eletriptan, frovatriptan, naratriptan, rizatriptan, and zolmitriptan), and dihydroergotamine (a serotonin agonist with additional actions on dopamine and adrenergic receptors) are first-line therapy for most severe migraines. Both the triptans and dihydroergotamine are equally effective in aborting migraine headaches. **Sumatriptan, 50 to 100 mg PO or 6 mg subcutaneously (SC),** may be given. Alternatively, sumatriptan may be given in combination with naproxen as **Treximet (sumatriptan 85 mg/naproxen 500 mg) PO once;** a second dose may be given to nonresponders after 2 or more hours—maximum is two doses per day. None of the other triptans has any advantage over sumatriptan. Alternatively, **dihydroergotamine, 0.5 to 1 mg IM, SC, or IV,** or by nasal spray (**Trudhesa 0.725 mg, one spray per nostril**), may be given and repeated in 1 hour if ineffective.

📖 These agents are contraindicated in the setting of uncontrolled hypertension, unstable coronary artery disease, coronary spasm, or pregnancy and in the presence of hemiplegic migraine.

Side effects of sumatriptan include chest or throat tightness, tingling in the head or limbs, and nausea. Dihydroergotamine is less likely to induce chest pain but more likely to cause nausea. A life-threatening condition called *serotonin syndrome* can occur when triptans and selective serotonin reuptake inhibitors (SSRIs) or selective serotonin-norepinephrine reuptake inhibitors (SNRIs) are used together. Triptans and dihydroergotamine should not be used within 24 hours of one another because of the risk of additive effects causing coronary spasm.

In patients with severe migraines in whom vasoconstrictors are contraindicated, one of the following dopamine antagonists may be tried:

- **Metoclopramide, 10 mg IV**
- **Chlorpromazine, 0.1 mg/kg IV over 20 minutes;** repeat after 15 minutes to a maximum dose of 37.5 mg (pretreatment with 5 mL/kg normal saline IV may prevent the hypotensive effects of chlorpromazine)
- **Prochlorperazine, 5 to 10 mg IV or IM or 25 mg per rectum**

Cluster Headache

Cluster headaches are difficult to treat. Most last less than 45 minutes, and oral treatment has minimal effect. If a cluster headache develops in the hospital and is severe, a parenteral narcotic, such as **codeine, 30 to 60 mg IM,** or **meperidine (Demerol), 50 to 100 mg IM,** may be tried. Alternatively, dihydroergotamine or sumatriptan may be effective in the same doses recommended for migraine headaches.

Postconcussion Headache

If intracranial hemorrhage has been ruled out by a CT scan of the head, postconcussion headache should be treated with an analgesic agent that is unlikely to cause sedation, such as acetaminophen or codeine. Aspirin is contraindicated in a postconcussion headache because it may predispose the patient to bleeding complications.

Hemorrhages and Space-Occupying Lesions

Patients with subdural, epidural, and subarachnoid hemorrhages and space-occupying lesions (brain abscess, tumor) that cause increases in intracranial pressure should be referred to a neurosurgeon as soon as possible. While neurosurgical consultation is pending, nimodipine, 60 mg PO every 4 hours, may improve the outcome in patients with subarachnoid hemorrhage.

Hypertensive Encephalopathy

Hypertensive encephalopathy should be managed by careful reduction of blood pressure (see Chapter 16, pages 174–175).

Benign Intracranial Hypertension

Benign intracranial hypertension (pseudotumor cerebri) is a syndrome of unknown cause. Intracranial pressure is increased (manifesting as headache and papilledema), but the patient has no evidence of a mass lesion or hydrocephalus. Refer the patient to a neurologist in the morning for further investigation and management.

Temporal Arteritis

Temporal arteritis should be treated immediately to prevent irreversible blindness. **Prednisone, 60 mg PO daily**, can be started immediately when this diagnosis is suspected and supported by an ESR higher than 60 mm/hour (Westergren method). Confirmation by temporal artery biopsy should be arranged within the next 3 days.

Glaucoma

A patient with acute angle-closure glaucoma should be referred to an ophthalmologist immediately.

Heart Rate and Rhythm Disorders

There are only three abnormalities in heart rate or rhythm that you will be called on to assess at night: too fast, too slow, and irregular. Remember that the main purpose of the heart rate is to keep cardiac output (CO) high enough to perfuse three vital organs: heart, brain, and kidneys. Your task is to find out why a patient's heart is beating too quickly, too slowly, or irregularly before it results in hypoperfusion of the patient's vital organs. Begin by asking whether the heart rate is too fast or too slow. (Rapid heart rates are discussed first; slow heart rates are addressed beginning on page 161 of this chapter.) Next, decide whether the rhythm is regular or irregular.

Rapid Heart Rates

PHONE CALL

Questions

1. What is the patient's heart rate?
2. Is the patient's heart rhythm regular or irregular?
3. Has this problem developed only since admission?
4. What is the patient's blood pressure (BP)?

   Remember that hypotension may be a cause of tachycardia (i.e., compensatory) or a result of tachycardia that does not allow adequate diastolic filling of the left ventricle to maintain CO.
5. Is the patient having chest pain or shortness of breath?

   Dysrhythmias are common in patients with underlying coronary artery disease. A rapid heart rate may be the result of myocardial ischemia or congestive heart failure (CHF), or it may precipitate ischemia or CHF in such a patient.
6. What is the patient's respiratory rate and pulse oximetry reading?

   Any illness causing hypoxia may result in tachycardia.
7. What is the patient's temperature?

Tachycardia, in proportion to the temperature elevation, is an expected finding in a febrile patient. However, you must examine the patient to ensure that there is no other cause for the rapid heart rate.

8. Does the patient have a pacemaker?
9. A wide-complexed tachycardia may occur in pacemaker patients as a result of a dual-chamber pacemaker tracking atrial arrhythmias, or as a result of a pacemaker-mediated tachycardia.

Orders

1. If the patient is experiencing tachycardia and *hypotension,* order a large-bore (size 16 if possible) intravenous line immediately.
2. If the patient is having *chest pain* or *shortness of breath,* order an intravenous line, ask the nurse to put the cardiac arrest cart in the room, and attach the electrocardiogram (ECG) monitor to the patient.
3. Order a stat 12-lead ECG and rhythm strip.

Informing the Registered Nurse

Tell the registered nurse (RN), "I will arrive at the bedside in … minutes."

If a patient has a rapid heart rate in association with chest pain (angina), shortness of breath (CHF), or hypotension, you must see the patient immediately.

ELEVATOR THOUGHTS

What causes rapid heart rates?

Rapid irregular heart rates:
1. Atrial fibrillation
2. Atrial flutter with variable block
3. Multifocal atrial tachycardia
4. Sinus tachycardia with premature atrial contractions (PACs) or premature ventricular contractions (PVCs)

Rapid regular heart rates:
1. Sinus tachycardia
2. Atrial flutter
3. Other supraventricular tachycardias (SVTs)
   a. Reentrant
      i. Atrioventricular nodal reentry
      ii. Accessory pathways (e.g., Wolff-Parkinson-White syndrome, concealed pathways)
      iii. Sinoatrial nodal reentrant tachycardia
      iv. Pacemaker-mediated tachycardia
   b. Nonreentrant
      i. Focal atrial tachycardia
      ii. Junctional tachycardia

4. Ventricular tachycardia

As electrophysiologic studies have enhanced knowledge about SVTs, their classification has become more mechanistic but sometimes less practical. Although sinus tachycardia, atrial fibrillation, and atrial flutter are tachycardias with a supraventricular origin, their mechanisms are sufficiently distinct from those of the other SVTs that they are often classified separately. The term *supraventricular tachycardia* is commonly reserved for (usually narrow-complex) tachycardia that is not clearly sinus, atrial fibrillation, or atrial flutter. Do not be distressed because you cannot differentiate an SVT due to atrioventricular (AV) nodal reentry from one resulting from orthodromic reentry using a concealed bypass tract. The precise mechanism of an SVT often is not apparent on the surface ECG, and in most cases the initial management is the same.

MAJOR THREAT TO LIFE

- Hypotension, which may lead to shock
- Angina, which may progress to myocardial infarction (MI)
- CHF, which may lead to hypoxia

It is useful to recall the determinants of BP, as expressed in the following two formulas:

$$BP = CO \times \text{total peripheral resistance}$$
$$CO = \text{heart rate} \times \text{stroke volume}$$

As demonstrated by the first equation, any decrease in CO results in a decrease in BP, unless it is accompanied by a compensatory increase in total peripheral resistance. In most instances a rapid heart rate increases CO; however, many types of rapid heart rates do not allow adequate time for diastolic filling of the ventricles, which results in a low stroke volume and, hence, decreased CO. The low CO may result in hypotension, in angina in a patient with underlying coronary artery disease, or in CHF in a patient with inadequate left ventricular reserve.

BEDSIDE

Quick-Look Test

Does the patient look well (comfortable), sick (uncomfortable or distressed), or critical (about to die)?

A patient with SVT or ventricular tachycardia may look deceptively well if adequate BP is maintained. Patients with tachycardia that is sufficiently severe to cause hypotension, angina, or pulmonary edema usually look sick or critically ill and are likely to be unstable.[1]

Airway and Vital Signs

What is the patient's heart rate? Is it regular or irregular?
 Read the ECG and rhythm strip.
 What is the patient's BP?
 If the patient is hypotensive (systolic BP < 90 mm Hg), you must decide the following quickly:

1. Whether the tachycardia is a result of the hypotension (i.e., compensatory tachycardia)
   or
2. Whether the hypotension is a result of the tachycardia (i.e., inadequate diastolic filling, which leads to low CO with low BP)
   📖 Three types of rapid heart rhythms occasionally cause hypotension because of decreased diastolic filling, resulting in hypoperfusion of vital organs: atrial fibrillation (or flutter) with rapid ventricular response, SVT, and ventricular tachycardia (Figs. 15.1 to 15.3). If the patient is hypotensive, it is important to recognize these rhythms immediately, because prompt treatment is needed to restore adequate CO.
 What is the patient's respiratory rate?
 A patient with tachypnea may have pulmonary edema—an important determination. If pulmonary edema is present, the patient qualifies as unstable and is probably in need of cardioversion.

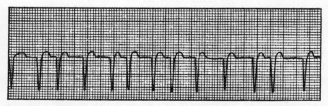

FIG. 15.1 Electrocardiographic tracing of atrial fibrillation with rapid ventricular response.

---

[1]The term *"unstable tachycardia"* is used in the 2010 American Heart Association's emergency cardiovascular care guidelines to refer to a situation in which the heart beats too fast for the patient's cardiovascular condition. In this situation, the patient displays serious symptoms (shortness of breath, chest pain, altered mental status) or is hypotensive or in pulmonary edema, and the symptoms can be attributed to the tachycardia. The term *"unstable tachycardia"* more accurately refers to the whole unstable condition of the patient rather than an unstable rhythm disorder.

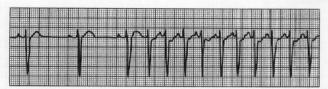

FIG. 15.2 **Electrocardiographic tracing of SVT**.

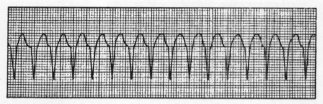

FIG. 15.3 **Electrocardiographic tracing of ventricular tachycardia**.

Management

Evaluation of Rapid Heart Rates in the Patient in Unstable Condition

If the patient is hypotensive and has atrial fibrillation (or flutter) with a rapid ventricular response, SVT, or ventricular tachycardia, emergency cardioversion may be required.

- Ask the RN to call immediately for your resident and an anesthetist.
- Ask the RN to bring the cardiac arrest cart into the room and attach the ECG monitor to the patient.
- Measure pulse oximetry levels, and give oxygen to maintain oxygen saturation ≥94%.
- Ensure that an intravenous line is in place.
- Ask the RN to have available **intravenous midazolam, 5 mg**.

Premedication to alleviate the pain of electrical shocks is required whenever possible. Your anesthesia team may have its own protocols or preferences for conscious sedation. Unless the situation is life-threatening, it is best to await the arrival of your resident and the anesthetist before administering premedication or proceeding to electrical cardioversion.

- If the patient has an SVT, you may attempt carotid sinus massage (see pages 157–158) or instruct the patient in a vagal maneuver (see page 157) while you await the arrival of more experienced help.

On occasion, these maneuvers break an SVT, obviating the need for pharmacologic or electrical conversion of the arrhythmia. If these maneuvers are unsuccessful, you must proceed to pharmacologic or electrical cardioversion.

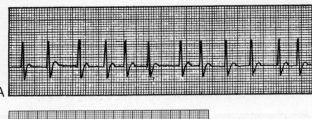

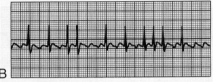

FIG. 15.4 **Electrocardiographic tracings of rapid irregular rhythms.**
A, Atrial fibrillation. *B,* Atrial flutter with variable block.

- If the patient has an SVT, ask the registered nurse to draw intravenous adenosine, 6 mg, into a syringe.

    📖 Adenosine has a very brief half-life, may be given to a patient in unstable condition, and may terminate an SVT such as atrioventricular nodal reentry without the need for electrical cardioversion. It can result in excess vasodilation due to activation of vascular adenosine receptors, cardiac arrhythmias including AV block and asystole, as well as cardiac ischemia. It should not be given without the guidance of your resident.

    If the patient is hypotensive and none of these three rhythms is present, the tachycardia is probably *secondary* to hypotension. You must perform a selective physical examination to decide which of the four major causes of hypotension is resulting in compensatory tachycardia:
1. Cardiogenic cause
2. Hypovolemic causes
3. Sepsis
4. Anaphylaxis

(Refer to Chapter 18 for the investigation and management of hypotension.)

Evaluation of Rapid Heart Rates in the Patient in Stable Condition

Fortunately, most of the patients you will see with rapid heart rates are not unstable. These cases are not life-threatening emergencies. Look at the ECG and rhythm strip, and decide which rapid rhythm the patient is experiencing.

    Rapid irregular rhythms:
- Atrial fibrillation (Fig. 15.4A)
- Atrial flutter with variable block (see Fig. 15.4B)

- Multifocal atrial tachycardia (Fig. 15.5)
- Sinus tachycardia with PACs (Fig. 15.6)
- Sinus tachycardia with PVCs (Fig. 15.7)
  Rapid regular rhythms:
- Sinus tachycardia (Fig. 15.8)
- Atrial flutter (Fig. 15.9)
- SVT: for example, focal atrial tachycardia (Fig. 15.10), atrioventricular nodal reentry, Wolff-Parkinson-White orthodromic tachycardia (Fig. 15.11)
- Ventricular tachycardia (Fig. 15.12)
- Pacemaker-mediated tachycardia (Fig. 15.13)

Note: A wide-complex regular tachycardia, such as that shown in Fig. 15.4, may represent monomorphic ventricular tachycardia,

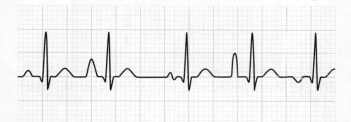

FIG. 15.5 Electrocardiographic tracing of rapid irregular rhythm: multifocal atrial tachycardia.

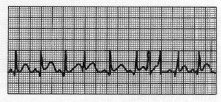

FIG. 15.6 Electrocardiographic tracing of rapid irregular rhythm: sinus tachycardia with PACs.

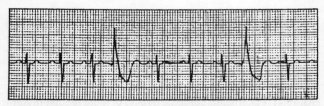

FIG. 15.7 Electrocardiographic tracing of rapid irregular rhythm: sinus tachycardia with PVCs.

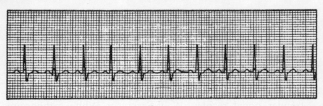

FIG. 15.8 Electrocardiographic tracing of rapid regular rhythm: sinus tachycardia.

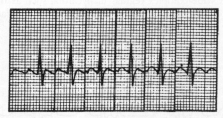

FIG. 15.9 Electrocardiographic tracing of rapid regular rhythm: atrial flutter.

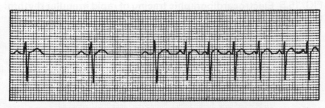

FIG. 15.10 Electrocardiographic tracing of rapid regular rhythm: SVT, focal atrial tachycardia.

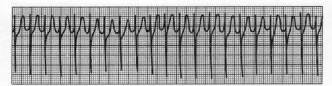

FIG. 15.11 Electrocardiographic tracing of rapid regular rhythm: SVT, atrioventricular nodal reentry, Wolff-Parkinson-White orthodromic tachycardia.

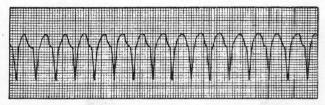

FIG. 15.12 **Electrocardiographic tracing of rapid regular rhythm: ventricular tachycardia**.

SVT with aberrancy, an SVT with QRS prolongation due to antiarrhythmic drugs or severe electrolyte abnormalities, or an antidromic AV nodal reentry rhythm. Most cases of wide-complex tachycardia in hospitalized patients are ventricular tachycardia, particularly if they occur in a patient with known or suspected coronary artery disease or cardiomyopathy. Do not assume that a wide-complex tachycardia is SVT with aberrancy just because the rhythm is well tolerated by the patient or because the patient is young. If you are uncertain, call your resident for help. If the wide-complexed tachycardia is regular and monomorphic, a trial of **adenosine, 6 mg intravenously (IV)**, may help differentiate SVT with aberrancy (which may terminate with this maneuver) from ventricular tachycardia. Verapamil can be dangerous in this situation: it may cause cardiovascular collapse in a patient with ventricular tachycardia.

Management of Rapid Irregular Rhythms

ATRIAL FIBRILLATION

If the patient is in unstable condition—that is, the patient is hypotensive, has chest pain (as in angina), or has shortness of breath (as in CHF)—and if atrial fibrillation is of recent onset (<2 days), the treatment of choice is cardioversion, beginning with 120 to 200 J biphasic or 200 J monophasic.

Atrial fibrillation with rapid ventricular rates and without evidence of hemodynamic compromise (no hypotension, angina, or CHF) can be treated with rate control agents. The decision whether to give the agents orally or IV depends on whether the patient looks unwell or is completely asymptomatic. A patient who looks unwell may be on the way to becoming unstable or may be having symptoms that do not technically qualify as *unstable* (e.g., anxiety, diaphoresis, palpitations); in this case, intravenous administration of one of these medications may be warranted. *Continuous electrocardiographic monitoring is required when any of these agents is given intravenously.* If the patient is completely asymptomatic, rate can be controlled at a more leisurely (and safer) pace with oral agents

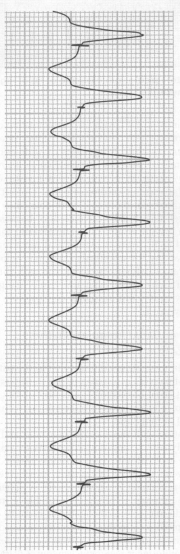

FIG. 15.13 Pacemaker-mediated tachycardia.

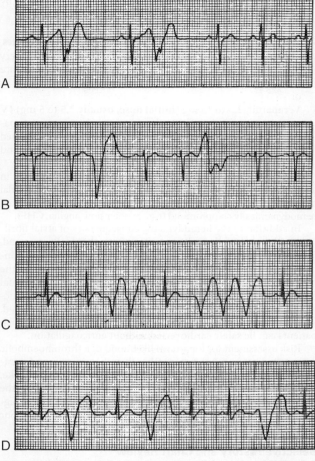

FIG. 15.14 Electrocardiographic tracings of examples of PVCs. *A,* R onT phenomenon. *B,* Multifocal. *C,* Couplets or salvos. *D,* Frequent.

that slow conduction through the atrioventricular node. Although intravenous digoxin was once the traditional choice for rate control, β-blockers and calcium channel blockers are safer and more effective. One of the following may be used to achieve rate control:

- **Metoprolol tartrate, 1 to 2 mg/minute IV**, up to a total of 5 mg if necessary. The initial oral dose is 25 to 50 mg twice a day, and this can be switched to a longer acting preparation (metoprolol succinate) once dosing requirements and tolerability are established; or

- **Esmolol, 0.5 mg/kg per minute IV over 1 minute, followed by an infusion of 0.05 to 0.2 mg/kg per minute;**
  or
- **Diltiazem, 0.25 mg/kg (usual dose, 15 to 25 mg) IV over 2 minutes.** The oral dose of the short-acting preparation is 30 to 90 mg every 6 hours, and this can be switched to a longer-acting preparation once dosing requirements and tolerability are established;
  or
- **Verapamil, 2.5 to 15 mg (initial dose, usually 2.5 to 5 mg) IV over 1 to 2 minutes.** The oral dose of the short-acting preparation is 80 to 120 mg every 8 hours, and this can be switched to a longer-acting preparation once dosing requirements and tolerability are established.

Atrial fibrillation with ventricular rates lower than 100/minute in an untreated patient is suggestive of underlying atrioventricular nodal dysfunction. Such patients rarely require cardioversion unless they are hemodynamically compromised (e.g., hypotension, angina, CHF).

In addition to the hemodynamic consequences of atrial fibrillation, the risk of thromboembolic events should be assessed. This risk is not acutely affected by measures directed at rate control, but cardioversion may precipitate an embolic event in the non-anticoagulated patient, particularly if the duration of atrial fibrillation is 48 hours or longer. If urgent cardioversion is anticipated, pre-cardioversion anticoagulation should be considered, and a transesophageal echocardiogram may help identify which patients can be safely cardioverted without anticoagulation.

Risk assessment for long-term likelihood of a thromboembolic event takes into account factors other than the presence and duration of atrial fibrillation, such as age, sex, history of previous stroke, and other comorbidities. A popular tool for risk stratification is the CHA2DS2VASc score. The decision to begin long-term anticoagulation and which agent to choose should be discussed with your resident and the patient's attending physician.

Selective History and Chart Review

Once the ventricular rate is controlled, perform a selective history and chart review, looking for the following associations and triggers of atrial fibrillation:

- Coronary artery disease
- Hypertension
- Hyperthyroidism (check thyroxine [T4] and thyroid-stimulating hormone [TSH] levels)
- Pulmonary embolism (check for risk factors; see page 293)
- Mitral or tricuspid valve disease (stenosis or regurgitation)
- Cardiomyopathy

- Congenital heart disease (e.g., atrial septal defect)
- Pericarditis or recent cardiac surgery
- Recent alcohol ingestion (holiday heart syndrome)
- Hypoxia

Selective Physical Examination

Look for specific causes of atrial fibrillation. Note that this process takes place after you have already begun to treat the patient.

Vitals	Repeat measurements now.
Head, ears, eyes, nose, throat (HEENT)	Exophthalmos, lid lag, lid retraction (hyperthyroidism)
Respiratory system (Resp)	Tachypnea, cyanosis, wheezing, pleural effusion (pulmonary embolus)
Cardiovascular system (CVS)	Murmur of mitral regurgitation or mitral stenosis (mitral valve disease)
Extremities (Ext)	Swelling, erythema, calf tenderness (deep vein thrombosis [DVT])
	Tremor, hyperactive deep tendon reflexes (hyperthyroidism)

MULTIFOCAL ATRIAL TACHYCARDIA

Specific management is not always required for this rhythm. The underlying cause should be treated; this is usually pulmonary disease, which is probably already being treated. Check for other underlying causes as follows:

- Pulmonary disease (especially chronic obstructive pulmonary disease [COPD])
- Hypoxia, hypercapnia
- Hypokalemia
- CHF
- Drugs: theophylline toxicity
- Caffeine, tobacco, alcohol use

Multifocal atrial tachycardia can be a forerunner of atrial fibrillation. If no remediable causes can be found, **short-acting verapamil, 80 to 120 mg PO three times daily, or short-acting diltiazem, 30 to 90 mg PO four times daily,** may provide rate control and diminish the frequency of focal rhythms. These drugs can be switched to a long-acting preparation once dosing requirements and tolerability are established.

Sinus Tachycardia With Premature Atrial Contractions. Treatment is the same as for multifocal atrial tachycardia. Although PACs may be forerunners of multifocal atrial tachycardia or atrial fibrillation, they do not need to be treated unless atrial fibrillation develops.

Sinus Tachycardia With Premature Ventricular Contractions. Certain features of PVCs have been described as "malignant": for example, R on T phenomenon (a premature ventricular complex near the peak of the T wave), multifocal PVCs, couplets or salvos (three or more PVCs in a row), and frequent PVCs (more than 5/ minute). Although these features have some relevance (Fig. 15.14), it is more important to consider the patient's condition and determine the context in which the PVCs are occurring. If the patient has myocardial ischemia, is hemodynamically unstable, has a serious metabolic or electrolyte abnormality, or is taking proarrhythmic medications (see page 161), and the patient is having very frequent PVCs or runs of nonsustained ventricular tachycardia, they should be transferred to a telemetry ward or the intensive care unit (ICU)/cardiac care unit (CCU) for further investigation and continuous electrocardiographic monitoring.

Look for the following common causes of PVCs in the hospital:
- *Myocardial ischemia* (symptoms or signs of angina or MI). This is the most important cause of PVCs to identify, if they are present. PVCs are not generally associated with an increased risk of death unless they occur in the setting of myocardial ischemia or MI.
- *Hypokalemia or hypomagnesemia.* Look for a recent serum potassium and magnesium value in the chart, and order repeated measurements if recent ones are not available. Check the 12-lead ECG for evidence of hypokalemia (Fig. 15.15). Determine whether the patient is taking diuretics that may cause hypokalemia (refer to Chapter 34 for treatment) or hypomagnesemia.
- *Hypoxia.* Obtain pulse oximetry measurements if hypoxia is suspected clinically.
- *Acid–base imbalance.* Check the chart for a recent HCO_3^- determination. Obtain arterial blood gas measurements if acidosis or alkalosis is suspected.
- *Cardiomyopathy.* Patients with cardiomyopathy that is sufficiently severe to cause PVCs are almost always already under the care of a cardiologist and have an established diagnosis of cardiomyopathy before you see them. Consult the patient's cardiologist for guidance in treating cardiomyopathy-related PVCs.
- *Drugs.* Drugs such as digoxin and other antiarrhythmic agents may actually cause PVCs.

Conditions such as *mitral valve prolapse* and *hyperthyroidism* can also cause PVCs, but these arrhythmias are not common presenting signs of these disorders in the hospital.

Try to identify whether any of the preceding factors are responsible for the PVCs, and correct them if possible. Hypokalemia,

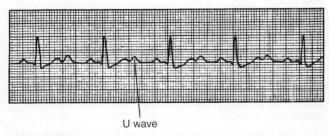

U wave

FIG. 15.15 Electrocardiographic features of hypokalemia.

hypoxia, and acid–base disturbances can usually be identified and corrected at the patient's bedside. However, if myocardial ischemia, cardiomyopathy, digoxin toxicity, or hyperthyroidism is suspected, the patient should be transferred to a telemetry ward or the ICU/CCU for continuous electrocardiographic monitoring and initiation of antiarrhythmic agents if indicated.

After the PVCs have been treated, the patient may still have *sinus tachycardia*. Investigation and management of the underlying sinus tachycardia should be undertaken as follows.

Management of Rapid Regular Rhythms

SINUS TACHYCARDIA

There is no specific drug for the treatment of sinus tachycardia. It is important to find the *underlying cause* of this dysrhythmia. The most common causes of persistent sinus tachycardia in hospitalized patients are as follows:
- Hypovolemia
- Hypotension (cardiogenic, hypovolemic, septic, anaphylactic; refer to Chapter 18 for the investigation and management of hypotension)
- Hypoxia of any cause (CHF, pulmonary embolism, pneumonia, bronchospasm [COPD, asthma]; refer to Chapter 24 for the investigation and management of shortness of breath)
- Fever
- Anxiety or pain
- Hyperthyroidism
- Drugs

    Management of sinus tachycardia always consists of treatment of the underlying causes.

SUPRAVENTRICULAR TACHYCARDIA: ATRIAL FLUTTER

The treatment of atrial flutter is similar to that of atrial fibrillation. If the patient is in *unstable* condition, synchronized cardioversion may be required; if the patient is in *stable* condition, he or she may be treated with β-blockers or calcium channel blockers IV or PO (see page 149). Often, the doses of digoxin necessary to slow the ventricular rate are higher for atrial flutter than for atrial fibrillation. Look for causes in the chart that may predispose the patient to atrial flutter; for the most part, these are the same diseases that can cause atrial fibrillation (see page 152).

SUPRAVENTRICULAR TACHYCARDIA: ATRIOVENTRICULAR NODAL REENTRY AND FOCAL ATRIAL TACHYCARDIAS

Patient in Unstable Condition. If the patient is in *unstable* condition (has hypotension, angina, CHF, or impaired mentation), prepare for immediate cardioversion as follows:

- Ask the RN to call immediately for your resident and an anesthetist.
- Ask the RN to bring the cardiac arrest cart into the room. Attach the ECG monitor to the patient. Attach the cardioversion pads (shave the chest and back if necessary to ensure good pad contact). Set the defibrillator to 50 J, in the "synchronize" mode.
- Attach a pulse oximeter. If necessary, give the patient O_2 by mask to maintain an oxygen saturation level >94%.
- Ensure that an intravenous line is in place.
- Ask the RN to have available **intravenous midazolam, 5 mg.**

📖 Premedication to alleviate the pain of electrical shocks is required whenever possible. Your anesthesia team may have its own protocols or preferences for conscious sedation. Unless you are faced with a life-threatening situation, it is best to await the arrival of your resident and the anesthetist before administering premedication or proceeding to electrical cardioversion.

- Ask the RN to draw **intravenous adenosine, 6 mg,** into a syringe.

📖 Adenosine has a very brief half-life, may be given to a patient in unstable condition, and may terminate an SVT such as atrioventricular nodal reentry without the need for cardioversion. Adenosine *should not be given,* however, without the guidance of your resident.

- If the patient has an SVT, you may attempt Valsalva maneuvers or carotid sinus massage (see discussion below) while you await the arrival of more experienced help.

📖 On occasion, these maneuvers *break* an SVT, obviating the need for pharmacologic or electrical conversion of the arrhythmia. If these maneuvers are unsuccessful, you must proceed to pharmacologic or electrical cardioversion.

- While you wait for your resident to arrive, try nonelectrical means to convert the rhythm, such as a Valsalva maneuver or carotid sinus massage (see later discussion).

Patient in Stable Condition. If the patient is hemodynamically stable, you may try one or more of the following measures to break the tachycardia:

- Valsalva maneuver. Ask the patient to hold his or her breath and to "bear down as if you are going to have a bowel movement." This maneuver increases vagal tone and may terminate an SVT.
- Carotid sinus massage. This maneuver is an effective form of vagal stimulation and may thereby terminate some SVTs. It should always be performed with intravenous atropine available and with continuous electrocardiographic monitoring, both for safety reasons (some patients have developed asystole) and to document the results.

Listen over the carotid arteries for bruits, and if they are present, do not perform carotid sinus massage. If no bruit is heard, proceed as follows. Turn the patient's head to the left. Locate the carotid sinus just anterior to the sternocleidomastoid muscle at the level of the top of the thyroid cartilage (Fig. 15.16). Feel the carotid pulsation at this point, and apply steady pressure to the carotid artery with two fingers for 5 to 10 seconds. Try the right side, and if this is not effective, try the left side. The carotid sinus must never be massaged on both sides simultaneously, because you will cut off cerebral blood flow.

📖 Carotid sinus massage has resulted, rarely, in cerebral embolization of an atherosclerotic plaque from carotid artery

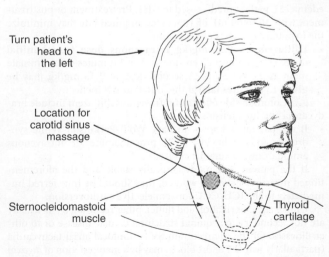

Turn patient's head to the left

Location for carotid sinus massage

Sternocleidomastoid muscle

Thyroid cartilage

FIG. 15.16 Carotid sinus massage.

compression. Although this is a rare complication, you can minimize the chances of its occurrence by first listening over the carotid
artery for a bruit. If you hear a bruit, do not perform carotid sinus
massage on that side.

- **Adenosine.** Administer **6 mg as a rapid intravenous bolus,**
  followed by a saline flush. If this is ineffective, increase to a
  12 mg intravenous push. Because of the very short half-life of
  adenosine, the doses can be administered at intervals of 60 seconds, if required.

  📖 Intravenous adenosine should be used with caution in patients with asthma and COPD. Lower doses may be required in patients who take dipyridamole or carbamazepine, in patients who have
  undergone cardiac transplantation, and when administered through
  a central line. Common side effects are transient and include facial
  flushing, dyspnea, and chest pressure. Some SVTs, particularly focal
  atrial tachycardia, may not be responsive to adenosine, in which case
  intravenous verapamil may be effective.

- **Verapamil.** Begin with **2.5 to 5 mg IV over 1 to 2 minutes.** If
  ineffective, the dose may be repeated in 5 to 10 minutes.
  Verapamil slows atrioventricular nodal conduction time and
  may thereby slow ventricular rate. Its advantage over intravenous digoxin is its more rapid onset of action (1 to 2 minutes,
  in contrast to 5 to 30 minutes for digoxin).

  📖 Verapamil may cause hypotension if injected too rapidly. It
  is essential to administer the dose slowly over 2 minutes. Verapamil is also a negative inotropic agent and may precipitate pulmonary
  edema in a patient predisposed to CHF. Pretreatment or posttreat-
  ment with **30 to 60 mL of 10% calcium gluconate** may minimize
  the hypotensive effects of verapamil.

- **Diltiazem.** A **0.25-mg/kg intravenous dose (usual initial
  dose, 15 to 20 mg)** given slowly over 2 minutes will terminate
  many reentrant SVTs. A second dose of **0.35 mg/kg may be
  given 15 minutes later** if the initial dose is ineffective.

  📖 Common side effects of intravenous diltiazem include bradycardia and hypotension.

- If the patient is known to have Wolff-Parkinson-White syndrome and is having SVT, procainamide or intravenous
  amiodarone is a suitable choice.

  If the patient is hemodynamically stable and the aforementioned measures have not worked, they should be transferred immediately to the ICU/CCU for semielective cardioversion.

  Unlike atrial fibrillation and flutter, other reentrant SVTs usually
  are not secondary to acquired structural cardiac disease or to other illnesses. Of the nonreentrant SVTs, unifocal atrial tachycardia
  (particularly with 2:1 or 3:1 block) may be a manifestation of *digoxin
  toxicity,* and junctional tachycardia may be seen with digoxin toxicity or after *acute MI* or *aortic or mitral valve surgery.*

SUSTAINED VENTRICULAR TACHYCARDIA

If the patient has no BP or pulse, call for the cardiac arrest team and proceed with resuscitation.

Patient in Unstable Condition. If the patient is in unstable condition (has hypotension, angina, CHF, or impaired mentation), do the following:

- Call for the cardiac arrest cart, your resident, and an anesthetist, and order a 12-lead ECG immediately.
- Attach the ECG monitor to the patient.
- Make sure that an intravenous line is in place.
- Attach a pulse oximeter. If necessary, give the patient O₂ by mask to maintain an oxygen saturation level >94%
- Prepare for *electrical cardioversion or defibrillation*. Attach the cardioversion pads (shave the chest and back if necessary to ensure good pad contact). Monomorphic ventricular tachycardia in an unstable patient should be cardioverted using 100 J in the synchronized mode. Polymorphic ventricular tachycardia in the unstable patient should be "defibrillated" using 200 J (biphasic) or 360 J (monophasic) in the unsynchronized mode.

Patient in Stable Condition. If the patient is *stable* (no hypotension, angina, CHF, or impaired mentation), do the following:

- Call for the cardiac arrest cart, your resident, and an anesthetist, and order a 12-lead ECG immediately.
- Attach the ECG monitor to the patient.
- Make sure that an intravenous line is in place.
- Attach a pulse oximeter. If necessary, give the patient O₂ by mask to maintain an oxygen saturation level >94%.
- Prepare for *electrical cardioversion*. Attach the cardioversion pads (shave the chest and back if necessary to ensure good pad contact). Monomorphic ventricular tachycardia in a stable patient should be cardioverted using 100 J in the synchronized mode.

If, despite cardioversion, the monomorphic ventricular tachycardia is recurrent, order one of the following:

Amiodarone, 150 mg intravenous bolus, over 10 minutes

or

Lidocaine, 1 to 1.5 mg/kg IV, to be given by syringe as rapidly as possible. At the same time, begin a **maintenance infusion of lidocaine at a rate of 1 to 4 mg/minute**. In elderly patients and in patients with liver disease, CHF, or hypotension, give half the maintenance dose. Additional boluses of lidocaine in doses of **0.5 to 0.75 mg/kg may be given every 5 to 10 minutes** after the initial bolus, to a **maximum total dose of 3 mg/kg.**

📖 Lidocaine may cause drowsiness, confusion, slurred speech, and seizures, especially in the elderly and in patients with heart failure or liver disease. Once your patient has been transferred to the ICU/CCU, the staff there must watch carefully for these signs of lidocaine toxicity.

or

procainamide, 20 to 50 mg/minute IV (until the arrhythmia is suppressed, hypotension occurs, or the QRS complex widens by >50 milliseconds) may also be tried. The **maximum total dose of procainamide should not exceed 17 mg/kg**. This may be followed by a **maintenance infusion of 1 to 4 mg/minute**.

Although procainamide is often more effective than lidocaine in breaking ventricular tachycardia, the patient must be monitored carefully for hypotension.

VENTRICULAR TACHYCARDIA IS POLYMORPHIC, PATIENT IS KNOWN TO HAVE A NORMAL BASELINE QT INTERVAL

If, despite cardioversion, the polymorphic ventricular tachycardia is recurrent, and the patient is known to have a normal baseline QT interval, intravenous amiodarone, lidocaine, or β-blockers may be used.

VENTRICULAR TACHYCARDIA IS POLYMORPHIC, PATIENT IS KNOWN TO HAVE A PROLONGED QT INTERVAL

If the baseline QT interval is prolonged, torsades de pointes should be suspected. This arrhythmia resembles a corkscrew pattern in the ECG and rhythm strip, with complexes rotating above and below the baseline (see Fig. 15.17). **Magnesium sulfate, 1 to 2 g IV**, is often effective in terminating this type of ventricular tachycardia, but overdrive pacing at about 100 beats/minute and isoproterenol can also be tried.

A patient with an episode of ventricular tachycardia should be transferred to the ICU/CCU for continuous electrocardiographic monitoring.

After immediate resuscitation, look for the following precipitating or potentiating causes of ventricular tachycardia:
1. Myocardial ischemia or MI
2. Hypoxia
3. Electrolyte imbalance (hypokalemia, hypomagnesemia, hypocalcemia)
4. Hypovolemia
5. Valvular heart disease

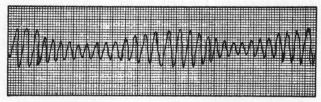

FIG. 15.17 **Electrocardiographic tracing of torsades de pointes**.

6. Acidemia
7. Cardiomyopathy, CHF
8. Drugs:
   - Antiarrhythmic drugs (e.g., dofetilide, ibutilide, quinidine, procainamide, disopyramide, sotalol, amiodarone)
   - Gastrointestinal drugs (e.g., ondansetron, droperidol)
   - Antimicrobials (e.g., macrolides, fluoroquinolones, antifungals)
   - Opioids (e.g., methadone, loperamide)
   - Antidepressants (e.g., selective serotonin reuptake inhibitors, tricyclics, mirtazapine)
   - Haloperidol
   - Arsenic trioxide

The drugs listed (and others) may prolong the QT interval to produce a characteristic type of ventricular tachycardia known as *torsades de pointes*. These drugs should be discontinued if such a rhythm develops.

PACEMAKER-RELATED TACHYCARDIAS

In patients with a dual-chamber pacemaker, a wide-complexed tachycardia can sometimes occur due to tracking of an atrial arrhythmia such as fibrillation or flutter, or due to a pacemaker-mediated tachycardia. With the former, the rhythm may be regular or irregular, and the clue is a rapid wide-complexed tachycardia with pacing spikes preceding each QRS complex. In a pacemaker-mediated tachycardia, a ventricular depolarization causes a retrograde atrial impulse that is then sensed, producing a new ventricular stimulation, resulting in an "endless loop" tachycardia. Magnet placement over the pacemaker will disable the ability of the pacemaker to sense, thereby preventing tracking of atrial depolarizations. This maneuver will aid in the diagnosis, and a more permanent solution can be achieved by reprogramming the pacemaker.

Slow Heart Rates

PHONE CALL

Questions

1. What is the patient's heart rate?
2. What is the patient's BP?
3. Is the patient taking digoxin, a β-blocker, a calcium channel blocker, or another antiarrhythmic drug?
4. Has the patient had a recent cardiac procedure?

Drugs such as digoxin, β-blockers, diltiazem, and verapamil possess both sinus and atrioventricular nodal suppressant properties and may cause profound sinus bradycardia or heart block. Other antiarrhythmic drugs that slow the ventricular rate, such as sotalol or amiodarone, possess β-blocking properties and may also cause bradycardia, and antiarrhythmic drugs that modulate the sodium channel (e.g., quinidine, procainamide, disopyramide) can cause atrioventricular block.

Some cardiac procedures such as transcatheter aortic valve replacement, arrhythmia ablations, open heart valve surgery, and others may damage the atrioventricular node and result in atrioventricular block.

Orders

1. If the patient is hypotensive (systolic BP <90 mm Hg), order an intravenous line to be inserted immediately and ask the RN to place the patient in the Trendelenburg position (foot of the bed up).

   Intravenous access is essential for delivering medications to increase the heart rate. Placing the patient in the Trendelenburg position achieves an autotransfusion of 200 to 300 mL of blood.

2. If the heart rate is lower than 40 beats/minute, ask the RN to have a premixed syringe of atropine, 1 mg, ready at the bedside.

3. Obtain a stat ECG and rhythm strip.

4. Ask the RN to bring the cardiac arrest cart into the room, and attach the ECG monitor to the patient.

Informing the Registered Nurse

Tell the RN, "I will arrive at the bedside in … minutes."

If a patient has bradycardia plus hypotension, or any heart rate slower than 50 beats/minute, you must see the patient immediately.

ELEVATOR THOUGHTS

What causes slow heart rates?

Sinus Bradycardia (Fig. 15.18)

Drugs	β-Blockers
	Calcium channel blockers
	Digoxin
	Other antiarrhythmic agents (amiodarone, sotalol)
	Others (e.g., methyldopa, clonidine, cimetidine, opioids and sedatives, lithium)
	Chemotherapy drugs (e.g., thalidomide, lenalidomide, paclitaxel)

Cardiac	Sinus node dysfunction
	Acute MI (usually of inferior wall)
	Vasovagal attack
Infections	Lyme disease, Chagas disease, Legionella, and others
Miscellaneous	Hypothyroidism
	Healthy young patients
	Well-conditioned athletes
	Increased intracranial pressure in association with hypertension
	Obstructive sleep apnea
	Hypothermia
	Anorexia nervosa

Second-Degree Atrioventricular Block: Type I (Wenckebach) (Fig. 15.19) and Type II (Fig. 15.20); and Third-Degree Atrioventricular Block (Fig. 15.21)

Drugs	β-Blockers
	Digoxin
	Calcium channel blockers
	Other antiarrhythmic agents (amiodarone, sotalol, quinidine, procainamide, disopyramide)
Cardiac	Acute MI
	Atrioventricular node dysfunction
	Cardiomyopathy
	Cardiac procedures (e.g., open heart surgery involving aortic or mitral valve replacement or VSD closure, transcatheter aortic valve implantation (TAVR) or VSD closure, arrhythmia ablation, alcohol septal ablation)
	Infections (e.g., myocarditis, Lyme disease)
Electrolyte abnormality	Hyperkalemia
Endocrine	Severe hyper- or hypothyroidism

Atrial Fibrillation With Slow Ventricular Rate (Fig. 15.22)

Any of the conditions that cause atrioventricular block (see above) can slow the ventricular response in a patient in atrial fibrillation.

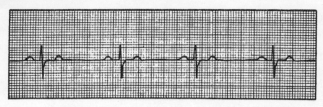

FIG. 15.18 Electrocardiographic tracing of slow heart rate: sinus bradycardia.

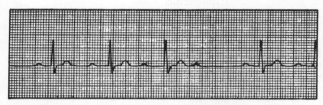

FIG. 15.19 Electrocardiographic tracing of slow heart rate: second-degree atrioventricular block (type I).

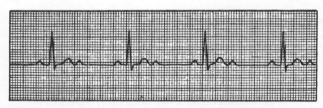

FIG. 15.20 Electrocardiographic tracing of slow heart rate: second-degree atrioventricular block (type II).

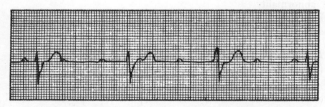

FIG. 15.21 Electrocardiographic tracing of slow heart rate: third-degree atrioventricular block.

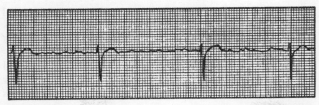

FIG. 15.22 Electrocardiographic tracing of atrial fibrillation with slow ventricular rate.

MAJOR THREAT TO LIFE

- Hypotension
- MI

Two major threats to life exist in a patient with bradycardia. First, if the heart rate is sufficiently low, hypotension resulting from inadequate CO causes hypoperfusion of vital organs. Second, if the bradycardia is caused by MI, the patient is prone to even more ominous dysrhythmias such as ventricular tachycardia, ventricular fibrillation, or asystole.

BEDSIDE

Quick-Look Test

Does the patient look well (comfortable), sick (uncomfortable or distressed), or critical (about to die)?

If the patient looks sick or critically ill, ask the RN to bring the cardiac arrest cart to the bedside and attach the ECG monitor to the patient. The ECG may provide a diagnosis of the patient's rhythm, continuous monitoring is enabled, and feedback about the effects of your interventions is provided instantly.

Airway and Vital Signs

What is the heart rate?

Read the ECG to identify which slow rhythm is occurring.

What is the BP?

Most causes of hypotension are accompanied by a compensatory reflex tachycardia. If hypotension exists with any type of bradycardia, proceed as follows:

- Notify your resident as soon as possible.
- Elevate the patient's legs. This is a temporary measure that shifts blood volume from the legs to the central circulation.
- Begin a 250- to 500-mL intravenous bolus of normal saline.
- Give **atropine, 0.5 mg IV,** as rapidly as possible. If there is no response after 3 to 5 minutes, give an **additional 0.5 mg**

of atropine IV every 3 to 5 minutes, not to exceed a total dose of 3 mg. If there is still no improvement, begin transcutaneous pacing, if available, or try **dopamine, 2 to 10 mcg/kg/minute IV** (must be given through a central line), or **epinephrine, 2 to 10 mcg/minute** (must be given through a central line). The patient should be transferred to the ICU/CCU for further monitoring and possible placement of a transvenous pacemaker.

Selective History and Chart Review

Look for the cause of bradycardia.

Drugs	β-Blockers
	Calcium channel blockers
	Digoxin
	Other antiarrhythmic agents (amiodarone, sotalol)
Cardiac	History of angina or ischemia or previous MI
	Any hint (chest pain, shortness of breath, nausea, vomiting) that a cardiac ischemic event occurred within the past few days
	Other evidence of atherosclerosis (previous stroke, transient ischemic attacks [TIAs], peripheral vascular disease) that may be a clue to the concomitant presence of coronary artery disease
	Current risk factors (hypertension, diabetes mellitus, smoking, hypercholesterolemia, family history of coronary artery disease) that may suggest that this is the first episode of cardiac ischemia
	Recent cardiac surgery or transcatheter procedure (e.g., open heart valve surgery, TAVR, arrhythmia ablation, alcohol septal ablation)
Vasovagal	History of pain, straining, or other Valsalva-like maneuver immediately before the occurrence of the bradycardia
Infections	History Lyme disease, Legionella, Chagas disease

If there is any evidence that the bradycardia is caused by an acute MI, cardiac markers should be drawn, and the patient should go to the ICU/CCU for electrocardiographic monitoring.

Selective Physical Examination

Look for a cause of bradycardia.

Vitals	Bradypnea (hypothyroidism)
	Hypothermia (hypothyroidism)
	Hypertension (risk factor for coronary artery disease)
HEENT	Coarse facial features (hypothyroidism)
	Loss of lateral third of eyebrows (hypothyroidism)
	Periorbital xanthomas (coronary artery disease)
	Unilateral periorbital edema (Chagas disease)
	Conjunctivitis (Lyme disease)
	Fundi with hypertensive or diabetic changes (coronary artery disease)
	Carotid bruits (cerebrovascular disease with concomitant coronary artery disease)
CVS	New S_3, S_4, or mitral regurgitant murmur (nonspecific but common findings in acute MI)
Lungs	Rales, consolidation (Legionella pneumonia)
Abdomen (ABD)	Renal, aortic, or femoral bruits (signs of atherosclerosis, suggesting possible concomitant coronary artery disease)
Ext	Poor peripheral pulses (signs of peripheral vascular disease, suggesting possible concomitant coronary artery disease)
Neurologic system	Delayed return phase of deep tendon reflexes (hypothyroidism)
	Cranial nerve palsies and peripheral neuropathy (Lyme disease)
Skin	Erythema migrans lesions (Lyme disease)
	Chagoma (Chagas disease)

Management

Sinus Bradycardia

- No immediate treatment is required if the patient is not hypotensive.
- If the patient is taking digoxin and has a heart rate lower than 60 beats/minute, further digoxin doses should be withheld until the heart rate exceeds 60 beats/minute.
- If the patient is taking medications that depress conduction, no immediate treatment is required, as long as the patient is not hypotensive. However, with very slow heart rates (<40 beats/

minute), subsequent doses of these medications should be withheld until the heart rate exceeds 60 beats/minute. Further maintenance doses can be determined in consultation with the attending physician.

Second-Degree Atrioventricular Block (Types I and II) and Third-Degree Block

For patients with either second- or third-degree atrioventricular block, any drugs that are known to prolong atrioventricular conduction should be temporarily withheld, and the patient should be transferred to a bed where continuous electrocardiographic monitoring is available.

Atrial Fibrillation With Slow Ventricular Response

This dysrhythmia does not necessitate treatment unless the patient is hypotensive or has symptoms (syncope, confusion, angina, CHF) suggestive of vital organ hypoperfusion. Definitive treatment includes discontinuation of drugs that depress atrioventricular conduction and, in some cases, transfer to the ICU/CCU for pacemaker placement. An assessment of long- and short-term risk for thromboembolic events should be made, and decisions regarding anticoagulation discussed with your resident and the patient's attending physician (see page 152).

REMEMBER

1. Abrupt discontinuation of some β-blockers may result in rebound hypertension, angina, or MI. Observe the patient closely over the next several days. When the heart rate rises above 60 beats/minute, the β-blocker may be reinstituted at a lower dosage. When bradycardia is treated in this manner, rebound hypertension or cardiac ischemia is seldom a problem.
2. On occasion, digoxin overdose causes life-threatening dysrhythmias that are unresponsive to conventional measures. In these instances, digoxin-specific antibodies may be effective in reversing the toxic effects of digoxin.

High Blood Pressure

Calls concerning high blood pressure (BP) are frequent at night. Drugs that rapidly reduce the pressure are rarely required. The level of the BP itself is of less importance than the rate of the rise and the setting in which the high BP is occurring. The risk of abruptly lowering BP is that blood flow to the brain or myocardium, or both, may be compromised; this risk is highest in patients with preexisting compromised blood supply.

PHONE CALL

Questions

1. Why was the patient admitted?
2. Is the patient pregnant?

    Hypertension in a pregnant patient may indicate the development of preeclampsia or eclampsia and should be assessed immediately.
3. Is the patient taking antidepressant drugs?

    If hypertension occurs in a patient who is taking monoamine oxidase (MAO) inhibitors or tricyclic antidepressants, a catecholamine crisis may be resulting from food or drug interaction.
4. Is the patient in the emergency department?

    Hypertension in a young individual in the emergency department may be catecholamine hypertension caused by cocaine, amphetamine, or phencyclidine (PCP) abuse.
5. How high is the patient's BP, and what has the BP been previously?
6. Does the patient have symptoms suggestive of a hypertensive emergency?
    a. Back and chest pain (aortic dissection)
    b. Chest pain (myocardial ischemia)
    c. Shortness of breath (pulmonary edema)
    d. Headache, neck stiffness (subarachnoid hemorrhage)
    e. Headache, vomiting, confusion, seizures (hypertensive encephalopathy)
7. What antihypertensive medication has the patient been taking?

Orders

If the patient has any symptoms of a hypertensive emergency, order intravenous saline lock for venous access.

Informing the Registered Nurse

Tell the registered nurse (RN), "I will be at the bedside in ... minutes."

Immediate assessment and possibly prompt lowering of BP are required in the following situations:

- Eclampsia
- Aortic dissection
- Pulmonary edema resistant to other emergency treatment (see Chapter 24, pages 289–292)
- Myocardial ischemia
- Catecholamine crisis
- Hypertensive encephalopathy
- Uncontrolled bleeding anywhere, including worsening vision secondary to retinal hemorrhage

ELEVATOR THOUGHTS

The diagnosis of *preeclampsia* can be made in a previously normotensive obstetric patient after 20 weeks of gestation with new onset of systolic blood pressure ≥140 mmHg or diastolic blood pressure ≥90 mmHg on at least two occasions at least 4 hours apart or systolic blood pressure ≥160 mmHg or diastolic blood pressure ≥110 mmHg taken at least twice within a few minutes, *and* proteinuria (≥300 mg per 24-hour urine collection, or protein:creatinine ratio ≥0.3, or urine dipstick reading ≥2+). In the absence of proteinuria, preeclampsia is diagnosed by new-onset hypertension with other end-organ damage such as new thrombocytopenia (platelet count <100,000/microL), renal insufficiency (serum creatinine of >1.1 mg/dL [97 micromol/L] or a doubling of the serum creatinine concentration in the absence of other renal disease), impaired liver function, pulmonary edema, or persistent cerebral or visual symptoms.

Superimposed preeclampsia may occur in patients with preexisting hypertension who develop worsening hypertension with either proteinuria or end-organ damage, or both, after 20 weeks of gestation.

Aortic dissection is potentiated by high shearing forces determined by the rate of rise of the intraventricular pressure and of the systolic pressure.

Elevation of afterload (increased systemic vascular resistance and elevated BP) may be a readily correctable detrimental factor in *myocardial ischemia* and *pulmonary edema*.

Catecholamine crisis can be caused by the following:

Illicit drug use	Cocaine, amphetamines, phencyclidine
Drug interaction	MAO inhibitors with indirect-acting catechols such as wine, cheese; ephedrine
	Tricyclics, direct-acting catecholamines (epinephrine, pseudoephedrine, norepinephrine)
Drug withdrawal	Abrupt withdrawal from antihypertensive agents such as β-blockers, centrally acting α-agonists, and angiotensin-converting enzyme (ACE) inhibitors may result in a rebound hypertensive crisis.
Pheochromocytoma	May produce a hypertensive crisis through overproduction of epinephrine or norepinephrine
Burns	Some patients with second- or third-degree burns develop a transient hypertensive crisis, usually resolving within 2 weeks, as a result of high circulating levels of catecholamines, renin, and angiotensin II

Hypertensive encephalopathy is a rare complication of hypertension and is unusual in hospitalized patients. Vomiting developing over several days, headache (particularly an occipital headache or neck ache), lethargy, and confusion are suggestive symptoms and are caused by cerebral edema that results from cerebral hyperperfusion that, in turn, results from a sudden, severe rise in BP. Focal neurologic deficits are uncommon in the early course of encephalopathy.

BP fluctuates in normal individuals and more so in hypertensive individuals. Excitement, fear, and anxiety from unrelated medical conditions or procedures can cause marked transient increases in BP. To measure BP, you must use care with regard to proper cuff size and placement, and the measurements should be repeated to confirm the readings.

MAJOR THREAT TO LIFE

The major immediate threat to life is a marked increase in BP with the following:

- Eclampsia
- Aortic dissection
- Pulmonary edema

- Myocardial infarction
- Hypertensive encephalopathy

BEDSIDE

Quick-Look Test

Does the patient look well (comfortable), sick (uncomfortable or distressed), or critical (about to die)?

Unless the patient is having seizures (eclampsia, hypertensive encephalopathy) or is markedly short of breath (pulmonary edema), the severity of the situation cannot be assessed from the initial appearance. The patient may have hypertensive encephalopathy and yet look deceptively well.

Airway and Vital Signs

What is the patient's BP?

Measure the BP again in both arms.

📖 A lower pressure in one arm may be a clue to aortic dissection but may also be seen in cases of subclavian artery stenosis. Too small a cuff (e.g., on an obese patient or a patient with rigid arteriosclerotic peripheral vessels) may yield readings that are factitiously high in relation to the intra-arterial pressure.

What is the patient's heart rate?

Bradycardia and hypertension in a patient not taking β-blockers may indicate increasing intracranial pressure.

Tachycardia and hypertension can occur in catecholamine crisis.

Selective History

Can the patient further elucidate the duration of hypertension?

Lowering BP precipitously in a patient with long-standing hypertension may result in acute underperfusion of brain, heart, kidneys, and other organ systems; knowledge of the duration and severity of hypertension is helpful in determining the rate at which BP should be lowered.

Does the patient have any symptoms suggestive of a hypertensive emergency?

- Headache (an occipital headache or neck ache), lethargy, or blurred vision may be suggestive of hypertensive encephalopathy).
- Chest pain may be suggestive of myocardial ischemia.
- Shortness of breath can be a sign of pulmonary edema.
- Back or chest pain can be indicative of aortic dissection.
- Unilateral weakness or sensory symptoms could be signs of a stroke; such an episode in a previously hypertensive patient may be associated with a transient increase in BP.
- Nausea and vomiting may be a symptom of increased intracranial pressure.

Selective Physical Examination

Does the patient have evidence of a hypertensive emergency?

Head, ears, eyes, nose, throat (HEENT)	Assess the fundi for hypertensive changes (generalized or focal arteriolar narrowing, flame-shaped hemorrhages near the disk, dot-and-blot hemorrhages, exudates).
	Papilledema is an ominous finding in patients with hypertension. Hypertensive encephalopathy can occur without papilledema, but retinal hemorrhages and exudates are almost always present.
Respiratory	Crackles, pleural effusion (congestive heart failure)
Cardiovascular system (CVS)	Elevated jugular venous pressure, presence of a third heart sound (congestive heart failure)
Neurologic system	Confusion, delirium, agitation, or lethargy (hypertensive encephalopathy)
	Localized deficits (stroke)

Management

Most often, elevated BP is an isolated finding in an asymptomatic patient known to have hypertension. Although long-term control of hypertension in such patients is of proven benefit, acute lowering of BP is not. Remember that in the acute situation, there is a risk of lowering BP too quickly in patients with long-standing hypertension and a decreased ability to autoregulate cerebral blood flow. Do not treat the BP reading. Treat the condition associated with it.

📖 In hypertensive emergencies, oral and sublingual agents should generally be avoided because they are more likely to have a slow onset of action and/or cause precipitous and uncontrollable falls in BP. In general, IV agents, administered in a monitored setting, are preferred.

True emergencies necessitate special management. These situations include the following:
- Hypertensive encephalopathy
- Eclampsia
- Subarachnoid or cerebral hemorrhage
- Aortic dissection
- Hypertension and pulmonary edema or myocardial ischemia
- Catecholamine crisis

In most instances a prompt lowering of BP by 10% to 15% in the first hour should be the goal, with cautious further reductions thereafter, so that a total reduction of 25% is achieved by the end of 24 hours. Call your resident for help if you are unfamiliar with the management of these conditions.

Hypertensive Encephalopathy

Hypertensive encephalopathy is almost always accompanied by retinal exudates and hemorrhages and is often accompanied by papilledema. Focal neurologic deficits are unusual early on; their presence suggests that the elevated pressure is probably associated with a stroke. Remember the risk of lowering pressure too quickly in patients with atherothrombotic cerebrovascular disease; you can precipitate a stroke! For lowering pressure in patients with compromised cerebral blood flow, select agents that lower BP but protect cerebral blood flow through cerebral arterial vasodilation.

1. Transfer the patient to the intensive care unit/cardiac care unit (intensive care unit [ICU]/coronary care unit [CCU]) for electrocardiographic (ECG) monitoring and intra-arterial BP monitoring. Remember that oral and sublingual agents should generally be *avoided* in this situation because they have a slower onset of action and cannot control the rate and degree of BP reduction. Your goal is to get the patient to the ICU/CCU so that intravenous agents can be instituted in a monitored setting as soon as possible. Once the patient is in the ICU/CCU, the goal is to reduce the BP by about 10% to 20% within the first hour of treatment, with more gradual reduction thereafter so that a total reduction of 25% is achieved by the end of 24 hours. Two intravenous agents are commonly used in this situation:
   a. **Labetalol** is a combined α- and β-blocking agent that may be given intravenously (IV) without intra-arterial monitoring. It may be given as a **20-mg IV push over 2 minutes and may be repeated or increased to 40 or 80 mg IV every 10 minutes**, depending on effect, to a **maximum cumulative dose of 300 mg**. Alternatively, after the 20 mg IV bolus, start a labetalol infusion at 0.5 to 2 mg/minute, titrating to response up to a maximum of 10 mg/minute to a maximum cumulative dose of 300 mg. Labetalol is not as useful in lowering BP if the patient is already taking a β-blocker. Side effects include bronchoconstriction, heart block, and bradycardia.
   b. **Nitroprusside** is an arteriolar and venous dilator with an onset of action of a few seconds and a duration of 2 to 5 minutes, so if its use is necessary, its effect can be rapidly reversed simply by discontinuing the infusion. The usual starting dose is **0.1 to 0.5 mcg/kg/minute** and may be titrated to effect, to a maximum dose of 10 mcg/kg/min. Side effects include headache, nausea, abdominal cramps, thiocyanate toxicity, and CO_2 retention. Nitroprusside carries a theoretical risk of intracranial shunting of blood and

therefore should be avoided in the presence of raised intracranial pressure.

c. Nicardipine and clevidipine are dihydropyridine calcium
channel blockers administered by infusion. Nicardipine is
given beginning at 5 mg/hour, increasing by 2.5 mg/hour
every 15 minutes to a maximum dose of 15 mg/hour.
Consider reducing the dose to 3 mg/hour once a response is
achieved. Side effects may include tachycardia, nausea, vomiting, headache, and increased intracranial pressure. Clevidipine is given beginning at 1 to 2 mg/hour, increasing by 1
to 2 mg/hour every 90 seconds and by smaller increments
as target BP is approached. The usual dosage range is 4 to
6 mg/hour. Side effects may include atrial fibrillation, nausea, vomiting, headache, and acute renal injury.

d. Fenoldopam is a dopamine D1 agonist that can be given IV
beginning at 0.1 mcg/kg/min and increasing by 0.05 to 0.1
mcg/kg/min every 15 minutes until target BP is reached;
maximum dose is 1.6 mcg/kg/min. It primarily affects the
renal capillaries reducing peripheral resistance. Side effects
may include nausea, vomiting, headaches, tachycardia,
myocardial ischemia, and hypokalemia.

2. Once BP control is achieved through parenteral means, the
patient should begin an appropriate oral regimen to maintain
satisfactory BP control.

Preeclampsia and Eclampsia

Treatment of preeclampsia and eclampsia is complicated by the risk
to the fetus and the mother from both the disorder and the treatment.
The treatment of choice near term is magnesium sulfate until the
baby can be delivered. Treatment should be initiated only in consultation with the patient's obstetrician. Magnesium sulfate is given as
an intravenous infusion: administer a loading dose of 4 to 6 g IV over
20 minutes, followed by a maintenance infusion of 1 to 2 g/hour. A
reduced maintenance dose may be necessary in persons with renal
insufficiency. Order a measurement of serum magnesium level every
4 hours; the aim is for a serum magnesium level of 2.0 to 3.5 mmol/L.

Note that magnesium sulfate does not lower BP. It is given to prevent seizures. Local practice may include giving other drugs, such as
intravenous labetalol, hydralazine, nicardipine, or PO nifedipine. Diuretics should be avoided, because affected patients usually have volume depletion already, with an activated renin-angiotensin system.

Subarachnoid or Cerebral Hemorrhage

Although there is no proof that lowering BP alters the outcome
of subarachnoid or cerebral hemorrhage, many neurologists administer drugs to control elevated BP in these situations. Unless

you are familiar with the local practice, a neurologist should be consulted.

Aortic Dissection

1. Transfer the patient to the ICU/CCU immediately for intra-arterial BP monitoring and control of BP with parenteral drugs.
2. First-line treatment for aortic dissection is a β-blocker, which reduces the rate of rise of intraventricular pressure and hence the shearing force. These should be given parenterally, and high doses may be required, as follows:
   a. **Esmolol, 0.25 to 0.5 mg/kg for 1 minute, followed by a continuous infusion of 0.25 to 0.05 mg/kg/minute (maximum of 0.3 mg/kg/minute). The only advantage of esmolol is its short half-life, which provides a rapid onset and a rapid offset of action.**
   b. **Metoprolol 5 mg IV every 5 minutes for 3 doses, then 5 to 10 mg IV q6h PRN.**
   c. **Propranolol, 1 to 3 mg by slow IV push, repeating every 2 to 5 minutes to a total of 5 mg.**
   d. **Labetalol** alone may be used for aortic dissection in the same regimen as for hypertensive encephalopathy (see page 174).
3. Intravenous diltiazem or verapamil may be given in patients who do not tolerate beta blockers.
4. If blood pressure is not controlled by IV beta blockers, then the addition of **nitroprusside, at an initial dose of 0.1 0.25 to 0.5 mcg/kg/minute, titrating to effect, up to a maximum dose of 10 mcg/kg/minute,** may be used. Nitroprusside should not be used for the treatment of aortic dissection without an accompanying beta blocker.
5. Intravenous nicardipine, clevidipine, nitroglycerine, enalaprilat, and fenoldopam are vasodilators that can be used as alternatives to nitroprusside.

Hypertension and Pulmonary Edema or Myocardial Ischemia

1. In addition to BP control, pulmonary edema should be treated with the measures outlined in Chapter 24, pages 289–292.
2. Transfer the patient to the ICU/CCU for continuous ECG and intra-arterial BP monitoring.
3. Notify the ICU/CCU staff that the patient requires an intravenous nitroglycerin infusion. Experimental evidence suggests that intravenous nitroglycerin is preferable to intravenous nitroprusside for the control of BP in a patient with myocardial ischemia, because nitroprusside may cause a coronary steal phenomenon, resulting in extension of the ischemic zone. In a patient with cardiac disease, it is therefore preferable to attempt

BP control with intravenous nitroglycerin; if nitroglycerin is unsuccessful, nitroprusside can be used.

4. If the patient is hypertensive and tachycardic and has myocardial ischemia but no evidence of pulmonary edema, β-adrenergic blockade is helpful in addition to intravenous nitroglycerin. Any of the following agents may be used acutely:

   a. **Propranolol,** 1 to 3 mg by slow IV push, repeating every 2 to 5 minutes to a total of 5 mg.
   b. **Esmolol,** 0.5 mg/kg for 1 minute, followed by a continuous infusion of 0.05 mg/kg/minute (maximum, 0.3 mg/kg/minute).
   c. **Metoprolol,** 1.5 to 5 mg IV, rarely up to 15 mg IV.

Catecholamine Crisis

Pheochromocytoma (pallor, palpitations, perspiration) is the classic condition associated with intermittent alarmingly high BP. Other conditions associated with sudden and severe increases in BP include *cocaine, amphetamine, and phencyclidine* abuse; major second- or third-degree *burns;* abrupt antihypertensive drug *withdrawal;* and food (cheese), drug (ephedrine), and drink (wine) *interactions* with MAO inhibitors (antidepressants). Currently used MAO inhibitors include tranylcypromine sulfate (Parnate), phenelzine sulfate (Nardil), and isocarboxazid (Marplan). If sudden increases in BP are observed in patients who take these drugs, the most likely cause is an interaction with a substance that is releasing catecholamine stores, which are overabundant because one of the catecholamine-metabolizing enzymes (i.e., MAO) has been inhibited.

1. Transfer the patient to the ICU/CCU for ECG and intra-arterial BP monitoring.
2. Notify the ICU/CCU staff that the patient requires special parenteral antihypertensive drugs.
3. In cases of known or suspected pheochromocytoma, **phentolamine mesylate,** a direct α-blocker, may be administered IV for marked elevation of BP. This drug acts directly on vascular smooth muscle and thereby causes a decrease in peripheral resistance and an increase in venous capacity. This effect may be accompanied by cardiac stimulation, with tachycardia greater than can be explained by a reflex response to peripheral vasodilation. In an emergency, **phentolamine mesylate 2.5 to 5 mg IV may be given, followed by an infusion of 1 mg/minute, titrating up to 40 mg/hour if required.** Alternatively, **nitroprusside** or **nicardipine** can be used.
4. In *cocaine-induced hypertension,* labetalol, phentolamine, or nitroprusside may be used in the same dosages as described previously. Propranolol and β-blockers other than labetalol should be avoided because of the risk of unopposed α-adrenergic stimulation.

5. In *amphetamine-induced hypertension,* phentolamine or nitroprusside may be used in the same dosages as described previously. Propranolol and β-blockers should be avoided because of the risk of unopposed α-adrenergic stimulation.

Ecstasy (3,4-methylenedioxymethamphetamine) is structurally related to methamphetamine, with hallucinogenic and amphetamine-like effects, but it has greater central stimulatory effects than amphetamine does. Its cardiovascular effects include an increase in systolic and diastolic pressure and a reflex slowing of heart rate. Nitroprusside or an α-adrenergic-blocking drug is the agent of choice to control BP.

6. In *catecholamine crisis* associated with MAO inhibition, phentolamine, labetalol, or nitroprusside may be effective.

High Blood Pressure in the Absence of a Hypertensive Emergency

New antihypertensive medication, in the absence of one of the hypertensive emergencies, is best initiated in consultation with your resident. It is not a matter of simply choosing one of the myriad of oral agents available; you must consider the patient's age, the degree of hypertension, other comorbid conditions, and concomitant medications. For instance, an ACE inhibitor may be a good choice as initial therapy for a hypertensive patient with coronary artery disease, together with a β-blocker if the patient has had a recent myocardial infarction. An ACE inhibitor or angiotensin receptor blocker is a good choice for a hypertensive patient with a reduced left ventricular ejection fraction. An ACE inhibitor is also a good choice for a hypertensive patient with proteinuric chronic kidney disease. In most cases, if the hypertension is not associated with one of the hypertensive emergencies, initiation of new oral agents at night is not necessary and may cause more harm than good. Remember to treat the patient, not just the condition.

Hypnotics, Laxatives, Analgesics, and Antipyretics

Telephone calls regarding the ordering of hypnotic, laxative, analgesic, and antipyretic medications are frequent. The majority of these requests can be managed over the telephone.

Hypnotics

Questions

1. Why is a hypnotic drug being requested? The majority of requests for nighttime sedation are related to insomnia. Sleeping pills should not be prescribed for restless or agitated patients who have not been examined.
2. Has the patient received hypnotics before?
3. What are the patient's vital signs?
4. What was the reason for the patient's hospital admission?
5. Does the patient have any of the following conditions in which hypnotics are contraindicated?
   a. Depression (an antidepressant is the drug of choice if insomnia is a manifestation of depression)
   b. Confusion
   c. Hepatic or respiratory insufficiency
   d. Sleep apnea
   e. Myasthenia gravis
6. Is the patient taking other centrally active drugs that may interact, such as alcohol, antidepressants, antihistamines, and narcotics?
7. Does the patient have any drug allergies?
   The major contraindication to a specific hypnotic is a known allergy to the drug.

Orders

A benzodiazepine is the drug of choice for short-term treatment of insomnia. Sedative effects are comparable among all benzodiazepines; only the onset and duration of effect differ. Table 17.1 lists the drug doses of various benzodiazepines.

Informing the Registered Nurse

Tell the registered nurse (RN), "I will arrive at the bedside in . . . minutes."

Agitated, restless patients should be assessed before hypnotics are prescribed.

REMEMBER

1. All benzodiazepines and the specific benzodiazepine-receptor agonists (see Table 17.1) have hypnotic properties. Those with a short duration of action, such as triazolam, carry a higher risk of adverse effects, such as early morning insomnia and rebound daytime anxiety, whereas those with a long half-life are associated with more hangover effects. Temazepam (Restoril) is therefore a reasonable choice, providing a rapid onset of action and duration to cover the usual sleep period. Oxazepam (Serax) is a reasonable alternative, although it should be given 60 to 90 minutes before bedtime because of its relatively slow absorption. Both temazepam and oxazepam are available in generic formulations.
2. The newer benzodiazepine-receptor agonists provide no advantage over temazepam and are more expensive.
3. Benzodiazepines should not be prescribed on a nightly basis; they should be discontinued temporarily once acceptable sleep has been achieved for 1 or 2 nights. The use of benzodiazepines for less than 14 consecutive nights helps prevent the development of drug tolerance and dependence.
4. Be aware of the adverse effects of any drug you prescribe. The adverse effects of benzodiazepines are central nervous system depression (tiredness, drowsiness, feelings of detachment), headache, dizziness, ataxia, confusion, disorientation in elderly patients, and psychological dependence.
5. Barbiturates and nonbarbiturate hypnotics other than benzodiazepines usually carry more risks than advantages and should be avoided.

Laxatives

Constipation is frequently aggravated or caused by drugs (e.g., iron supplements, calcium channel blockers, aluminum-containing antacids) or medical conditions (e.g., hypothyroidism, diabetes

TABLE 17.1	Characteristics of Benzodiazepines, Benzodiazepine-Receptor Agonists, Melatonin-Receptor Agonists and Antidepressants Used as Hypnotics

Drug	Trade Name	Usual Adult Dose (mg PO)	Time of Peak Effect (Hours)	Approximate Half-Life Drug and Metabolites (Hours)
Benzodiazepines				
Estazolam	Prosom	1-2	0.5-6	10-24
Triazolam	Halcion	0.125-0.25	1-2	1.5-5
Temazepam	Restoril	30	2-3	10-20
Nitrazepam	Mogadon	5-10	2-3	16-55
Flurazepam	Dalmane	15-30	0.5-1	50-100
Lorazepam	Ativan	0.5-2	2-4	10-20
Quazepam	Doral	7.5-15	1	39-73
Oxazepam	Serax	15-30	2-4	5-15
Specific Benzodiazepine-Receptor Agonists				
Eszopiclone	Lunesta	2-3	1-2	6
Zalpione	Sonata	5-10	1	1
Zolpidem	Ambien	2.5-10	1.5	2.5
Zopiclone	Imovane	3.75-7.5	1-2	5
Melatonin-Receptor Agonists				
Ramelteon	Rozerem	8	45 min	1-2.6
Suvorexant	Belsomra	10	2	12
Antidepressants				
Trazadone	Oleptra	25-100	1-2	5-9
Doxepine	Selinor	25-150	3-5	6-8
Mirtazapine	Remeron	15-45	2-3	20-30

mellitus, Parkinson's disease, diverticular disease). Hospitalized patients commonly require laxatives, particularly after acute myocardial infarction to limit straining, during the administration of narcotics, during prolonged bed rest, and during evacuation of the bowels before abdominal surgery and some gastrointestinal diagnostic procedures. The solutions used in enemas have either hypertonic properties to stimulate rectal peristalsis or surfactant properties to soften impacted feces.

PHONE CALL

Questions

1. Why is a laxative being requested? The frequency of bowel movements is highly variable in the normal population, rang-

ing from twice daily to once every 3 days. Make certain you know what a particular patient's normal bowel pattern is before you prescribe a laxative.
2. Has the patient received laxatives before? If so, which ones have been tried so far?
3. What are the patient's vital signs?
4. What was the reason for admission?
5. When was a rectal examination last performed? Fecal impaction, which must be diagnosed (and sometimes treated) by means of a rectal examination, is a relative contraindication to oral laxative use.
6. Does the patient have nausea, vomiting, or abdominal pain? These symptoms are suggestive of an acute gastrointestinal disorder.

Orders

Table 17.2 lists the drug doses of selected laxatives, and Table 17.3 lists the drug doses of enemas. Bowel movements can be increased in frequency if the stool is liquefied. Both bulk and osmotic laxatives increase the water content in the intestine. An increase in the frequency of bowel movements can also be induced by stool softeners and colon-irritating drugs that increase peristalsis.

Informing the Registered Nurse

Tell the RN, "I will arrive at the bedside in . . . minutes."

When a laxative has been requested, you need to assess the patient only when the patient has associated nausea, vomiting, or abdominal pain or when fecal impaction is suspected. (See Chapter 5 for the assessment and management of abdominal pain.)

REMEMBER

1. When a patient is constipated (unless there is fecal impaction), an oral laxative is the treatment of choice. If the oral laxative fails, a stronger-acting laxative can be used; if that is not effective, a suppository is prescribed. Finally, enemas can be used as follows: first, a hypertonic enema solution (e.g., Fleet) should be tried; if that is unsuccessful, an oil-retention enema can be tried.
2. When fecal impaction is present, an oil-based enema is the treatment of choice.
3. Soapsuds enemas are used primarily for preoperative bowel cleansing. They are quite uncomfortable because of the large volumes used and are rarely required in the treatment of constipation.

TABLE 17.2	Characteristics of Selected Laxatives	
Drug	**Dosage**	**Comments**
Bulk Forming		
Psyllium hydrophilic (Metamucil and others)	3-6.5 g PO once/day to tid	Cellulose binds drugs (e.g., digoxin); not useful for acute constipation
Surface Active		
Docusate (sodium dioctyl sulfosuccinate; Colace)	100 mg PO tid; 50 mg/90 mL enema fluid	Stool softener; lowers surface tension
Lubricant		
Mineral oil	Emulsion 15 mL bid	Impairs the absorption of fat-soluble vitamins
Osmotic		
Lactulose	15-30 mL PO	—
Glycerin	2.67-g suppository	Onset in 30 min
Milk of magnesia	15-30 mL PO	Do not administer magnesium preparations to patients with renal impairment
Magnesium citrate oral solution	15 g/300-mL solution, or 7-21 mL of a 70% solution	—
Stimulant		
Anthraquinones	Variable	Onset in 6 h; urine (cascara, senna) may be brown
Diphenylmethanes (e.g., bisacodyl)	5-15 mg PO or 10 mg PR	See page 482
Castor oil	15-60 mL	May produce voluminous evacuation

Analgesics

Most hospital pharmacies do not allow narcotic medication orders to stand indefinitely. Narcotic medications need to be reordered every 3 to 5 days, depending on the individual medical institution. Consequently, if the house staff fails to reorder these medications during the day, you may be called to do so at night.

PHONE CALL

Questions

1. Why is an analgesic being requested? The majority of requests are for reordering of medications.

TABLE 17.3   Characteristics of Selected Enemas

Preparation	Onset	Caution	Usual Adult Dosage	Use
Sodium phosphate and sodium biphosphate (Fleet)	Immediate	Do not administer when patient has nausea, vomiting, or abdominal pain	60-120 mL (6 g sodium phosphate and 16 g sodium biphosphate/100 mL)[a]	Acute evacuation of the bowel before diagnostic procedures; acute constipation
Bisacodyl (Fleet Bisacodyl)	Immediate	Do not administer when patient has nausea, vomiting, or abdominal pain. Avoid in pregnant patients and patients with myocardial infarction; may worsen orthostatic hypotension, weakness, and incoordination in elderly patients	37.5 mL (10 mg/30 mL)[a]	Acute evacuation of the bowel before diagnostic procedures; acute constipation
Mineral oil (Fleet mineral oil)	Immediate	Do not administer when patient has nausea, vomiting, or abdominal pain	60-120 mL[a]	Impacted feces
Microlax (sodium citrate, 450 mg; sodium alkylsulfoacetate, 45 mg; sorbic acid, 5 mg)	5-15 min	Do not administer when patient has nausea, vomiting, or abdominal pain	5 mL	Fecal impaction when hard stool is present in the rectum; not useful if rectum is empty

[a]Available in disposable plastic containers.

2. How severe is the patient's pain? This question helps determine whether a nonnarcotic analgesic may be sufficient.

3. Is this pain a new problem? For the new onset of undiagnosed pain, you must assess the patient at the bedside before you order an analgesic medication.

4. What are the patient's vital signs? The onset of fever in association with pain is suggestive of a localized infectious process.

5. Why was the patient admitted?

6. Does the patient have any drug allergies?

Orders

Tables 17.4 and 17.5 provide the drug dosages of selected analgesics.

TABLE 17.4	Characteristics of Commonly Used Analgesics for Mild to Moderate Pain		
Drug	**Duration of Effect (Hours)**	**Usual Adult PO Dosage**	**Comments**
Acetaminophen, paracetamol (Tylenol)	4	325-975 mg q4h	Has practically no anti-inflammatory or platelet effects
Aspirin, acetyl-salicylic acid	4	650-975 mg q4h	Equal analgesia to acetaminophen, except more effective in inflammatory arthritis; has an irreversible platelet effect
Diclofenac (Voltaren)	6-8	25-50 mg q6-8h	Can cause an increase in hepatic enzymes
Diflunisal (Dolobid)	8-12	1000 mg, then 500 mg q12h	Salicylate derivative but has no antiplatelet effect at lower doses
Ibuprofen (Motrin, Advil)	4	400 mg q4-6h	More effective than 650 mg of aspirin as an analgesic
Indomethacin (Indocin)	8-12	25-50 mg q8-12h	High incidence of gastrointestinal and renal side effects; not indicated for routine use as an analgesic
Naproxen (Naprosyn)	6	500 mg, then 250 mg q6-8h	—

TABLE 17.5	Characteristics of Selected Narcotic Drugs		
Drug	**PO**	**SC or IM**	**Comments**
Codeine	2-4	30-60 mg q4-6h	More effective than propoxyphene and less addicting than oxycodone
Oxycodone with acetaminophen or aspirin (Percocet, Percodan)	2-4	—	**Not recommended because of high abuse potential**
Morphine Sulfate Preparations			
MSIR (immediate release)	5-30 mg q4-6h[a]	—	Available in oral solution or tablet form
MS Contin (sustained release)	15-120 mg q12h	—	Because it is difficult to titrate sustained-release doses, it is best to initiate morphine treatment with an immediate-release preparation
Morphine injection	—	5-15 mg q4-6h[a]	—
Tramadol (Ultram)	100-300 mg PO daily	—	Originally released as a noncontrolled drug—since 2014 placed under controlled drug status because of its abuse potential and severe withdrawal reactions
Tramadol/Acetaminophen (Tramacet)	37.5 mg tramadol/325 mg acetaminophen	PO q4-6 h	—
Other Drugs			
Anileridine (Leritine)	25-50 mg q4-6h[a]	25-50 mg q4-6h[a]	—
Hydromorphone (Dilaudid)	2-4 mg q4h[a]	2 mg q4h[a]	—
Meperidine (Demerol)	50-150 mg q4h[a]	50-150 mg q4h[a]	—

[a]The duration of action tends to be longer with oral than with parenteral administration.

Informing the Registered Nurse

Tell the RN, "I will arrive at the bedside in . . . minutes."

If a patient has any undiagnosed pain, new onset of severe pain, or change in character of previous pain, you must assess the patient at the bedside before you order an analgesic.

Mild pain and most moderate to severe pain can be alleviated with nonopioid analgesics such as acetaminophen and nonsteroidal anti-inflammatory drugs (NSAIDs). NSAIDs are more effective but have more side effects. A combination of an NSAID with acetaminophen may be as effective as an opioid/acetaminophen combination.

Acetylsalicylic acid (aspirin) is effective in treating mild to moderate pain either alone or in combination with other OTC or prescription analgesics. It is usually avoided because it irreversibly inhibits platelet function for the 8- to 10-day life of the platelet.

Severe pain may require an opioid agonist. A short-acting opioid should be selected and used for the shortest time possible. Codeine is preferred over oxycodone because of the lower risk of abuse. However, physical dependence on codeine can occur if taken for 7 to 10 days.

Neuropathic pain (diabetic neuropathy, postherpetic neuralgia, fibromyalgia) can be treated with centrally acting neurotransmitter inhibitors. Opioids should not be used since these conditions tend to be long lasting (Table 17.6).

REMEMBER

If reversal of a narcotic overdose is required, the following actions are recommended:

1. *Reversal of postoperative narcotic depression.* Administer **naloxone (Narcan), 0.2 to 2 mg intravenously every 5 minutes,** until the desired improved level of consciousness is achieved (maximum total dose, 10 mg). Doses every 1 to 2 hours may be necessary to maintain reversal of central nervous system depression. *Naloxone is also available by nasal spray as Narcan 2, 4, or 8 mg or Kloxxado 8 mg.*

2. *Reversal of suspected narcotic overdose.* If the patient is comatose, intubation for airway protection should be undertaken before overdose reversal. Abrupt reversal may induce nausea and vomiting, with the attendant risk of aspiration pneumonia. Administer **naloxone, 0.2 mg intravenously, subcutaneously, or intramuscularly, every 5 minutes** for several doses. If the initial doses are ineffective, the dosage may be increased incrementally up to a maximum total dose of 10 mg.

TABLE 17.6	Drugs for Neuropathic Pain				
Drug	**Trade Name**	**Action**	**Dosage**	**Side Effects**	**Uses**
Cycloben- zaprine	Flexeril	Related to tricyclics 5-HT2 receptor antagonist	5-10 mg PO tid	Drowsi- ness, dry mouth, dizziness	Centrally acting muscle relaxant— relieves muscle spasm
Duloxatine	Cymbalta	Serotonin- norepineph- rine uptake inhibitor	30-60 mg PO once daily	Anaphy- lactic reactions	Neuropathic pain fibromy- algia
Gabapentin	Neurontin	Binds to calcium channels in the CNS inhibiting the release of excitatory neurotrans- mitters	300 mg PO once daily to a maximum of 1800 mg od	Dizziness, somno- lence	Post-herpetic neuralgia, diabetic neuropathy, anticonvul- sant
Pregabalin	Lyrica	Binds to calcium channels in the CNS inhibiting the release of excitatory neurotrans- mitters	50 mg PO tid	Anaphy- lactic reactions, panic attacks, anxiety	Post-herpetic neuralgia, diabetic neuropathy, anticonvul- sant

3. *Adverse effects of abrupt narcotic reversal.* Nausea and vomiting, if provoked in a patient with an unprotected airway, may result in aspiration pneumonia. Hypertension and tachycardia can occur during narcotic reversal and may result in congestive heart failure in a patient with reduced left ventricular function.

Antipyretics

Antipyretics should not be prescribed for an adult patient with fever unless the cause of the fever is known or the fever itself is causing symptoms. (Refer to Chapter 12 for the approach to the febrile patient. See Table 17.4 for the dosages and side effects of acetaminophen and aspirin.)

Hypotension and Shock

Hypotension is a problem that commonly requires attention at night. Do not panic. Remember that hypotension does not progress to shock until tissue perfusion becomes inadequate. Blood pressure (BP) must be adequate for perfusion of three vital organs: brain, heart, and kidneys. Some patients normally have systolic BPs in the range of 85 to 100 mm Hg. The BP is usually adequate as long as the patient is not confused, disoriented, or unconscious; is not having angina; and is passing urine. In a patient who is normally hypertensive, however, a BP of 105/70 mm Hg may result in serious hypoperfusion.

PHONE CALL

Questions

1. What is the patient's BP?
2. What is the patient's heart rate?
3. What is the patient's temperature?

    Fever in addition to hypotension is suggestive of impending septic shock.
4. Is the patient conscious?
5. Is the patient having chest pain?
6. Is the patient wheezing or having trouble breathing?

    📖 Wheezing is suggestive of anaphylaxis.
7. Does the patient have evidence of bleeding?
8. Has the patient been given intravenous contrast material or any new medication within the past 6 hours?

    If you are called to see a hypotensive patient in the x-ray department or a patient who has recently returned to the room after undergoing an x-ray procedure involving the administration of intravenous contrast material, your primary thought should be that the patient might be having an anaphylactic reaction.
9. What was the admitting diagnosis?

Orders

1. If *anaphylaxis* is suspected, ask the registered nurse (RN) to have available a premixed syringe of intravenous epinephrine from the cardiac arrest cart.
2. If the information provided over the telephone supports the possibility of impending or established hypovolemic shock, order the following:
   a. Two large-bore (size 16, if possible) intravenous lines immediately, if not already in place. Intravenous access is a high priority in a hypotensive patient.
   b. Place the patient in the reverse Trendelenburg position (i.e., head of the bed down and foot of the bed up). Hypotension should be assessed immediately, but if you are unable to get to the patient's bedside for 10–15 minutes, also ask the RN to administer **500 mL of normal saline intravenously (IV)**, as rapidly as possible.
   c. Take a pulse oximetry reading and have an arterial blood gas tray at the patient's bedside. Identification and correction of hypoxia and acidemia are essential in the management of shock.
   d. Administer oxygen by high-flow nasal cannula at a rate to maintain a pulse oximetry reading of ≥94%.
3. If the admitting diagnosis is *gastrointestinal bleeding,* or if there is visible evidence of blood loss, take the following actions:
   a. Ensure that blood is available and on hold for the patient. If not, order a stat crossmatch for 2, 4, or 6 U of packed red blood cells, depending on your estimate of blood loss.
   b. Order a hemoglobin measurement stat.
   📖 *Caution:* The hemoglobin value may be normal during an acute hemorrhage and may drop only with correction of the intravascular volume by a shift of fluid from the interstitial and intracellular spaces, or by fluid therapy. (Refer to Chapter 13 for further investigation and management of gastrointestinal bleeding.)
4. If an arrhythmia or ischemic myocardial event is suspected, order a stat electrocardiogram (ECG) and rhythm strip.
   These may help you identify an arrhythmia or an acute myocardial infarction, which may be responsible for hypotension.

Informing the Registered Nurse

Tell the RN, "I will arrive at the bedside in … minutes."

If a patient has hypotension, you must see the patient immediately.

ELEVATOR THOUGHTS

What causes hypotension or shock?
- Cardiogenic causes

- Hypovolemia
- Peripheral vasodilation
  - Sepsis
  - Anaphylaxis
  - Neurogenic causes (e.g., traumatic brain or spinal cord injury)
  - Endocrine causes (e.g., Addisonian crisis, severe hypothyroidism)
- Obstructive causes

Two formulas are useful to remember when you consider the causes of hypotension:

$$BP = \text{cardiac output} \times \text{total peripheral resistance (TPR)}$$
$$\text{Cardiac output} = \text{heart rate} \times \text{stroke volume}$$

These formulas demonstrate that hypotension results from a fall in either cardiac output or TPR. *Cardiogenic causes* result from a fall in cardiac output that, in turn, results from either a fall in heart rate (e.g., heart block) or a fall in stroke volume (e.g., acute myocardial infarction, ruptured papillary muscle with severe mitral regurgitation, ruptured interventricular septum with new ventricular septal defect). *Hypovolemia* reduces stroke volume; hence, cardiac output falls. *Obstructive causes* reduce stroke volume by impairing venous return to the heart (e.g., cardiac tamponade, superior vena cava obstruction, tension pneumothorax) or obstructing outflow (e.g., massive pulmonary embolism). Profound *peripheral vasodilation* (e.g., sepsis, anaphylaxis, traumatic brain or spinal cord injury, and, less commonly, Addisonian crisis or severe hypothyroidism) cause hypotension by lowering TPR. In many conditions, there is overlap in pathological mechanisms—for example, septic shock is mediated predominantly by a fall in TPR, but sepsis may also reduce CO by depressing myocardial contractility.

MAJOR THREAT TO LIFE

- Shock

Remember that hypotension does not progress to shock until tissue perfusion becomes inadequate. Shock is relatively easy to diagnose. Your goal is to identify and correct the cause of hypotension before it results in hypoperfusion of vital organs.

BEDSIDE

Quick-Look Test

Does the patient look well (comfortable), sick (uncomfortable or distressed), or critical (about to die)?

A patient with hypotension but adequate tissue perfusion usually looks well. However, once perfusion of vital organs is compromised, the patient looks sick or critically ill.

Airway and Vital Signs

Is the patient's airway clear?

If the patient is obtunded and cannot protect his or her airway, endotracheal intubation is required. Ask the RN to notify the intensive care unit/cardiac care unit (ICU/CCU) immediately. Roll the patient onto the left side to avoid aspiration until intubation is achieved.

Is the patient breathing?

Assess respiration by checking the respiratory rate, the position of the trachea, and chest expansion and by performing auscultation. All patients in shock should receive high-flow oxygen. If acute respiratory distress and marked respiratory effort accompany shock, intubation and ventilation may be necessary.

What is the status of the patient's circulation?

If hypotension is not severe, examine the patient for postural changes.

On standing, a postural rise in heart rate of more than 15 beats per minute, a fall in systolic BP of more than 15 mm Hg, or any fall in diastolic BP is indicative of significant hypovolemia.

Measure the heart rate. Most causes of hypotension are accompanied by a compensatory reflex sinus tachycardia. If the patient is experiencing bradycardia, refer to the discussion of bradycardia (later in this chapter) for further evaluation and management.

Determine whether the patient is in shock. This should take less than 20 seconds.

Vitals	Repeat measurements now.
Cardiovascular system (CVS)	Pulse volume, jugular venous pressure (JVP)
	Skin temperature and color
	Capillary refill (normal, <2 seconds)
Neurologic system	Mental status

📖 Shock is a clinical diagnosis: systolic BP usually less than 90 mm Hg with evidence of inadequate tissue perfusion, such as inadequate perfusion of the skin (which may be cold, clammy, or cyanotic) and of the central nervous system (manifested by agitation, confusion, lethargy, or coma). In fact, the kidney is a sensitive indicator of shock (urine output <20 mL/h), but the immediate placement of a Foley catheter should not take priority over resuscitation measures.

What is the patient's temperature?

An elevated temperature or hypothermia (<36.8°C) is suggestive of sepsis. However remember that sepsis may occur in some
patients, especially elderly patients, who have a normal temperature. Therefore the absence of fever does not rule out the possibility
of septic shock.

What do the patient's pulse and ECG reveal?

Bradycardia

If the resting heart rate is <50 beats per minute in the presence of
hypotension, suspect one of three disorders:

* *Vasovagal attack.* If this is the case, the patient is usually normotensive by the time you arrive. Look for retrospective evidence of
straining, the Valsalva maneuver, pain, or some other stimulus to
vagal outflow. If vasovagal attack is suspected and bradycardia persists despite leg elevation, administer **atropine, 0.5 mg IV**, every 3
to 5 minutes as needed, not to exceed a total dose of 3 mg.
* *Autonomic dysfunction.* The patient may have been given too
much of a prescribed β-blocker or calcium channel blocker,
which can result in hypotension, or the patient may be hypotensive for some other reason but is unable to generate a
tachycardia because of β-blockade, calcium channel blockade,
underlying sick sinus syndrome, or autonomic neuropathy. If
the systolic BP is lower than 90 mm Hg, administer **atropine,
0.5 mg IV**, every 3 to 5 minutes as needed, not to exceed a total
dose of 3 mg.
* *Heart block.* The patient may have a profound sinus bradycardia or a heart block (e.g., after acute myocardial infarction).
Obtain a stat ECG to document the dysrhythmia. If systolic
BP is lower than 90 mm Hg, atropine may be helpful for a sinus bradycardia (with or without a first-degree AV block) or
a second-degree AV block, type I, but is usually ineffective in
a second-degree AV block type II and in a third-degree AV
block. The dosage is **atropine, 0.5 mg IV**, every 3 to 5 minutes
as needed, not to exceed a total dose of 3 mg. Refer to Chapter
15 for further investigation and management of heart block.

Tachycardia

A compensatory sinus tachycardia is an expected, appropriate response in a hypotensive patient. Look at the ECG to ensure that
the patient does not have one of the following three rapid heart
rhythms, which may cause hypotension as a result of inadequate
diastolic filling, with or without loss of the atrial kick:

* Atrial fibrillation with rapid ventricular response (Fig. 18.1)
* Supraventricular tachycardia (Fig. 18.2)
* Ventricular tachycardia (Fig. 18.3)

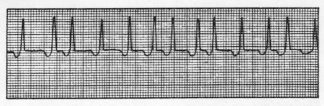

FIG. 18.1 Electrocardiographic representation of atrial fibrillation with rapid ventricular response.

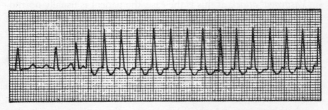

FIG. 18.2 Electrocardiographic representation of supraventricular tachycardia.

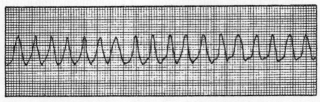

FIG. 18.3 Electrocardiographic representation of ventricular tachycardia.

If any of these three rhythms is present in a hypotensive patient, emergency electrical cardioversion may be required. Prepare for cardioversion as follows:

- Ask the RN to notify your resident and an anesthetist immediately.
- Ask the RN to bring the cardiac arrest cart into the room.
- Attach the electrocardiographic monitor to the patient.
- Ask the RN to draw **midazolam, 5 mg IV**, into a syringe.
- Ensure that an intravenous line is in place. (Refer to Chapter 15, pages 142–146, for further treatment of rapid heart rates associated with hypotension.)
- If the patient has a supraventricular tachycardia, also ask the RN to draw **adenosine, 6 mg IV**, into a syringe. Intravenous

adenosine may terminate some supraventricular tachycardias, obviating the patient's need for electrical cardioversion.

Selective Physical Examination

Determine the cause of hypotension or shock by assessing the *volume status.*

Cardiogenic shock and shock due to obstruction of venous inflow or arterial outflow may result in a clinical picture of volume overload. Hypovolemic, septic, or anaphylactic shock results in a clinical picture of volume depletion.

Vitals	Repeat measurements now.
Head, eyes, ears, nose, and throat	Elevated JVP (congestive heart failure [CHF], tamponade, right ventricular [RV] failure secondary to pulmonary embolism), flat neck veins (volume depletion)
Respiratory system	Stridor (anaphylaxis) Crackles, pleural effusions (CHF) Wheezes (anaphylaxis, CHF)
Cardiovascular system	Cardiac apex displaced laterally, third heart sound (S_3) (CHF)
Abdomen	Hepatomegaly with positive hepatojugular reflux (CHF)
Extremities	Presacral or ankle edema (CHF)
Skin	Urticaria (anaphylaxis)
Rectal	Melena or hematochezia (gastrointestinal bleeding)

Remember that *wheezing* may be present with both CHF and anaphylaxis. The administration of epinephrine may save the life of someone with anaphylaxis but may kill someone with CHF. Anaphylactic shock comes on relatively suddenly, and an inciting factor (e.g., intravenous contrast material, penicillin) can almost always be identified. Usually, other signs, such as angioedema or urticaria, are present.

Management

What immediate measures need to be taken to correct shock or prevent it from occurring?

Normalize the intravascular volume. All forms of shock can initially be managed with volume expansion. In the case of cardiogenic shock that results from suspected myocardial infarction, allow the intravenous normal saline bolus to run through, as long as there is no overt evidence of pulmonary edema; this helps optimize preload until the patient's condition stabilizes or a decision is made to use invasive hemodynamic monitoring to further guide fluid therapy. If overt pulmonary edema is or becomes evident, then stop the intravenous normal saline. Proper management also requires preload and afterload reduction and further investigation, as outlined in Chapter 24.

All *other forms of shock* necessitate more aggressive volume expansion. This can be achieved quickly through elevation of the legs (i.e., reverse Trendelenburg position) and the repeated administration of small volumes (200 to 300 mL over 15 to 30 minutes) of an intravenous fluid that will remain at least temporarily in the intravascular space, such as **normal saline or Ringer's lactate**. Reassess volume status after each bolus of intravenous fluid, aiming for a JVP of 2 to 3 cm H_2O above the sternal angle and concomitant normalization of heart rate, BP, and tissue perfusion.

If the patient is in *anaphylactic shock,* treat rapidly, as follows:
1. Epinephrine
Two strengths of epinephrine are available for injection. Make sure that you are using the correct strength.

For *profound anaphylactic shock* that is immediately life-threatening, use the intravenous route: **epinephrine, 1 mg (10 mL of the 0.1 mg/mL solution), administered every 3 to 5 minutes.** Follow each dose with a 20-mL flush of normal saline (NS), and elevate the arm for 10 to 20 seconds after each dose. See page 426 for alternative doses and routes.

For *less severe situations,* epinephrine can be given intramuscularly (IM) (note the different concentration): **epinephrine, 0.5 mg (0.5 mL of the 1 mg/mL solution) IM**, repeated after 5 minutes in the absence of improvement or if deterioration occurs. Several doses may be necessary.

Epinephrine is the most important drug for any anaphylactic reaction. Through its α-adrenergic action, it reverses peripheral vasodilatation; through its β-adrenergic action, it reduces bronchoconstriction and increases the force of cardiac contraction. In addition it suppresses histamine and leukotriene release.
2. Intravenous normal saline wide open until the patient is normotensive.
3. **Hydrocortisone, 500 mg by slow intravenous or IM injection or orally**, followed by 100 mg IV, IM, or orally every 6 hours to help avert late sequelae.
This is particularly necessary for patients with asthma who have been treated previously with corticosteroids.
4. **Salbutamol, 250 mcg/kg IV over 2 minutes or 2.5 mg/3 mL normal saline by nebulizer.**
This is an adjunctive measure if bronchospasm is a major feature.

Correct *hypoxia* and *acidemia.* If the patient is in shock, obtain arterial blood gas measurements and administer oxygen. If the arterial pH is lower than 7.2 in the absence of respiratory acidosis, order $NaHCO_3$, 0.5 to 1 ampule (44.6 mmol) IV. Monitor the effects of treatment by repeat arterial blood gas measurements every 30 minutes until the patient is stabilized.

What is the specific cause of hypotension or shock (determined while the intravascular volume is restored)?

Cardiogenic Shock

This is commonly a result of acute myocardial infarction, which results in an abrupt reduction of stroke volume as a consequence of either sudden pump failure or rupture of the interventricular septum, LV free wall, or papillary muscle. Order a stat ECG, portable chest radiograph, and cardiac enzyme tests. However, any of the causative factors of CHF listed on page 287 may be operative.

Obstructive Shock

Do not conclude that the patient with hypotension, impaired tissue perfusion, and elevated JVP is in cardiogenic shock without considering obstructive causes of shock. Four obstructive conditions can cause hypotension and elevated JVP:

- *Cardiac tamponade* may cause elevated JVP, arterial hypotension, and soft heart sounds (Beck triad). Suspect this as the diagnosis if there is a pulsus paradoxus with pressure higher than 10 mm Hg during relaxed respirations (see pages 284–288).
- A massive *pulmonary embolus* can cause hypotension, elevated JVP, and cyanosis and may be accompanied by additional evidence of acute right ventricular overload (e.g., positive hepatojugular reflux, right ventricular heave, loud P_2, right-sided S_3, murmur of tricuspid insufficiency). If pulmonary embolism is suspected, call your resident immediately, and treat as outlined in Chapter 24, pages 293–299.
- *Superior vena cava obstruction* may cause hypotension and elevated JVP that does not vary with respiration. Additional features may include headache, facial plethora, conjunctival injection, and dilation of collateral veins in the upper thorax and neck. Obstruction is usually caused by a tumor; therefore consider this diagnosis in oncology patients.
- *Tension pneumothorax* can also cause hypotension and elevated JVP by means of positive intrathoracic pressure that decreases venous return to the heart. Look for severe dyspnea, unilateral hyperresonance, and decreased air entry, with tracheal shift away from the involved side. If a tension pneumothorax is suspected, do not wait for radiographic confirmation. Call for your resident and get a 14- to 16-gauge needle ready to aspirate the pleural space at the second intercostal space in the midclavicular line on the affected side. This is a medical emergency!

Hypovolemia

If you suspect that gastrointestinal bleeding or other *acute blood loss* (e.g., ruptured abdominal aortic aneurysm) is responsible for hypotension, consult a surgeon immediately.

Excess fluid losses via sweating, vomiting, diarrhea, and polyuria and third-space losses (e.g., pancreatitis, peritonitis) respond to simple intravascular volume expansion with normal saline or Ringer's lactate and correction of the underlying problem.

Drugs are common causes of hypotension, resulting from relative hypovolemia with or without bradycardias as a result of their effects on the heart and peripheral circulation. Common offenders are morphine, meperidine, nitroglycerin, β-blockers, calcium channel blockers, angiotensin-converting enzyme (ACE) inhibitors, angiotensin receptor blockers (ARBs), and antihypertensive agents. In these instances, hypotension is seldom accompanied by evidence of inadequate tissue perfusion and can usually be avoided by reducing the dose or altering the schedule of drug administration.

In most cases, the reverse Trendelenburg position or a small volume (300 to 500 mL) of normal saline or Ringer's lactate usually suffices to support the BP until the effect of the drug wears off. The hypotension of narcotics (morphine, meperidine) can be reversed by **naloxone hydrochloride, 0.4 to 2 mg (maximum total dose, 10 mg) IV, SC or IM every 5 minutes**, until the desired degree of reversal is achieved. A higher dose naloxone is available as Zimhi (Naloxone-Adamis) 5 mg IM or SC.

Sepsis

On occasion, intravascular volume repletion and appropriate antibiotics are sufficient to resolve hypotension associated with septic shock. For continuing hypotension despite intravascular volume repletion, however, the patient must be admitted to the ICU/CCU for vasopressor support.

Anaphylactic Shock

This must be recognized and treated immediately to prevent fatal laryngeal edema. Treat as described on page 196.

Neurogenic and Endocrine Shock

After initial resuscitation measures, neurogenic shock and endocrine shock are best managed by consultation with the neurosurgeon and endocrinologist, respectively.

REMEMBER

1. Consider *toxic shock syndrome* in any hypotensive premeno-pausal woman. Ask about tampon or menstrual cup use, or if the patient is obtunded, perform a pelvic examination and remove any tampon or menstrual cup that is present.

2. The skin is not a vital organ but gives valuable evidence of tissue perfusion. Remember that during the early stage of septic shock, the skin may be warm and dry as a result of abnormal peripheral vasodilation.

3. Adequate BP is required to perfuse three vital organs: *brain, heart,* and *kidneys.* After you have successfully rescued your patient from an episode of hypotension, look out for hypotensive sequelae during the next few days. Not surprisingly, the common sequelae involve these three vital organs:

    a. *Brain:* thrombotic stroke in a patient with underlying cerebrovascular disease

    b. *Heart:* myocardial infarction in a patient with preexisting atherosclerosis

    c. *Kidney:* acute tubular necrosis; monitor urine output and check urea and creatinine levels in a few days

4. Centrilobular hepatic necrosis (manifested by jaundice and elevated liver enzymes) and bowel ischemia or infarction may also be sequelae of hypotension in a critically ill patient.

Leg Pain

The easiest approach to leg pain in a nighttime case is to identify which part of the leg hurts. Most leg pain originates from the muscles, joints, bones, or vascular supply to the legs; however, several causes of referred leg pain also exist.

PHONE CALL

Questions

1. Which part of the leg hurts? Is the leg swollen or discolored?
2. What are the patient's vital signs?
3. Was the pain sudden in onset, or is it chronic?
4. Why was the patient admitted?
5. Has there been a recent leg injury or fracture? Does the patient have a leg cast on?

Leg pain after a leg injury, fracture, or casting raises the possibility of a compartment syndrome.

Orders

No orders are necessary.

Informing the Registered Nurse

Tell the registered nurse (RN), "I will arrive at the bedside in . . . minutes."

If an acutely ill patient has a pulseless limb, fever, or severe leg pain of any cause, you must see the patient immediately. If leg pain increases 24 to 48 hours after casting, you must also see the patient immediately.

ELEVATOR THOUGHTS

What causes leg pain?

Bone and Joint Disease

1. Lumbar disk disease (sciatica)

2. Arthritis
   a. Septic (*Staphylococcus aureus*, *Neisseria gonorrhoeae*, *Streptococcus pneumoniae*, *Haemophilus influenzae*, and gram-negative bacilli)
   b. Inflammatory (gout, pseudogout, rheumatoid arthritis, systemic lupus erythematosus)
   c. Degenerative (osteoarthritis)
3. Osteomyelitis
4. Rupture of Baker cyst
5. Skeletal tumor

Vascular Disease

1. Arterial disease
   a. Acute arterial insufficiency (e.g., thromboembolism, cholesterol embolism)
   b. Arteriosclerosis obliterans (chronic arterial insufficiency)
   c. Thromboangiitis obliterans (Buerger disease)
2. Venous disease
   a. Deep vein thrombosis (DVT)
   b. Superficial thrombophlebitis

Muscle, Soft Tissue, or Nerve Pain

1. Fasciitis, pyomyositis, or myonecrosis
2. Compartment syndrome
3. Cellulitis
4. Neuropathies (e.g., diabetes)
5. Reflex sympathetic dystrophy syndrome
6. Erythema nodosum
7. Nodular liquefying panniculitis
8. Benign nocturnal leg cramps

MAJOR THREAT TO LIFE

- Loss of limb from arterial insufficiency
- Pulmonary embolism from DVT
- Septic arthritis
- Fasciitis, pyomyositis, or myonecrosis
- Compartment syndrome

Acute arterial occlusion of the lower extremity, if left untreated, may result in gangrene in as little as 6 hours. DVT may result in severe respiratory insufficiency or death if pulmonary embolism occurs. Although *septic arthritis* is not likely to result in loss of life overnight, it can result in permanent joint damage if it is not recognized and managed promptly. Anaerobic infections resulting in *fasciitis, pyomyositis, or myonecrosis* may lead to septic shock. An unrecognized *compartment syndrome* can result in permanent ischemic muscle contractures within hours.

Although the list of possible diagnoses of leg pain is long, emergency treatment at night is necessary for only the five major conditions that pose a threat to life. You should perform a systematic inspection, looking for evidence of each of these conditions in a patient with leg pain.

Quick-Look Test

Does the patient look well (comfortable), sick (uncomfortable or distressed), or critical (about to die)?

Most patients with significant leg pain lie still, appear apprehensive, and are reluctant to move the affected extremity.

Airway and Vital Signs

Leg pain should not compromise the vital signs; however, abnormalities in the vital signs may provide clues to the cause of leg pain.

What is the patient's heart rate? Is it regular or irregular?

Pain from any cause may result in tachycardia. However, an irregular rhythm is suggestive of atrial fibrillation, which raises the possibility of an embolic event.

What is the patient's blood pressure?

Pain or anxiety from any cause may raise the blood pressure.

What is the patient's temperature?

Fever is a sign of infection or inflammation, as may be seen with DVT, septic arthritis, fasciitis, pyomyositis, or myonecrosis.

Acute Arterial Insufficiency

Selective History

Was the pain sudden in onset (which is suggestive of an arterial embolism)?

Does the patient have a history of underlying cardiac disease (e.g., atrial fibrillation, mitral stenosis, ventricular aneurysm, prosthetic heart valve) that might predispose to arterial embolization?

Does the patient have a history of intermittent claudication (which is suggestive of long-standing chronic arterial insufficiency)?

Is the patient receiving heparin?

Heparin-induced thrombocytopenia Type II may cause acute intravascular thrombosis as a result of platelet aggregation by heparin-dependent immunoglobulin G antibodies. Suspect this disorder in a patient receiving heparin if the platelet count is ≤ 150,000/mm^3, or there has been a 50% decrease in platelet count from previously; necrotic skin lesions at heparin injection sites are another clue. The condition usually occurs after about 5 days of heparin therapy, but it may be seen earlier in patients who have received heparin previously. It is more common in patients receiving unfractionated heparin, but may also occur with low-molecular-weight heparins.

Selective Physical Examination

Look for the Six P's:

1. Pain
2. Pallor
3. Pulselessness
4. Paresthesias
5. Paralysis
6. Poikilothermia (inability to regulate core body temperature)

The following findings are suggestive of a major arterial embolism:

Skin	Pallor
	Focal areas of gangrene
	Bilateral brawny discoloration (arterioscle-rosis obliterans)
	Diminished temperature, especially if unilateral
Cardiovascular system	Check the femoral, popliteal, and pedal pulses
	In acute or chronic arterial occlusion, pulses are absent distal to the site of occlusion.
Neurologic system	Paresthesias, diminished light touch in a stocking distribution

An *acute arterial embolism* tends to cause unilateral pain, pallor, pulselessness, paresthesias, paralysis, and poikilothermia (the Six P's), whereas *chronic arterial insufficiency* that results from arteriosclerosis obliterans usually involves both lower limbs to a variable extent, with bilateral diminished pulses, trophic skin changes, loss of limb hair, and dependent rubor. Do not be fooled, however: although the manifestation of arteriosclerosis obliterans is almost always chronic and progressive, new thrombosis on top of a fixed atherosclerotic plaque may completely obstruct arterial flow, resulting in an acute-on-chronic presentation.

Management

Acute arterial insufficiency is a surgical emergency. If you suspect that an arterial thromboembolism has occluded a major artery, take the following steps:

1. Immediately notify your resident and a vascular surgeon.
2. Draw a stat blood sample for a complete blood cell count (CBC) and measurement of activated partial thromboplastin time (aPTT).
3. Begin IV fluids, for example **0.9% normal saline 250 ml IV bolus over 1 hour, followed by 75 to 100 ml/hr thereafter**, with modifications made depending on the patient's volume status.
4. If heparin is not contraindicated, administer **heparin, 60 to 80 U/kg intravenous bolus, followed by a maintenance infu-**

sion of 12 to 18 U/kg/hour, in the lower range for patients with a higher risk of bleeding. (See page 298 for precautions in the use of heparin.)

5. If limb viability is threatened, the patient may require emergency thrombectomy, catheter-directed thrombolysis, or bypass. If limb viability is not a concern, direct intraarterial recombinant tissue-type plasminogen activator (r-TPA), urokinase, or streptokinase may achieve lysis of a thrombus, but this should be initiated *only* under the guidance of a vascular surgeon.

Acute arterial insufficiency resulting from *heparin-induced thrombocytopenia* is a complex situation; ask your resident and a hematologist for help. In most cases, heparin must be discontinued immediately. If continued parenteral anticoagulation is necessary (i.e., for the original indication for which heparin was prescribed), a non-heparin anticoagulant (e.g., argatroban, danaparoid, fondaparinux, or bivalirudin) is recommended. Alternatively, oral anticoagulation using a direct-acting oral anticoagulant (DOAC) such as dabigatran, rivaroxaban, apixaban, or edoxaban can be used.

Acute arterial insufficiency from a septic embolism (e.g., due to bacterial endocarditis) should be considered if the patient has cardiac valvular abnormalities or a prosthetic heart valve. If limb viability is threatened, emergency embolectomy should be organized. Blood cultures should be drawn and an echocardiogram arranged.

Chronic arterial insufficiency resulting from arteriosclerosis obliterans is not usually an emergency unless an acute thrombosis occurs on top of a long-standing fixed plaque. In this case, direct intraarterial r-TPA, urokinase, or streptokinase may result in clot lysis, but these agents should be administered only under the guidance of a vascular surgeon. The more common scenario is a complaint of pain at rest in a patient with chronic intermittent claudication. If limb viability is of no immediate concern, pain at rest can be treated with nonnarcotic analgesics, such as **acetaminophen, 325 to 975 mg orally (PO) every 4 hours** as needed, and placement of the affected extremity in the dependent position. More definitive therapy, including lumbar sympathectomy or direct arterial surgery, is seldom required on an emergency basis.

Deep Vein Thrombosis

Selective History

Look for predisposing causes:

1. Stasis
   a. Prolonged bed rest or hospitalization
   b. Immobilized limb (e.g., stroke)
   c. Congestive heart failure
   d. Pregnancy (particularly postpartum)

2. Vein injury
   a. Lower extremity trauma
   b. Recent surgery (especially abdominal, pelvic, and orthopedic procedures)
3. Hypercoagulability
   a. Congenital or inherited (factor V Leiden, protein C and S deficiency, antithrombin III deficiency, G20210A prothrombin gene mutation, dysfibrinogenemia, hyperhomocysteinemia)
   b. Acquired (after orthopedic surgery; antiphospholipid antibody; drugs, such as oral contraceptives or hormone replacement therapy, tamoxifen, raloxifene)
   c. Associated with systemic disease (malignancy, inflammatory bowel disease, nephrotic syndrome, polycythemia vera)
4. Older age (>50 years)
5. Obesity
6. Prior episode of venous thromboembolism

Selective Physical Examination

Look for the following signs involving the calf or thigh:
1. Tenderness
2. Erythema
3. Edema: subtle degrees of swelling may be appreciated by measuring and comparing the circumferences of both calves and thighs at several different levels.
4. Warmth
5. Distention of the overlying superficial veins
6. Homans sign: with the patient supine, flex the knee and then sharply dorsiflex the ankle; pain in the calf during ankle dorsiflexion is supportive evidence of a calf DVT, but its absence does not exclude the diagnosis.

Components of the selective history and physical examination help you assess the pretest probability that the patient has a DVT. A useful clinical tool for this assessment is the Wells score (Box 19.1).

Draw a blood sample for CBC, aPTT, prothrombin time, platelet count, and creatinine in anticipation of possible anticoagulation. A d-dimer test if available may also help in confirming or excluding the diagnosis. d-Dimer is a degradation product of cross-linked fibrin and is detectable at levels higher than 500 ng/mL of fibrinogen equivalent units in most patients with DVT or pulmonary embolism.

Management

DVT should be recognized and treated immediately to prevent pulmonary embolization and acute right ventricular failure.

BOX 19.1	Wells Score

- Paralysis, paresis, or recent orthopedic casting of a lower extremity (1 point)
- Recently bedridden for longer than 3 days or major surgery within the past 4 weeks (1 point)
- Localized tenderness in the deep vein system (1 point)
- Swelling of an entire leg (1 point)
- Calf swelling 3 cm greater than the other calf, measured 10 cm below the tibial tuberosity (1 point)
- Pitting edema greater in the symptomatic leg (1 point)
- Collateral nonvaricose superficial veins (1 point)
- Active cancer or cancer treated within the past 6 months (1 point)
- Alternative diagnosis more likely than deep vein thrombosis (DVT) (e.g., Baker cyst, cellulitis, muscle damage, postphlebitic syndrome, inguinal lymphadenopathy, external venous compression (–2 points)

    0 points = low probability of DVT
    1-2 points = moderate probability of DVT
    3-8 points = high probability of DVT

For patients with a *low-probability* Wells score and a negative d-dimer test result, DVT is effectively ruled out, and anticoagulation is not required. If the result of the d-dimer test is positive, then an ultrasound examination should be performed.

For patients with a *moderate-* or *high-probability* Wells score, an ultrasound examination should be performed immediately, if available, to confirm or rule out a DVT. If ultrasonography is not available at night in your institution, then it is reasonable to begin anticoagulation without further confirmation of the diagnosis at this point. However, before you order an anticoagulant, ensure that the patient has no active bleeding, no severe bleeding diathesis, a platelet count higher than 20,000/mm^3, hasn't had an acute intracranial hemorrhage, recent major trauma, and hasn't had high-bleeding-risk surgery or is about to undergo emergency high-bleeding-risk surgery—these conditions are absolute contraindications to anticoagulation. Relative contraindications include brain or spinal tumors, large abdominal aortic aneurysms in the context of severe hypertension, stable aortic dissection, recurrent bleeding from gastrointestinal telangiectasias, and recent or planned emergency low-bleeding-risk surgery. Patients with these conditions require confirmation of DVT by an imaging modality and, if DVT is documented, require consultation for possible interruption of the inferior vena cava by the insertion of a transvenous caval device.

If a patient has no contraindications, begin an anticoagulant. Initial use of low-molecular-weight heparin (LMWH) has largely supplanted IV unfractionated heparin because of its safety and ease of administration. Several formulations exist the different distributions of molecular weight result in differences in inhibitory activities against factor Xa and thrombin, the extent of plasma protein binding, and plasma half-lives. You should familiarize yourself with the LMWH formulation used in your hospital. Also, be careful to note that the dose of LMWH used in the treatment of DVT is considerably higher than that used for DVT prophylaxis.

One regimen is to use LMWH for 5 days, then transition to dabigatran or edoxaban. For example, begin treatment with Dalteparin (Fragmin) 200 IU/kg by deep SC injection once daily, or, for patients with an increased risk of bleeding, 100 IU/kg q12h SC or 100 IU/kg by continuous IV infusion over 12 h. After 5 days, transition to an oral anticoagulant such as dabigatran or edoxaban.

Alternatives to initial treatment with low-molecular-weight heparin include apixaban at a dose of 10 mg BID for 7 days, then reduced to 5 mg twice per day (BID); rivaroxaban can be used at 15 mg PO BID for 21 days, then 20 mg PO once daily thereafter.

After anticoagulation is begun, the diagnosis should be confirmed in the morning by compression ultrasonography, which is the noninvasive test of choice to diagnose a first episode of DVT. If this test is not available, impedance plethysmography, nuclear venography, contrast venography, and magnetic resonance venography are other options. Equipment for impedance plethysmography is not available in many institutions, but this method may be more useful in detecting *recurrent* DVT than is compression ultrasonography, because abnormal values obtained with impedance plethysmography normalize more quickly after a previous DVT episode than do values obtained with compression ultrasonography.

If you have used intravenous unfractionated heparin, monitor the aPTT every 4 to 6 hours, and adjust the maintenance dosage of heparin until the aPTT is in the therapeutic range (1.5 to 2.5 × control values). After this, daily aPTT measurements are sufficient. Initial measurements of aPTT are made only to ensure adequate anticoagulation. LMWH does not consistently modify aPTT or thrombin clotting time in the usual dosages given; therefore these tests cannot be used to modify doses. Anti–factor Xa activity has been used to assess the activity of LMWH but does not appear to be correlated with efficacy.

Write an order that the patient should receive no aspirin-containing or other antiplatelet drugs, sulfinpyrazone, dipyridamole, or thrombolytic agents, and no intramuscular injections while taking anticoagulants.

Ask the patient daily about signs of bleeding or bruising. Inform the patient that prolonged pressure is required after venipuncture to prevent local bruising while the patient is taking anticoagulants.

Septic Arthritis

Selective History

During evaluations, patients with septic arthritis most often point to the painful joint involved. Your job is to determine whether the joint in question is infected. Two rules can be helpful:

- If a single joint is swollen, red, and tender, it should be considered septic until proven otherwise.
- In a patient with multiple-joint involvement (as may occur with rheumatoid arthritis or other inflammatory arthritides), if a single joint is inflamed out of proportion to the other joints involved, the joint in question should be considered possibly infected.

Look for predisposing conditions:

1. Age older than 80 years
2. Diabetes
3. Rheumatoid arthritis
4. Prosthetic joint
5. Recent joint surgery
6. Cellulitis

Selective Physical Examination

Fever may be present. The knee joint is most commonly affected. The joint is swollen, tender, and erythematous, and its range of motion is restricted. These signs may be less marked, however, in an elderly patient or in a patient taking steroids.

Septic arthritis of the hip is often missed because of the deep location of the hip joint; swelling may not be detected easily. Conditions involving the hip joint sometimes manifest only through referred pain to the groin, buttocks, lateral thigh, or anterior aspect of the knee. The affected extremity is usually held in adduction, flexion, and internal rotation.

Management

Septic arthritis is a medical emergency. Any joint suspected of being septic should be aspirated without delay. You need your resident's help or the assistance of a rheumatologist to perform joint aspiration. The diagnosis of septic arthritis is made by demonstrating microorganisms on a Gram stain of synovial fluid. Treatment with appropriate antibiotics must be prompt; this should not await confirmation by culture and should be directed by the results of the Gram stain. When microorganisms are not seen on the synovial fluid sample, empirical antibiotics should be administered. The choice of antibiotics depends on the clinical setting (Table 19.1).

Synovial fluid should be analyzed for the following:

- White blood cell count and differential

TABLE 19.1	Recommended Antibiotics for the Empirical Treatment of Septic Arthritis, Based on Clinical Setting and Initial Gram Stain Results

Clinical Setting	Usual Organism	Recommended Antibiotics Before Culture and Sensitivity Results
Gram-Positive Cocci		
Adults	*Staphylococcus aureus*	Vancomycin, 30 mg/kg per day in two or four divided doses (total dose should not exceed 2 g/day)
Prosthetic joint	Group A streptococci *S. aureus*	
Rheumatoid arthritis	*S. epidermidis* *S. aureus*	
Gram-Negative Bacilli		
Adults	Gram-negative aerobes	Ceftazidime, 1-2 g IV q8h or
Healthy young adult, sexually active	*Neisseria gonorrhoeae*	Ceftriaxone, 2 g IV daily or Cefotaxime 2 g IV q8h or In cephalosporin-allergic patients: Azithromycin 500-2000 mg PO daily or Gemifloxacin 320 mg PO daily
Illicit intravenous drug use	*Pseudomonas* spp.	A third-generation cephalosporin as for adults, plus gentamicin, 5-7 mg/kg per day in two or three divided doses
Gram Stain Result: No Organisms Seen		
Immunocompetent patient		Vancomycin, 30 mg/kg per day in two or four divided doses (total dose should not exceed 2 g/day)
Immunocompromised patient or traumatic bacterial arthritis		Vancomycin, 30 mg/kg per day in two or four divided doses (total dose should not exceed 2 g/day) plus a third-generation cephalosporin

Modifications to the original antibiotic selection can be made when culture and sensitivity results are available.

- Glucose level determination
- Gram stain
- Aerobic and anaerobic cultures
- Gonococcal culture
- Tuberculosis stain and culture
  Blood samples should be sent for the following:
- Simultaneous serum glucose determination
- Aerobic and anaerobic cultures
- Gonococcal culture

In septic arthritis, the synovial fluid is usually cloudy or purulent, and the white blood cell count is $\geq$10,000/mm^3 with $\geq$90% neutrophils. The synovial glucose level is 50% or less of the glucose level of a simultaneously drawn serum sample.

Necrotizing Fasciitis, Pyomyositis, and Myonecrosis

This group of infections is usually caused by a mixture of organisms, including anaerobes, most often involving *Clostridium perfringens*.

Selective History

These infections usually arise as a complication of surgery or deep traumatic wounds. The diagnosis may be more elusive in cases that arise spontaneously without a history of obvious injury. Heroin addicts are predisposed to a localized form of pyomyositis that may involve the thigh.

Selective Physical Examination

Look for the following:
1. Pus or gas formation in soft tissues
2. Subcutaneous crepitance
3. Local swelling and edema over a wound site, sometimes with a *frothy* wound exudate
4. Dark patches of cutaneous gangrene (a late finding)
5. In patients with clostridial myonecrosis, the development of systemic toxemia, with tachycardia, hypotension, renal failure, and the patient's feelings of impending doom, followed by toxic delirium and coma

Management

These infections are surgical emergencies. If you think the patient has fasciitis, pyomyositis, or myonecrosis, consult a surgeon immediately. Systemic antibiotics (usually including high-dose penicillin) are also indicated in the treatment of these clostridial infections.

Compartment Syndrome

Some muscle groups in the leg are surrounded by well-fitted fascial sheaths, leaving no space for swelling, should an injury occur. The compartment syndrome develops as a result of compression from an injured, edematous muscle within its sheaths. The increased pressure interferes with the circulation to the nerves and muscles within the compartment, which results in further ischemia. A characteristic of the compartment syndrome is that the amount of pain is out of proportion to the injury.

Selective History

Look for predisposing causes:
1. Recent fractures of the tibia and fibula
2. Overly tight pressure bandages or casts
3. Blunt leg trauma
4. Prolonged, unaccustomed, vigorous exertion
5. Anticoagulant medication

Patients receiving anticoagulants are at risk for developing compartment syndrome as a result of bleeding within the enclosed fascial sheath, sometimes after relatively minor trauma.

Selective Physical Examination

The anterior compartment of the leg is affected most commonly. It contains the anterior tibial, extensor hallucis longus, and extensor digitorum longus muscles.

Look for the following:
1. Pain and tenderness over the involved compartment
2. Overlying skin that is possibly erythematous, glossy, and edematous
3. Sensory loss on the dorsum of the foot between the first and second toes
4. Increasing pain on passive stretching of the involved muscle groups
5. Weakness of dorsiflexion of the ankles and toes (foot drop)

📖 *Caution:* The pedal pulses are rarely obliterated by the compartment swelling and may be easy to feel despite progressive muscle and nerve damage within the compartment.

If the patient has a tibial fracture that has been casted, it may be difficult to properly examine the affected extremity. In any such patient who develops increasing pain 24 to 48 hours after casting, a compartment syndrome should be suspected, and the cast should be removed so that the leg can be properly examined.

Management

Once the diagnosis of compartment syndrome is confirmed, a decompressing fasciotomy must be performed immediately by a surgeon. A delay of more than 12 hours may lead to irreversible muscle necrosis and contracture formation. Conservative measures, which may involve ice packs and elevation, are only temporizing. Pressure dressings should be removed.

Less Urgent Conditions

If the five major threats to life have been ruled out, you can take a less rushed approach to the diagnosis and look for other, less urgent conditions.

Selective Physical Examination

Benign nocturnal leg cramps often occur in the absence of physical findings.

Skin	Localized skin and subcutaneous erythema, swelling, and warmth (cellulitis)
	Painful subcutaneous red nodules (erythema nodosum, nodular liquefying panniculitis)
	Tender superficial vein with surrounding erythema and edema (superficial thrombophlebitis)
	Blue toe syndrome or livedo reticularis (cholesterol emboli)
	Focal areas of gangrene from cholesterol emboli (usually from the thoracic or abdominal aorta) cause a bluish discoloration in one or more toes. *Livedo reticularis* refers to cyanotic mottling of the skin in a fishnet-like pattern.
	Erythema, swelling, dysesthesias, increased hair growth of one foot (reflex sympathetic dystrophy syndrome)
Musculoskeletal system	Posterior knee joint swelling (Baker cyst)
	Joint inflammation (rheumatoid arthritis, systemic lupus erythematosus, gout, pseudogout)
	Palpate the hip and test range of motion (hip joint disease may cause leg pain with little or no evidence of inflammation).
Neurologic system	If no visible abnormality is found, a complete neurologic examination is needed to look for lumbar disk disease (sciatica) or peripheral neuropathy (e.g., diabetes).

Management
Acute Gout

Acute gout results from the sudden release of monosodium urate crystals from the cartilage and synovial membranes into the joint space. The diagnosis is made by synovial fluid aspiration and demonstration of negatively birefringent monosodium urate crystals with the use of polarizing microscopy.

At night, your main goal is to terminate the acute attack as quickly as possible. You can accomplish this in one of several ways: indomethacin (Indocin), 100 mg PO, followed by 50 mg PO every 6 hours may be given until pain relief occurs. Alternatively, colchicine is effective in doses of 1 mg PO initially, followed by 0.5 mg PO every 2 hours, until the pain improves, until abdominal discomfort or diarrhea occurs, or until a total of 8 mg is administered. In some countries colchicine tablets contain 1.2 mg and 0.6 mg respectively. A third option is prednisone 30 to 40 mg PO daily with a gradual taper over 7 to 10 days. Intraarticular triamcinolone hexacetonide, 15 to 30 mg, or methylprednisolone acetate (Depo-Medrol), 20 to 40 mg, is occasionally required.

Pseudogout

Pseudogout is a result of the release of calcium pyrophosphate dihydrate crystals from the joint cartilage into the joint space. Diagnosis is made by means of joint aspiration and demonstration of weakly positive birefringent rods when viewed under polarized light. Acute inflammation usually responds to indomethacin, 25 to 50 mg PO three times daily for 10 to 14 days; aspiration of fluid; and steroid injection.

Lumbar Disk Disease

Initially, lumbar disk disease can be treated conservatively with bed rest, analgesics, and muscle relaxants.

Thromboangiitis Obliterans (Buerger Disease)

The primary treatment for this condition is complete abstinence from tobacco. Intermittent pneumatic compression may improve blood flow in persons with ischemic pain and calcium channel blockers may help reduce vasospasm.

Erythema Nodosum

Erythema nodosum should be considered a symptom of some other underlying disorder, including drug reaction (oral contraceptives, penicillin, sulfonamides, bromides), inflammatory bowel disease, tuberculosis, fungal infection, and sarcoidosis. Treatment of the underlying condition is required.

Nodular Liquefying Panniculitis

These nodules can be differentiated from those of erythema nodosum by their mobility with palpation. They occur in association with acute pancreatitis or pancreatic neoplasms. Treatment of the underlying condition is required.

Reflex Sympathetic Dystrophy Syndrome

This disorder is often precipitated by a myocardial infarction, stroke, or local trauma that occurs weeks to months before characteristic redness, swelling (usually of the entire foot), and burning pain develop. Increased sweating of the involved extremity also may occur, along with increased hair growth on the extremity. The condition may respond to analgesic agents and physical therapy. On occasion, surgical sympathectomy or a short course of steroids is required.

Baker Cyst

A Baker cyst is caused by extension of inflamed synovial tissue into the popliteal space, which results in pain and swelling behind the knee. A well-known complication is rupture of the synovial sac into the adjacent tissues. This may mimic a calf DVT with tenderness, swelling, and a positive Homans sign. The diagnosis can be confirmed with a popliteal ultrasonography or arthrography. Treatment involves drainage of the cyst or intraarticular steroid injection. On occasion, surgical synovectomy is required.

Superficial Thrombophlebitis

This condition manifests in the lower extremity with a tender vein and surrounding edema and erythema. Fever is often present. Superficial vein thrombosis seldom propagates into the deep venous system, and anticoagulation therapy is not recommended. Treatment involves local measures, such as leg elevation, heat, and nonsteroidal anti-inflammatory drugs (NSAIDs), such as **indomethacin, 25 to 50 mg PO three times daily**.

Cellulitis

Cellulitis is most often caused by *Staphylococcus* or *Streptococcus* organisms. Because it can be difficult to determine which one is responsible, treatment to cover both organisms is usual. Small, localized areas of cellulitis with intact skin can be treated with **cloxacillin or cephalexin 250 to 500 mg PO four times daily**. If the patient is febrile, the area of cellulitis is extensive or purulent, or if the patient is diabetic, methicillin-resistant *Staphylococcus aureus* or erythromycin-resistant *Streptococcus pyogenes* may be the causative organisms. Until culture and sensitivity results are available, treatment should be initiated with **ceftaroline, 600 mg IV every 12 hours or daptomycin, 4 mg/kg IV every 24 hours**.

For cellulitis associated with skin ulcers in a diabetic patient, swab samples should be obtained for Gram stain, culture, and sensitivity testing. In a diabetic patient, such infections are commonly caused by multiple organisms.

Benign Nocturnal Leg Cramps

The cause of this condition is unknown. They may respond to **quinine sulfate, 300 mg PO at bedtime as needed**. Use should be limited because of frequent side effects including headache, dizziness, blurred vision, tinnitus, nausea, and sweating.

Lines, Tubes, and Drains

Almost every patient admitted to the hospital has some form of intravenous (IV) line, tube, or drain inserted during their stay. These devices are useful in the care of patients, but on occasion they can clog, leak, or otherwise malfunction, and your expertise and common sense are needed to remedy the problem.

The corrective measures necessary to deal with problematic lines, tubes, and drains carry the risk of contact with blood and body fluids. Therefore, make sure you are familiar with and follow your institution's infection control guidelines.

This chapter describes some of the problems that can occur with commonly used lines, tubes, and drains.

CENTRAL LINES

CHEST TUBES

URETHRAL CATHETERS

T-TUBES, J-TUBES, AND PENROSE DRAINS

NASOGASTRIC AND ENTERAL FEEDING TUBES

1. Blocked nasogastric and enteral feeding tubes (page 253)
2. Dislodged nasogastric and enteral feeding tubes (page 254)

CENTRAL LINES

Blocked Central Lines

PHONE CALL

Questions

1. How long has the line been blocked?
2. What are the patient's vital signs?
3. Why was the patient admitted?

Orders

Ask the registered nurse (RN) to bring a dressing set, two pairs of sterile gloves in your size, chlorhexidine skin disinfectant, a 5-mL syringe, and a 20- or 21-gauge needle to the patient's bedside.

📖 You may need to remove the dressing that is securing the central line, and you must keep the site sterile. A second pair of sterile gloves is useful because gloves are easily contaminated.

Informing the Registered Nurse

Tell the RN, "I will arrive at the bedside in … minutes."

If a central line is blocked, you must see the patient immediately.

ELEVATOR THOUGHTS

What causes a central line to block?

1. Mechanical causes:
   - Clamp closed on external catheter
   - Kinked tubing (Fig. 20.1)
   - Too-tight suture
   - Catheter tip blocked by vessel wall
2. Thrombus at the catheter tip (Fig. 20.1)
3. Leaks or cracks at catheter or connecting sites
4. Precipitation of calcium and phosphorous or of medications incompatible with TPN infusions
5. Inadequate flushing after blood product administration
6. Infection, e.g., Malassezia Furfur associated with lipid infusions.

MAJOR THREAT TO LIFE

- Failure of delivery of medications

Interruption of the delivery of essential medications may temporarily deprive the patient of required treatment.

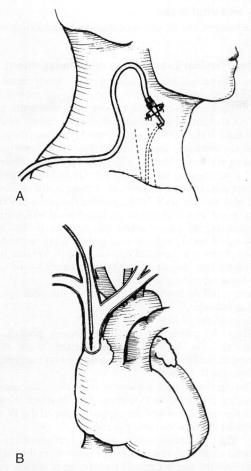

FIG. 20.1 Examples of causes of blocked central lines. *A,* Kinked tubing. *B,* Thrombosis at the catheter tip.

Quick-Look Test

Does the patient look well (comfortable), sick (uncomfortable or distressed), or critical (about to die)?

A blocked central line by itself should not cause the patient to look sick or critically ill. If the patient looks unwell, search for another cause.

Airway and Vital Signs

A blocked central line should not compromise the airway or other vital signs.

Selective Physical Examination and Management

1. Inspect the central line. Is the clamp inadvertently closed on the external catheter? If so, releasing the clamp will solve the problem. Is the line kinked? If so, remove the dressing that secures the line, straighten the line, and see whether there is now a flow of IV fluid. If the problem was a kinked line, clean the area, using sterile technique, and secure the line with a plastic occlusive dressing without re-kinking it. Is a too-tight suture obstructing flow? If so, snipping the offending suture and re-securing with a looser suture solves the problem. If there is still no flow of IV fluid with the line wide open, consider the possibility that the tip of the catheter is up against the blood vessel wall. Sometimes repositioning the patient solves this problem. If this does not work, withdraw the catheter 1 cm and see if this improves flow. If the catheter is a tunnelled line such as a Hickmann, Broviac, or dialysis line, this should NOT be attempted—the catheter may break off and embolize.

2. If there is still no flow of IV fluid with the line wide open, proceed as follows:

   a. Turn off the IV line.

   b. Place the patient in the Trendelenburg position (head down). Take the 5-mL syringe and the 20- or 21-gauge capped needle, and get ready to disconnect the central line from the IV tubing.

   c. During the expiration phase of respiration, disconnect the central line from the IV tubing. Quickly attach the syringe to the central line and the capped needle to the IV tubing. The latter keeps the tubing sterile.

   📖 The disconnection must be performed quickly to avoid an air embolus, which may result from the sucking of air into the line because of negative intrathoracic pressure generated during inspiration. The risk of an air embolus is diminished by clamping the IV tubing, placing the patient in the Trendelenburg position, and disconnecting the line only during expiration.

   d. Draw back gently on the syringe, because too much force will collapse the central line tubing. If the line is blocked with a small thrombus, this maneuver is often sufficient to dislodge the clot.

   e. Draw back 3 mL of blood if possible. During the expiratory phase of respiration, remove the capped needle from the end of the IV tubing, remove the syringe from the central line, and reattach the IV tubing to the central line. Turn the IV line on again.

📖 Blocked central lines should never be flushed. Flushing may dislodge a clot attached to the catheter tip, causing a pulmonary embolism.

3. If these maneuvers are unsuccessful in unblocking the central line, determine whether the central line is still necessary. Is the patient receiving medications that can be delivered only via a central line (e.g., amphotericin, dopamine, total parenteral nutrition)? Was the central line started because of lack of peripheral vein access? If so, reexamine the patient to see whether any peripheral veins are now suitable for IV access.

4. If central venous access is essential, the next step is to insert a new central line at a different site. A new central line should not be inserted over a guide wire placed through the blocked central line, because insertion of the guide wire may also dislodge a clot.

In situations in which central venous access is essential and no alternative sites are available, t-PA has been used to dissolve the obstructing clot. Significant risks accompany the use of t-PA in this situation.

5. Central line occlusion from suspected precipitation of medications or lipid emulsion requires specialized help, and, depending on the offending medication, may respond to administration of acid or base, or, in the case of lipid emulsion, ethanol. Call your resident or attending physician for help.

Bleeding at the Site of Entry of the Central Line

PHONE CALL

Questions

1. What are the patient's vital signs?
2. Why was the patient admitted?

Orders

Ask the RN to bring a dressing set, two pairs of sterile gloves in your size, and chlorhexidine skin disinfectant to the patient's bedside.

📖 You may need to remove the plastic occlusive dressing that is securing the central line, and you must keep the site sterile.

Informing the Registered Nurse

Tell the RN, "I will arrive at the bedside in … minutes."

If bleeding occurs at the central line site, you must see the patient immediately.

ELEVATOR THOUGHTS

What causes bleeding at the line insertion site?
1. Oozing of subcutaneous and cutaneous blood vessels (capillaries)
2. Coagulation disorders
   a. Drugs (anticoagulants, platelet inhibitors, fibrinolytic agents)
   b. Thrombocytopenia, platelet dysfunction
   c. Clotting factor deficiency

MAJOR THREAT TO LIFE

- Upper airway obstruction
  Bleeding into the soft tissues of the neck may cause tracheal compression, resulting in life-threatening upper airway obstruction.

BEDSIDE

Quick-Look Test

Does the patient look well (comfortable), sick (uncomfortable or distressed), or critical (about to die)?
  Patients who have bleeding at the line insertion site look well unless the upper airway is obstructed or excessive blood loss has occurred.

Airway and Vital Signs

Is the patient's airway clear? What is the patient's respiratory rate?
  Check the airway. If you find any evidence of an upper airway (inspiratory stridor or significant swelling of soft tissue of the neck), call your resident for help immediately.

Selective Physical Examination and Management

1. Remove the dressing, and try to identify a specific area of bleeding.
2. If you are unable to identify a specific site of bleeding, clean the site, using sterile technique, and reinspect the area. Usually, generalized oozing of blood is seen at the entry site, and no single skin vessel is identified as the culprit.
3. Apply continuous pressure to the entry site for 20 minutes. With a gloved hand, apply a folded, sterile 2 × 2-cm gauze dressing to the site with firm, continuous pressure. Do not release this pressure during the 20 minutes, because the platelet plug you are allowing to form may be broken (Fig. 20.2). A weighted sandbag may be used to provide pressure particularly for femoral catheters, but may be difficult to use on the neck or subclavian areas.
4. Reinspect the entry site. If the bleeding has stopped, clean the area, using sterile technique, and secure the line with a plastic occlusive dressing. If bleeding continues at the site, repeat the previous maneuver for an additional 20 minutes. If continuous pressure has

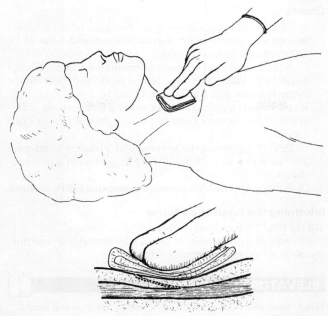

FIG. 20.2 Apply continuous, firm local pressure for 20 minutes to stop the oozing of blood from the central line entry site (*top*). Make sure the pressure is applied over the puncture site in the vein (*bottom*) and not at the skin entry site.

been applied, the bleeding should stop. In the unusual circumstance in which the bleeding has not stopped, a coagulation disorder should be suspected. (Refer to Chapter 32 for the management of coagulation problems.) Alternatively, a single suture may be placed at the site of bleeding in an attempt to provide hemostasis.

5. Removal and relocation of the central line should be considered if bleeding at the insertion site is excessive and persists despite the previous measures.

Shortness of Breath After Insertion of the Central Line

PHONE CALL

Questions

1. How long has the patient had shortness of breath?
2. What are the patient's vital signs?
3. Why was the patient admitted?

Orders

1. Ask the RN to bring a dressing set, two pairs of sterile gloves in your size, chlorhexidine skin disinfectant, and a size 16 IV catheter to the patient's bedside.

   If the patient has a tension pneumothorax, you must insert a size 16 IV catheter into the second intercostal space on the hyper-resonant side, with your resident's guidance.

2. If you suspect a pneumothorax, order a stat portable radiograph of the patient's chest in the upright position in expiration.

    Hypotension, tachypnea, and pleuritic chest pain after insertion of a central line are suggestive of a pneumothorax.

3. Order oxygen by mask to keep **oxygen saturation at 94% or above**.

Informing the Registered Nurse

Tell the RN, "I will arrive at the bedside in … minutes."

If a patient has shortness of breath after central line insertion, you must see the patient immediately.

ELEVATOR THOUGHTS

What causes shortness of breath after insertion of a central line?

The following causes are illustrated in Fig. 20.3:

1. Pneumothorax or tension pneumothorax
2. Massive soft tissue hematoma from inadvertent puncture of the carotid artery, which results in upper airway obstruction
3. Cardiac tamponade
4. Air embolus
5. Pleural effusion

MAJOR THREAT TO LIFE

- Upper airway obstruction
- Tension pneumothorax
- Cardiac tamponade
- Air embolus

Upper airway obstruction may result from a massive soft tissue hematoma (e.g., caused by inadvertent puncture of the carotid artery). A *tension pneumothorax* may develop minutes to days after the insertion of a central line if pleural perforation occurred during insertion. In rare cases, *cardiac tamponade* occurs as a result of perforation of the right atrium or right ventricle by the catheter. Air may inadvertently be introduced if the line is disconnected incorrectly, which results in an *air embolus*.

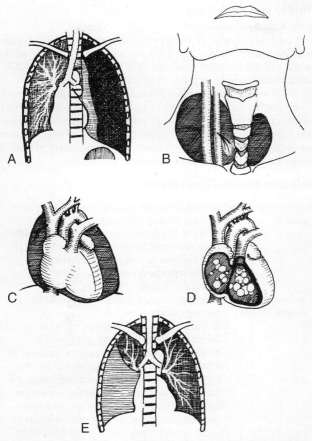

FIG. 20.3 Causes of shortness of breath after central line insertion.
A, Pneumothorax. *B,* Massive soft tissue hematoma from inadvertent carotid artery puncture, resulting in upper airway obstruction. *C,* Cardiac tamponade. *D,* Air embolus. *E,* Pleural effusion.

BEDSIDE

Quick-Look Test

Does the patient look well (comfortable), sick (uncomfortable or distressed), or critical (about to die)?

A patient with a tension pneumothorax, upper airway obstruction, cardiac tamponade, or air embolus looks sick or critically ill.

Airway and Vital Signs

Is the patient's airway clear?

Check the airway. If an upper airway obstruction is evident (i.e., inspiratory stridor or significant soft tissue swelling of the neck), call the intensive care unit (ICU)/cardiac care unit (CCU) team immediately for possible intubation of the patient.

What are the patient's blood pressure (BP) and respiratory rate?

Hypotension and tachypnea in a patient with a recently inserted central line may be indicative of a tension pneumothorax or cardiac tamponade, inadvertently caused at the time of line insertion. See pages 224–225 for the assessment and management of tension pneumothorax, and page 225 for cardiac tamponade.

Selective Physical Examination

Respiratory system	Tracheal deviation (tension pneumothorax or massive pleural effusion)
	Unilateral hyperresonance to percussion with decreased breath sounds (pneumothorax)
	Stony dullness to percussion, decreased breath sounds, decreased tactile fremitus (pleural effusion)
Cardiovascular system (CVS)	Pulsus paradoxus (cardiac tamponade or tension pneumothorax)
	📖 Pulsus paradoxus is present when the decrease in systolic BP with inspiration is more than 10 mm Hg (the normal variation in systolic BP with quiet respiration is 0-10 mm Hg). A pulsus paradoxus is definitely present if the radial pulse disappears during inspiration.
	Elevated jugular venous pressure (JVP) (cardiac tamponade or tension pneumothorax)
	Distant heart sounds (pericardial effusion or cardiac tamponade)
	Mill-wheel murmur, hypotension, elevated JVP (major air embolism)
Central line	Check all IV connections to ensure that they are not loose (air embolus).

Management

Tension Pneumothorax

Tension pneumothorax is a medical emergency that necessitates urgent treatment. You need supervision by your resident or attending physician.

1. Identify the second intercostal space in the midclavicular line on the affected (hyperresonant) side.

2. Mark this point with the pressure from a needle cap or ball-point pen cap.
3. Open the dressing set and pour the chlorhexidine into the appropriate space.
4. Put on the sterile gloves and clean the identified area.
5. Insert the size 16 IV catheter into the designated site. Remove the inner needle, leaving the plastic cannula in the chest. If a tension pneumothorax is present, you will hear air rushing out loudly through the catheter. You do not need to connect the catheter to suction; the lung will decompress itself.
6. Order a chest tube sent to the room immediately. Definitive treatment is insertion of a chest tube.

Pneumothorax Without Tension

Small pneumothoraces (<15%) are usually reabsorbed spontaneously over a few days.

For *large* or *symptomatic pneumothoraces,* chest tube drainage is required.

Cardiac Tamponade

Cardiac tamponade is a medical emergency.
1. Clamp the IV tubing, and turn off the IV line.
2. Call the ICU/CCU team immediately for possible urgent pericardiocentesis. An emergency echocardiogram, if available, will confirm the diagnosis before pericardiocentesis.
3. Volume expansion with normal saline through a large-bore IV catheter may be a useful temporizing measure to help maintain adequate cardiac output.

Air Embolism

Air embolism may be treated by the following procedure:
1. Place the patient in the left lateral decubitus head down position. The patient should be kept in this position until the air bubbles have been reabsorbed. (Some experts advocate aspiration of air bubbles from the right ventricle.) If the patient is unwell with dyspnea or looks "about to die" from shock, supportive measures such as high-flow oxygen, IV fluid resuscitation, vasopressors, and mechanical ventilation should be considered.
2. Reinspect all the IV connections, and make sure they are secure.
3. If necessary, a new central line may have to be inserted.

Massive Unilateral Pleural Effusion

Massive unilateral pleural effusion should be managed as follows:
1. Clamp the IV tubing, and turn off the IV line.
2. Perform thoracentesis if the patient has marked shortness of breath.

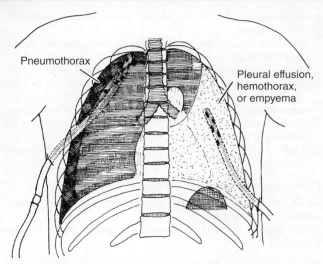

Pneumothorax

Pleural effusion,
hemothorax,
or empyema

FIG. 20.4 Chest tubes are inserted to drain air (pneumothoraces), blood (hemothoraces), fluid (pleural effusions), or pus (empyemas).

CHEST TUBES

Chest tubes are inserted to drain air (pneumothoraces); blood (hemothoraces); fluid (pleural effusions); or pus (empyemas) (Fig. 20.4). They should always be connected to an underwater seal. They may be left for straight drainage (no suction) or, more commonly, for suction. Fig. 20.5 illustrates the various equipment for chest tube drainage. Common chest tube problems are illustrated in Fig. 20.6.

Persistent Bubbling in the Drainage Container (Air Leak)

PHONE CALL

Questions

1. Why was the chest tube inserted?
2. What are the patient's vital signs?
3. Does the patient have shortness of breath?
4. Why was the patient admitted?

Orders

No orders are necessary.

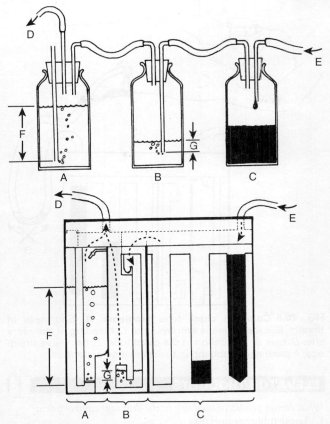

FIG. 20.5 **Chest tube apparatus.** *A,* Suction control chamber; *B,* underwater seal; *C,* collection chamber; *D,* exit toward suction; *E,* return from patient; *F,* height of liquid in suction control chamber, which equals the amount of suction in centimeters of water; *G,* height of underwater seal in centimeters of water.

Informing the Registered Nurse

Tell the RN, "I will arrive at the bedside in ... minutes."

Persistent bubbling in the drainage container is a potential emergency, and you must see the patient as soon as possible. If any malfunctioning of the chest tube is associated with shortness of breath, you must see the patient immediately.

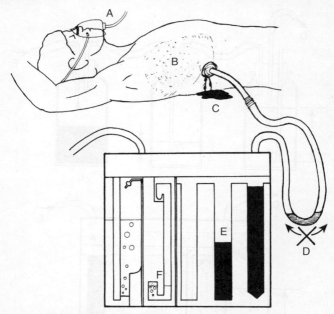

FIG. 20.6 Common chest tube problems. *A,* Shortness of breath; *B,* subcutaneous emphysema; *C,* bleeding at the entry site; *D,* loss of fluctuation in the chest tube; *E,* excessive drainage; *F,* persistent bubbling in the chest tube apparatus.

ELEVATOR THOUGHTS

What causes persistent bubbling in the drainage compartment?
1. Loose tubing connection
2. Air leaking into the chest around the chest tube at the insertion site
3. Traumatic tracheobronchial injury; a large, persistent air leak in a patient with traumatic pneumothorax is suggestive of a concomitant tracheobronchial injury
4. Persistent bronchopleural air leak
   a. Postlobectomy
   b. Ruptured bleb or bulla (e.g., asthma, emphysema)
   c. After intrathoracic procedures (e.g., needle biopsy, thoracentesis)

MAJOR THREAT TO LIFE

A persistent air leak is suggestive of either a pneumothorax from intrathoracic injury or a loose connection of the drainage apparatus.

Hence, the major threat to life is the underlying intrathoracic disease process responsible for the persistent air leak. As long as air continues to bubble through the collection chamber, you can be certain that excessive intrapleural air will not accumulate.

BEDSIDE

Quick-Look Test

Does the patient look well (comfortable), sick (uncomfortable or distressed), or critical (about to die)?

If a small air leak is the problem, the patient may look well. A patient who looks sick may be developing a larger pneumothorax or may look sick for unrelated reasons.

Airway and Vital Signs

If all tubing connections are snug and the chest tube dressing is airtight, a persistent air leak means that the patient has a pneumothorax. As long as air continues to bubble through the collection chamber, the pneumothorax should drain and thus not result in an alteration of vital signs.

Selective History and Chart Review

Why was the chest tube inserted?

If the chest tube was inserted to drain a pneumothorax, the liquid in the tube should be bubbling unless the lung is fully expanded and the leak has sealed. If the chest tube was inserted to drain a hemothorax, a pleural effusion, or an empyema with straight drainage (no suction), the new onset of bubbling in the collection chamber represents a loose tubing connection, air leaking into the chest from around the chest tube insertion site, or the development of a pneumothorax.

Selective Physical Examination and Management

If a pneumothorax is not present, a persistent air leak is indicated by air bubbles in the underwater seal section of the chest drainage system while the suction is turned off. If the air leak is small, it may be seen only if you increase intrapleural pressure (e.g., have the patient cough; Fig. 20.7).

Clamping of chest tubes before a radiograph is taken may be dangerous, especially if a persistent pneumothorax is present. Never leave a patient with a clamped chest tube unattended. A tension pneumothorax may develop rapidly if the chest drainage system has a ball-valve mechanism.

The following procedure is recommended when bubbling persists in the drainage compartment:

1. Inspect the tubing connections to ensure that all seals are airtight.

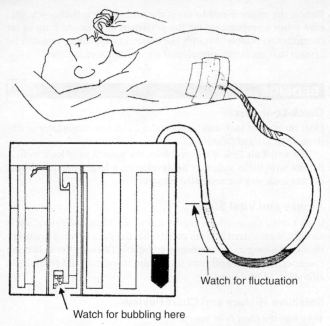

Watch for fluctuation

Watch for bubbling here

FIG. 20.7 Loss of fluctuation of the underwater seal. Ask the patient to cough, and observe for any fluctuation or bubbling in the chest tube apparatus.

2. Remove the dressing at the entry site of the chest tube, listen for sucking sounds, and observe the incision area. If the incision is too large and inadequately closed, insert one or two sterile 2-0 sutures to seal the opening. If the incision is adequately closed with sutures, reapply a pressure dressing, ensuring that the petrolatum (Vaseline) gauze occlusive dressing seals the incision.
3. Disconnect the suction from the chest drainage system. Persistent air leak (spontaneous or with coughing) is usually from the lung (persistent pneumothorax).
4. Obtain a chest radiograph to ensure correct tube placement. The chest tube holes should be inside the thorax, and the tip of the tube should be away from mediastinal and subclavicular structures.
5. If on chest radiograph the lung does not appear re-expanded, call surgeons for possible placement of a second chest tube and for management of the persistent air leak from the lung.

Bleeding Around the Site of Entry of the Chest Tube

PHONE CALL

Questions
1. Why was the chest tube inserted?
2. What are the patient's vital signs?
3. Does the patient have shortness of breath?
4. Why was the patient admitted?

Orders
Ask the RN to bring a dressing set, two pairs of sterile gloves in your size, and chlorhexidine skin cleanser to the patient's bedside. You must remove the dressing around the chest tube, and you must keep the site sterile.

Informing the Registered Nurse
Tell the RN, "I will arrive at the bedside in … minutes."

Bleeding around the chest tube entry site is a potential emergency, requiring you to see the patient as soon as possible. If any malfunctioning of the chest tube is associated with shortness of breath, you must see the patient immediately.

ELEVATOR THOUGHTS

What causes bleeding around the chest tube entry site?
1. Inadequate pressure bandage
2. Inadequate closure of the incision with suture
3. Coagulation disorders
4. Trauma to intercostal vessels or lung during insertion of the chest tube
5. Blockage of the chest tube or an inadequately sized chest tube with drainage of the hemothorax around the entry site

MAJOR THREAT TO LIFE

- Hemorrhagic shock
  Continuous oozing, if allowed to progress, may eventually lead to intravascular volume depletion and, in the extreme case, hemorrhagic shock.

BEDSIDE

Quick-Look Test
Does the patient look well (comfortable), sick (uncomfortable or distressed), or critical (about to die)?

If the amount of bleeding from the site of entry of the chest tube is small, the patient probably looks well. A patient who has lost more blood may look sick or critically ill.

Airway and Vital Signs

What are the patient's BP, heart rate, and respiratory rate?

Hypotension and tachycardia may indicate major loss of blood. Tachypnea may indicate a large hemothorax.

Selective History and Chart Review

Why was the chest tube inserted?

Check the following recent laboratory results: hemoglobin value, prothrombin time, activated partial thromboplastin time (aPTT), and platelet count.

Selective Physical Examination and Management

Remove the dressing at the chest tube entry site, and inspect the incision. If the incision is too large and inadequately closed, insert one or two sutures to seal the opening. If the incision is adequately closed with sutures, reapply a pressure dressing over the site, taking care to ensure that the pressure is maintained. Such maneuvers, when performed adequately, stop the bleeding in the majority of situations.

If the chest tube is obstructed, which results in blood draining around the entry site, try milking the chest tube. Reinspect to see whether this maneuver has reestablished fluctuation in the underwater seal. The connecting tube is made of rubber, and you can strip it carefully, using the chest tube strippers. These two maneuvers may help dislodge any blood clots and debris blocking the tube.

If the chest tube is too small, it may be unable to drain a large hemothorax adequately. A larger sized chest tube may be required.

Drainage of an Excessive Volume of Blood

PHONE CALL

Questions

1. Why was the chest tube inserted?
2. What are the patient's vital signs?
3. Does the patient have shortness of breath?
4. Why was the patient admitted?

Orders

No orders are necessary.

Informing the Registered Nurse

Tell the RN, "I will arrive at the bedside in … minutes."

Drainage of an excessive volume of blood via the chest tube is a potential emergency, and you must see the patient immediately. Also, if any malfunctioning of a chest tube is associated with shortness of breath, you must see the patient immediately.

ELEVATOR THOUGHTS

What causes excessive blood to drain via the chest tube?
1. Intrathoracic bleeding

MAJOR THREAT TO LIFE

- Hemorrhagic shock
  Hemorrhagic shock may result from excessive intrathoracic blood loss.

BEDSIDE

Quick-Look Test

Does the patient look well (comfortable), sick (uncomfortable or distressed), or critical (about to die)?

A patient with hemorrhagic shock looks pale, sweaty, and restless.

Airway and Vital Signs

What are the patient's BP and heart rate?

Hypotension and tachycardia may indicate hemorrhagic shock.

What is the patient's respiratory rate?

Tachypnea and hypotension may indicate a tension pneumothorax.

Management I

1. Administer supplemental O_2, in a dosage to keep oxygen saturation at 94% or above.
2. If the patient is hypotensive, draw 20 mL of blood and start a large-bore IV line (size 16 if possible). Administer normal saline or Ringer's lactate, 500 mL intravenously, as fast as possible.
3. Send blood for an immediate crossmatch for 4 to 6 U of packed red blood cells "on hold" and measure hemoglobin, prothrombin time, aPTT, and platelet count.
4. Order a stat radiograph of the patient's chest.

Selective Chart Review and Management II

Is the patient receiving anticoagulant medication (heparin, warfarin, direct-acting oral anticoagulants)?

If so, review the initial indication for anticoagulation. Can the anticoagulant be safely discontinued or reversed? Consult the hematology department for assistance in the management of this difficult and potentially life-threatening situation.

How much blood has the patient lost over the past 48 hours?

Estimate the amount of blood loss by reviewing the intake-output chart.

- If the patient has lost more than 500 mL over 8 hours, consultation with a thoracic surgeon is recommended. The patient may need an emergency thoracotomy to localize the site of hemorrhage and achieve hemostasis.
- If the patient has lost less than 500 mL over 8 hours, order hourly monitoring of the blood lost via the chest tube, and note that a physician needs to be informed if the blood loss is more than 50 mL/hour.

Loss of Fluctuation of the Underwater Seal

PHONE CALL

Questions

1. Why was the chest tube inserted?
2. What are the patient's vital signs?
3. Does the patient have shortness of breath?
4. Why was the patient admitted?

Orders

No orders are necessary.

Informing the Registered Nurse

Tell the RN, "I will arrive at the bedside in … minutes."

Loss of fluctuation of the underwater seal is a potential emergency, and you must see the patient as soon as possible. Also, if any malfunctioning of a chest tube is associated with shortness of breath, you must see the patient immediately.

ELEVATOR THOUGHTS

What causes loss of fluctuation of the underwater seal?

1. Kinked chest tube
2. Plugged chest tube
3. Improper chest tube positioning

The underwater seal is essentially a one-way, low-resistance valve. During expiration, the intrapleural pressure increases, becoming higher than atmospheric pressure and forcing air or fluid that is in the pleural space through the chest tube and underwater seal (see Fig. 20.7).

MAJOR THREAT TO LIFE

- Tension pneumothorax
  Inadequate drainage of a pneumothorax because of a blocked chest tube may lead to a tension pneumothorax (Figs. 20.8 and 20.9).

BEDSIDE

Quick-Look Test

Does the patient look well (comfortable), sick (uncomfortable or distressed), or critical (about to die)?

A patient who looks sick may be developing a tension pneumothorax or may look sick for unrelated reasons.

Airway and Vital Signs

What are the patient's BP and respiratory rate?

Hypotension and tachypnea may be signs of a tension pneumothorax.

Selective History and Chart Review

Why was the chest tube inserted?

How long ago did the chest tube stop fluctuating?

What has been draining from the chest tube? What volume has drained over the past 24 hours?

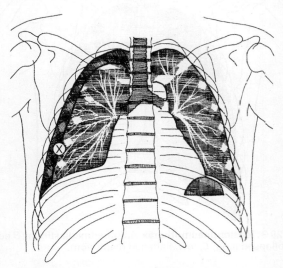

FIG. 20.8 Pneumothorax. *X*, edge of visceral pleura or lung.

Selective Physical Examination and Management

1. Inspect the underwater seal. Is there any fluctuation? Ask the patient to cough, and observe the tube for any fluctuation. A chest tube whose distal aperture is located within the pleural space fluctuates with respiration.

2. Inspect the chest tube for kinking. You may need to remove the dressing at the chest tube entry site. If the chest tube is kinked, reposition it and reinspect it for fluctuation of the underwater seal.

3. Try milking the chest tube. Reinspect it to see whether this maneuver reestablishes fluctuation in the underwater seal. The connecting tubing is rubber, and you can carefully strip it, using chest tube strippers. These two maneuvers help dislodge blood clots and debris that may be blocking the tube.

4. Order a portable radiograph of the patient's chest. Improper positioning of the chest tube may result in loss of fluctuation of the underwater seal.

5. If the tube is not fluctuating after all the aforementioned maneuvers have been attempted, a new chest tube may have to be inserted.

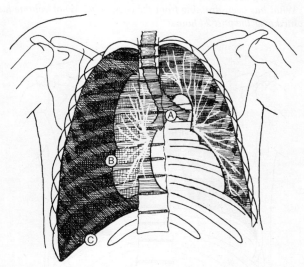

FIG. 20.9 Tension pneumothorax. *A*, Shifted mediastinum; *B*, edge of collapsed lung; *C*, low, flattened diaphragm.

Subcutaneous Emphysema

PHONE CALL

Questions
1. Why was the chest tube inserted?
2. What are the patient's vital signs?
3. Does the patient have shortness of breath?
4. Why was the patient admitted?

Orders
Ask the RN to bring a dressing set, two pairs of sterile gloves in your size, and chlorhexidine skin cleanser to the patient's bedside. You must remove the dressing around the chest tube, and you must keep the site sterile.

Informing the Registered Nurse
Tell the RN, "I will arrive at the bedside in … minutes."

Subcutaneous emphysema is a potential emergency, and you must see the patient immediately. Also, if any malfunctioning of a chest tube is associated with shortness of breath, you must see the patient immediately.

ELEVATOR THOUGHTS

What causes subcutaneous emphysema?
1. Chest tube size too small for the leak
2. Inadequate suction
3. Chest tube aperture in the chest wall
4. Chest tube in the chest wall or abdominal cavity

Insignificant localized subcutaneous emphysema around the entry site is not uncommon after chest tube insertion

MAJOR THREAT TO LIFE

- Upper airway obstruction

Subcutaneous emphysema extending up into the neck rarely results in tracheal compression.

BEDSIDE

Quick-Look Test
Does the patient look well (comfortable), sick (uncomfortable or distressed), or critical (about to die)?

A patient with upper airway obstruction looks sick or critical, and inspiratory stridor may be audible.

Airway and Vital Signs

Inspect and palpate the patient's neck for subcutaneous emphysema.

What is the patient's respiratory rate?

A patient with an upper airway obstruction is tachypneic.

What are the patient's BP and heart rate?

Subcutaneous emphysema may be accompanied by a tension pneumothorax. If it is, the patient is tachycardic.

Selective History and Chart Review

Why was the chest tube inserted?

Selective Physical Examination and Management

If there is significant upper airway obstruction (palpable sub-cutaneous emphysema over the trachea, inspiratory stridor, tachypnea), call the ICU/CCU team immediately for the patient's probable intubation and transfer to the ICU/CCU. Cardiothoracic surgery may be required if mediastinal decompression is indicated.

What size chest tube was inserted? Is the tube's diameter too small?

Multifenestrated vinyl chest tubes are available in two sizes: 20F and 36F. The 20F may not be large enough, and air may escape from the pleural cavity into the chest wall, which would result in subcutaneous emphysema. If the chest tube is too small, a larg-er one must be inserted. Sometimes, two large chest tubes are re-quired for adequate drainage.

Is the chest tube connected to suction equipment?

A large pneumothorax may not be drained adequately if it is connected only to an underwater seal, as opposed to suction equipment.

Remove the dressing at the chest tube site and inspect the chest tube. Are any of the drainage holes in the distal end of the chest tube visible?

None of the drainage lines should be visible. They should all be inside the pleural cavity. Subcutaneous emphysema may be caused by misplacement of the chest tube, with one of the drainage holes inadvertently in the soft tissue of the chest wall. A new chest tube should be inserted. Do not reinsert the partially extruded chest tube because you may introduce infection into the pleural space.

Shortness of Breath

PHONE CALL

Questions

1. Why was the chest tube inserted?

2. What are the patient's vital signs?
3. Why was the patient admitted?

Orders

Ask the RN to bring a dressing set, two pairs of sterile gloves in your size, chlorhexidine skin cleanser, and a size 16 IV catheter to the patient's bedside.

 A tension pneumothorax, if present, is treated most effectively by the insertion of a size 16 IV catheter into the pleural space on the affected side.

Informing the Registered Nurse

Tell the RN, "I will arrive at the bedside in … minutes."

Shortness of breath in a patient with a chest tube in place is a potential emergency, and you must see the patient immediately.

ELEVATOR THOUGHTS

What causes shortness of breath in a patient with a chest tube?

Causes Related to the Chest Tube

1. Tension pneumothorax, which may occur because of any of the following conditions:
   a. Inadequate suction
   b. Misplaced tube (i.e., chest tube not in the pleural cavity)
   c. Blocked or kinked tube
   d. Bronchopulmonary bronchopleural fistula
2. Increasing pneumothorax (which may result from the same causes of tension pneumothorax)
3. Subcutaneous emphysema
4. Increasing pleural effusion or hemothorax
5. Re-expansion pulmonary edema (which sometimes occurs after rapid expansion of a pneumothorax, drainage of pleural fluid, or both)

Causes Unrelated to the Chest Tube

See Chapter 24.

MAJOR THREAT TO LIFE

- Tension pneumothorax
- Upper airway obstruction

Inadequate drainage of a pneumothorax produced through a ball-valve mechanism may result in a life-threatening tension pneumothorax. Tracheal compression from interstitial emphysema rarely causes upper airway obstruction.

BEDSIDE

Quick-Look Test

Does the patient look well (comfortable), sick (uncomfortable or distressed), or critical (about to die)?

A sick- or critical-looking patient may have a tension pneumothorax or may have an unrelated reason for shortness of breath (see Chapter 24).

Airway and Vital Signs

Inspect and palpate the neck for subcutaneous emphysema.

What is the patient's respiratory rate?

Rates faster than 20/minute are suggestive of hypoxia, pain, or anxiety. Look for thoracoabdominal dissociation, which may be a sign of impending respiratory failure. Remember that the rib cage and abdominal wall normally move in the same direction during inspiration and expiration.

What are the patient's BP and heart rate?

Hypotension and tachycardia may indicate a tension pneumothorax or another unrelated cause of shortness of breath (see Chapter 24).

Selective Physical Examination

Does the patient have a tension pneumothorax?

Vitals	Tachypnea
	Hypotension
Head, ears, eyes, nose, throat (HEENT)	Tracheal deviation away from the hyperresonant side
Respiratory system	Unilateral hyperresonance
	Decreased air entry on hyperresonant side
CVS	Elevated JVP
Chest tube	Is there bubbling in the collection chamber?
	📖 Absence of bubbling is suggestive of malposition or malfunction of the chest tube.

Selective Chart Review

Why was the chest tube inserted?

Management 🖉

1. If *upper airway obstruction* is significant (palpable subcutaneous emphysema over the trachea, inspiratory stridor, tachypnea), call the ICU/CCU team immediately for the patient's probable intubation and transfer to the ICU/CCU.

2. *Tension pneumothorax* is a medical emergency that necessitates urgent treatment. You need supervision by your resident or attending physician.
   a. Identify the second intercostal space in the midclavicular line on the affected (hyperresonant) side.
   b. Mark this point by using pressure from a needle cap or ballpoint pen cap.
   c. Open the dressing set and pour the chlorhexidine into the appropriate container.
   d. Put on the sterile gloves and clean the identified area.
   e. Insert the size 16 IV catheter into the designated site. Remove the inner needle, leaving the plastic cannula in the chest. If a tension pneumothorax is present, you will hear air rushing out loudly through the catheter. You do not need to connect the catheter to suction; the lung space will decompress itself.
   f. Order a chest tube sent to the patient's room immediately. Definitive treatment is insertion of a chest tube.
3. If a pneumothorax is increasing but you find no evidence of a tension pneumothorax, order a stat upright radiograph of the patient's chest in expiration. Meanwhile, look for any correctable causes, such as kinked or blocked tubing, inadequate suction, or a dislodged chest tube.
4. For the management of other causes of shortness of breath (i.e., causes unrelated to chest tubes), see Chapter 24.

URETHRAL CATHETERS

There are five types of urethral catheters, four of which are shown in Fig. 20.10:

1. The Foley (balloon retention) catheter is the most commonly used. It consists of a double-lumen tube. The larger lumen drains urine, and the smaller lumen admits 5 to 30 mL of water to inflate the balloon tip.
2. Straight (Robinson) catheters are used to obtain in-and-out collections of urine, to obtain sterile specimens in patients who are unable to void voluntarily, and to obtain postvoiding residual urine volume measurements.
3. A coudé catheter has a curved tip that facilitates insertion when a urethral obstruction (e.g., benign prostatic hypertrophy) hampers the passage of a Foley catheter.
4. Three-way irrigation catheters have—in addition to a lumen for urine drainage and one for balloon inflation—a third lumen for bladder irrigation. These catheters are commonly used after transurethral prostate resection to facilitate bladder irrigation and drainage of blood clots.
5. A Silastic catheter is similar to a Foley catheter but is made of softer, less reactive plastic. It is used when a urethral catheter is required on a long-term basis.

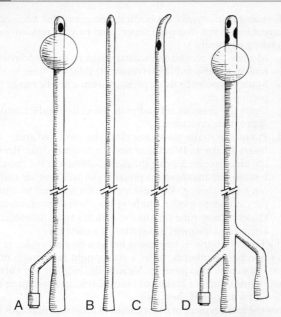

FIG. 20.10 **Urethral catheters.** *A,* Foley catheter. *B,* Straight (Robinson) catheter. *C,* Coudé catheter. *D,* Three-way irrigation catheter.

Blocked Urethral Catheter

PHONE CALL

Questions

1. How long has the catheter been blocked?
2. What are the patient's vital signs?
3. Does the patient have suprapubic pain?

   Urinary retention secondary to a blocked catheter can result in bladder distention and thus suprapubic pain.
4. Why was the patient admitted?

Orders

Ask the RN to try flushing the catheter with 30–40 mL of sterile normal saline if this has not been done.

Informing the Registered Nurse

Tell the RN, "I will arrive at the bedside in … minutes."

If the patient does not have suprapubic pain (bladder distention), assessment of a blocked urinary catheter can be delayed an hour or two if higher priority problems require your attention.

ELEVATOR THOUGHTS

What causes blocked urethral catheters?
1. Urinary sediment
2. Blood clots
3. Kinked catheter (look under the bed sheets)
4. Improperly placed or dislodged catheter

MAJOR THREAT TO LIFE

1. Bladder rupture
2. Progressive renal insufficiency

   Bladder rupture may occur if bladder distention progresses without decompression. Because bladder distention is painful, bladder rupture from this cause usually occurs only in unconscious or paraplegic patients. Persistent lower urinary tract obstruction may lead to hydronephrosis and *renal failure*.

BEDSIDE

Quick-Look Test

Does the patient look well (comfortable), sick (uncomfortable or distressed), or critical (about to die)?

   Most patients with blocked urethral catheters look well. However, patients with acute bladder distention may look distressed because of abdominal pain.

Airway and Vital Signs

A blocked urethral catheter is not usually responsible for alterations in vital signs unless pain from bladder distention causes tachypnea or tachycardia.

Selective Physical Examination and Management

1. Percuss and palpate the abdomen to determine whether the bladder is distended. Suprapubic dullness and tenderness suggest a distended bladder.
2. Examine the tubing for kinking of the catheter, blood clots, or sediment.
3. Order a sterile dressing tray, a 50-mL bulb syringe (or a 50-mL syringe and an adapter), and two pairs of sterile gloves in your size. Aspirate and irrigate the catheter with 30 to 40 mL of sterile normal saline as follows:

a. Ask an assistant to hold the distal part of the catheter close to the connection between the tubing and urinary drainage bag.

b. Put on sterile gloves, and clean the distal catheter and the proximal connecting tubing with chlorhexidine.

c. Disconnect the drainage tubing from the catheter. Ask an assistant to hold the connecting tubing in the air to maintain a sterile tip.

d. Using a 50-mL syringe, aspirate the catheter vigorously to dislodge and extract any blood clots or sediment. If the maneuver is unsuccessful, flush the catheter with 30 to 40 mL of sterile normal saline. Several attempts at aspiration should be made before you abandon this technique.

e. Using sterile technique, reconnect the catheter to the connecting tubing.

   The majority of blocked Foley catheters become unplugged with this maneuver.

4. If flushing of the catheter fails to relieve the obstruction, a new catheter should be inserted if one is still required.

Gross Hematuria

PHONE CALL

Questions

1. Why was the urethral catheter inserted?
2. What are the patient's vital signs?
3. Is the patient receiving anticoagulant drugs or cyclophosphamide?
4. Why was the patient admitted?

Orders

No orders are necessary.

Informing the Registered Nurse

Tell the RN, "I will arrive at the bedside in … minutes."

   If a patient receiving anticoagulants has gross hematuria, you must see the patient immediately.

ELEVATOR THOUGHTS

What causes gross hematuria in a catheterized patient?

1. Urethral trauma
   a. Inadvertent or partial removal of the catheter with the balloon still inflated
   b. Trauma during catheter insertion (false passage)

2. Drugs
   a. Anticoagulants (heparin, warfarin, direct-acting oral anti-coagulants)
   b. Fibrinolytic agents (streptokinase, tissue plasminogen activator [tPA], urokinase)
   c. Cyclophosphamide
3. Coagulation abnormalities
   a. Disseminated intravascular coagulation
   b. Specific factor deficiencies
   c. Thrombocytopenia
4. Unrelated problems
   a. Renal stones
   b. Carcinoma of the kidney, bladder, or prostate
   c. Glomerulonephritis
   d. Prostatitis
   e. Rupture of a bladder vein

MAJOR THREAT TO LIFE

- Hemorrhagic shock
  Although gross hematuria is dramatic and distressing to the patient, it is rare for bleeding to be significant enough to result in hemorrhagic shock. Only 1 mL of blood in 1 L of urine will change the color from yellow to red.

BEDSIDE

Quick-Look Test

Does the patient look well (comfortable), sick (uncomfortable or distressed), or critical (about to die)?

It is unusual for a patient with gross hematuria to look other than well. If a patient looks sick or critically ill, search for a separate unrecognized problem.

Airway and Vital Signs

What is the patient's BP?

Hypotension in a patient with gross hematuria may be a sign of hemorrhagic shock.

What is the patient's heart rate?

A resting tachycardia, though a nonspecific finding, may be indicative of hypovolemia if significant blood loss has occurred.

Selective History and Chart Review

Is the patient receiving any of the following medications?

Heparin, warfarin, direct-acting oral anticoagulants

Streptokinase, tPA, urokinase
Cyclophosphamide
Is any abnormality present in the coagulation profile?
Prothrombin time
aPTT
Platelet count
Does the patient have a history of urethral trauma?
Recent inadvertent removal of a Foley catheter with the balloon still inflated (especially in an elderly, confused patient)
Recent genitourinary surgery
Recent difficulty inserting a urethral catheter
Has the hemoglobin value decreased recently? How much blood has the patient lost?
Bleeding via the urinary tract is unlikely to cause significant hemodynamic changes unless the patient has recently undergone genitourinary surgery.

Management

1. If the patient is receiving anticoagulants, review the initial indication for the anticoagulation. Decide, in consultation with your resident and attending physician, whether the anticoagulation is still warranted, in view of the risks.
2. If a coagulation abnormality is identified, refer to Chapter 32 for a discussion of investigation and management.
3. If the patient has a history of recent urethral trauma, continued significant blood loss is unlikely. Have the patient's vital signs measured every 4 to 6 hours for the next 24 hours. Significant bleeding may be manifested by tachycardia and orthostatic hypotension.

Inability to Insert a Urethral Catheter

PHONE CALL

Questions

1. Why was the urethral catheter ordered?
2. What are the patient's vital signs?
3. Does the patient have suprapubic pain?
4. How many attempts have been made to catheterize the patient?
5. Why was the patient admitted?

Orders

Ask the RN to bring a catheter insertion set, two pairs of sterile gloves in your size, and chlorhexidine skin disinfectant to the patient's bedside.

Informing the Registered Nurse

Tell the RN, "I will arrive at the bedside in … minutes."

If the patient does not have suprapubic pain (bladder distention), insertion of a urethral catheter can be delayed an hour or two if higher priority problems require your attention.

ELEVATOR THOUGHTS

What causes difficulty in urethral catheterization?

1. Urethral edema
   a. Multiple insertion attempts
   b. Inadvertent removal of a Foley catheter with the balloon still inflated
2. Urethral obstruction
   a. Benign prostatic hypertrophy
   b. Carcinoma of the prostate
   c. Urethral stricture
   d. Anatomic anomaly (diverticulum, false passage)

MAJOR THREAT TO LIFE

- Bladder rupture
- Progressive renal insufficiency

Bladder rupture may occur if bladder distention is not relieved by placement of a urinary catheter. A suprapubic catheter may be required if urethral catheterization is impossible. Persistent bladder obstruction may lead to hydronephrosis and *renal failure*.

BEDSIDE

Quick-Look Test

Does the patient look well (comfortable), sick (uncomfortable or distressed), or critical (about to die)?

Patients with acute bladder distention may look distressed because of abdominal pain.

Airway and Vital Signs

Inability to insert a urethral catheter should not compromise the vital signs.

Selective History and Chart Review

Have multiple attempts at catheterization been made, or has a catheter been removed with the balloon still inflated (urethral edema)?

Does the patient have a history of benign prostatic hypertrophy, carcinoma of the prostate, urethral stricture, or an anatomic abnormality of the urethra?

What was the original indication for urethral catheter placement? Does the indication still exist?

Selective Physical Examination and Management

1. Percuss and palpate the abdomen to determine whether the bladder is distended. Suprapubic tenderness and dullness are suggestive of bladder distention.
2. If urethral edema is suspected, try inserting a smaller catheter.
3. If the patient has a history of urethral obstruction, try inserting a coudé catheter.
4. If you are unable to accomplish catheterization, consult the urology department for assistance.

T-TUBES, J-TUBES, PENROSE DRAINS, AND PIGTAIL DRAINS

T-tubes are usually used for postoperative drainage of the common bile duct after exploration or choledochotomy of the common bile duct (Fig. 20.11). A T-tube cholangiogram is commonly obtained

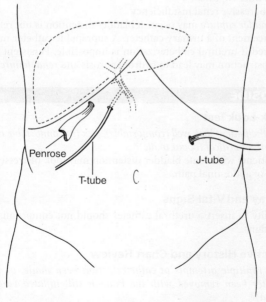

FIG. 20.11 T-tube, J-tube, and Penrose drain.

on the 7th to 10th postoperative day. If the cholangiogram is normal, the T-tube is removed. If a blockage (stricture, tumor, retained common duct stones) exists, the T-tube is left in place.

J-tubes, or jejunostomy tubes, are surgically inserted to provide enteral nutrition on a long-term basis. They are particularly useful for patients with gastroesophageal reflux and aspiration.

Gastrostomy tubes may be inserted percutaneously under direct-vision imaging (e.g., gastroscopy or fluoroscopy) and are used for long-term feeding in patients who have no gastroesophageal reflux.

Penrose drains are flat rubber drains inserted into wounds or operative sites with potential dead spaces to prevent the accumulation of pus, intestinal contents, blood, bile, or pancreatic juice.

Pigtail drains are typically placed percutaneously by an interventional radiologist in a Seldinger-technique as opposed to openly placed drains by the surgeon. The indication can be given pre- or postoperatively to drain collections without the need for open surgery (e.g., pancreatic pseudocyst, localized intraabdominal/pelvic abscess). After insertion via a wire, the tip of the drain is curled by pulling attached strings that are then wrapped around and anchored at the end of the drain. Pigtail drains are often smaller in diameter than other drainage tubes and tend to obstruct easier. This may require flushing as described on page 250. To remove a pigtail drain, the anchored pulling strings need to be cut first.

Closed suction (Davon or Jackson-Pratt) drains are used in operative sites with large potential dead spaces, where bacterial ingress may contaminate sterile cavities.

Sump drains have filters incorporated to prevent airborne bacteria from entering. They are usually used to drain peripancreatic fluid collections. Interventional radiologists sometimes insert various percutaneous drains into the biliary tree and intraabdominal abscesses. Problems with these drains should be referred to the radiologist or surgeon.

Blocked T-Tubes and J-Tubes

PHONE CALL

Questions

1. How long has the tube been blocked?
2. What type of tube is in place?
3. Has the tube been dislodged?
4. What operation was performed, and how many days ago?
5. What are the patient's vital signs?
6. Why was the patient admitted?

Orders

Ask the RN to bring a dressing set, two pairs of gloves in your size, and chlorhexidine skin disinfectant to the patient's bedside. You must remove the dressing around the drainage tube, and you must keep the site sterile.

Informing the Registered Nurse

Tell the RN, "I will arrive at the bedside in … minutes."

If you are certain that the tube has not been dislodged, assessment of blocked T-tubes and J-tubes can be delayed an hour or two if higher priority problems require your attention.

ELEVATOR THOUGHTS

What causes blockages in T-tubes, J-tubes, Penrose, and pigtail tubes?
1. Blood clots in the tube
2. Debris in the tube
3. Failure to irrigate the tube regularly

MAJOR THREAT TO LIFE

- Sepsis with blocked T-tubes

Blockages in T-tubes may lead to postoperative infection, with resultant abscess formation or systemic sepsis. If they are not dislodged, blocked J-tubes present no immediate threat to life. The risk for further surgery exists if the tube must be replaced.

BEDSIDE

Quick-Look Test

Does the patient look well (comfortable), sick (uncomfortable or distressed), or critical (about to die)?

A patient with a blocked T-tube or J-tube looks well unless the underlying problem causes the patient to look sick or critically ill.

Airway and Vital Signs

A blocked T-tube or J-tube should not compromise the airway or vital signs.

Selective Physical Examination and Management

Aspirate and irrigate the tube as follows:
1. Ask an assistant to hold the distal part of the T-tube or J-tube close to the connection between the tube and the drainage bag.

2. Put on sterile gloves and clean the distal end of the T-tube or J-tube and the proximal connecting tubing with chlorhexidine.
3. Disconnect the tube from the connecting tubing, and give the connecting tubing to the assistant to maintain a sterile field.
4. Using a 5-mL syringe, aspirate very gently (i.e., withdraw the syringe plunger) to dislodge and extract the obstruction.
5. If this maneuver is unsuccessful, fill a second 5-mL syringe with 3 mL of sterile normal saline and very gently flush the T-tube or J-tube by applying slow, careful pressure to the syringe plunger. After you flush with saline, attempt to aspirate gently. If this maneuver fails, do not try again.
6. Maintaining sterile technique, reconnect the T-tube, J-tube, Penrose, or pigtail tube and the drainage bag.

If aspiration and irrigation are unsuccessful, the surgeon should be informed immediately. The surgeon will decide whether to use T-tube cholangiography to visualize the problem or perform a closed exploration of the obstructed tube with a Fogarty catheter. Closed exploration should be performed only by a surgeon experienced in the procedure and only when a large, intact T-tube has been used or when the back wall of the T-limb has been cut away. An adequately functioning T-tube usually drains 100 to 250 mL over 8 hours.

Dislodged T-Tubes, J-Tubes, and Penrose Drains

PHONE CALL

Questions

1. How long ago was the tube or drain dislodged?
2. What type of tube is in place?
3. What operation was performed, and how many days ago?
4. What are the patient's vital signs?
5. Why was the patient admitted?

Orders

Ask the RN to bring a dressing set, two pairs of gloves in your size, and chlorhexidine skin cleanser to the patient's bedside. You must remove the dressing around the drainage tube, and you must keep the site sterile.

Informing the Registered Nurse

Tell the RN, "I will arrive at the bedside in … minutes."

If T-tubes and J-tubes are dislodged, you must see the patient immediately, because urgent replacement is mandatory if the tube was inserted recently. If examination is delayed, emergency surgery may be necessary to replace the tube.

ELEVATOR THOUGHTS

What causes dislodgment of tubes and drains?
1. Failure to secure the tube or drain adequately
2. Confused, uncooperative patient

MAJOR THREAT TO LIFE

- Sepsis

  Dislodgment of T-tubes and Penrose drains may lead to post-operative sepsis, with resultant abscess formation or systemic sepsis. If dislodged J-tubes and T-tubes cannot be replaced early, surgical replacement may be required; this increases the risk of morbidity and mortality from a second anesthetic.

BEDSIDE

Quick-Look Test

Does the patient look well (comfortable), sick (uncomfortable or distressed), or critical (about to die)?

A patient with a recently dislodged T-tube, J-tube, or Penrose drain looks well unless the underlying problem causes the patient to look sick or critically ill.

Airway and Vital Signs

A dislodged T-tube, J-tube, or Penrose drain should not compromise the vital signs acutely.

Selective Physical Examination and Management

Dislodged T-Tube

Dislodgment of a T-tube that drains the common bile duct is a potentially life-threatening situation, because septic shock can follow rapidly. If dislodgment is suspected, order immediate T-tube cholangiography, and inform the surgeon. If dislodgment is confirmed by the cholangiogram, the patient needs surgery to reestablish drainage.

Dislodged J-Tube

A dislodged J-tube (enterostomy tube) must be reinserted immediately, as follows:
1. Put on sterile gloves, and clean and drape the tube exit site.
2. If the tube is only partially dislodged, carefully clean the exposed tubing and gently advance the tube to the appropriate (previous) depth.
3. If the tube has been completely dislodged, select a similar sterile tube and introduce it gently through the track left by the previous tube. Do not force the tube in.

4. If this maneuver is successful, secure the tube well by suturing it in place with a 3-0 suture.
5. Order radiography with water-soluble radiocontrast to confirm correct positioning of the replaced or repositioned tube.

   If replacement of the J-tube is unsuccessful, notify the surgeon, who will decide whether an urgent reoperation is indicated.

Dislodged Penrose Drain

Dislodged Penrose drains should not be reinserted into the wound because of the risk of introducing bacteria into the site. Secure the Penrose drain in the position in which you find it, and examine the area daily for abscess formation (heat, tenderness, swelling) for the next few days. Inform the surgeon that the Penrose drain has become dislodged.

NASOGASTRIC AND ENTERAL FEEDING TUBES

Blocked Nasogastric and Enteral Feeding Tubes

PHONE CALL

Questions

1. How long has the tube been blocked?
2. What type of tube is in place?
3. Has the tube been dislodged?
4. What are the patient's vital signs?
5. Why was the patient admitted?

Orders

Ask the RN to bring a 50-mL syringe, sterile normal saline, and a bowl to the patient's bedside.

Informing the Registered Nurse

Tell the RN, "I will arrive at the bedside in … minutes."

Blockage of a nasogastric or enteral tube is not an emergency. Assessment can be delayed an hour or two if higher priority problems require your attention.

ELEVATOR THOUGHTS

What causes blockage of nasogastric or enteral feeding tubes?
1. Debris in the tube
2. Blood clots in the tube
3. Failure to irrigate the tube regularly

MAJOR THREAT TO LIFE

Aspiration pneumonia

If the nasogastric tube is blocked and thus fails to drain the stomach, gastric contents can be aspirated into the lungs.

BEDSIDE

Quick-Look Test

Does the patient look well (comfortable), sick (uncomfortable or distressed), or critical (about to die)?

If a blocked nasogastric tube fails to drain the gastric contents, the patient may experience nausea and vomiting and thus look sick.

Airway and Vital Signs

What is the patient's respiratory rate?

A blocked nasogastric tube should not compromise the airway unless gastric contents accumulate and are aspirated into the lungs.

Selective Physical Examination and Management

1. Irrigate the tube with 25 to 50 mL of normal saline. As the tube is being irrigated, listen over the stomach region for the gurgling of fluid, which indicates that the tube is in the stomach.
2. If the previous maneuver is unsuccessful, remove the tube and replace it with a new tube if gastric stasis persists, with the potential for aspiration.
3. Ensure that the usual nursing protocols are being followed for regular irrigation of the tube.

Dislodged Nasogastric and Enteral Feeding Tubes

PHONE CALL

Questions

1. How long has the tube been dislodged?
2. What type of tube is in place?
3. What are the patient's vital signs?
4. Why was the patient admitted?

Orders

No orders are necessary.

Informing the Registered Nurse

Tell the RN, "I will arrive at the bedside in ... minutes."

Assessment of a dislodged nasogastric or enteral feeding tube can be delayed an hour or two if higher priority problems require your attention. With a diabetic patient who has received insulin, however be careful to restore caloric intake before too long, if necessary by IV glucose infusion.

ELEVATOR THOUGHTS

What causes a nasogastric or enteral feeding tube to become dislodged?
1. Failure to secure the tube adequately
2. Behavior of a confused, uncooperative patient

MAJOR THREAT TO LIFE

- Aspiration pneumonia

If the nasogastric tube is dislodged and thus fails to drain the stomach, gastric contents may accumulate and can be aspirated into the lung. When an enteral feeding tube is dislodged or misplaced, the danger is that the enteral feeding solution will be infused into the lung.

BEDSIDE

Quick-Look Test

Does the patient look well (comfortable), sick (uncomfortable or distressed), or critical (about to die)?

Patients who have aspirated because of a dislodged nasogastric tube or a malpositioned feeding tube may appear tachypneic and unwell.

Airway and Vital Signs

Dislodgment of a nasogastric or enteral feeding tube should not compromise the vital signs unless the patient has aspirated the gastric contents or enteral feeding solutions.

Selective Physical Examination and Management

1. Inspect the tube, looking for markings that indicate how far in it is. If you are not familiar with these markings, ask the RN to bring a similar tube to the bedside so that you can estimate how far in the patient's tube is.
2. Aspirate the patient's tube to see whether gastric contents can be obtained. Using the 50-mL syringe, instill 25 to 50 mL of air while you listen over the stomach region with your stethoscope. If the tube is properly positioned, you should hear a gurgling swoosh as air is introduced into the stomach.
3. A small-bore enteral feeding tube should not be pushed farther down if it has been dislodged. Do not insert the guide

wire down the tube blindly, because the esophagus, stomach, or duodenum may be lacerated or perforated if the tip of the guide wire exits from one of the distal apertures in the tube. Dislodged enteral feeding tubes must be removed and replaced. The same tube can be reused; insert the guide wire into the tube under direct vision ex vivo. The tube, stiffened by the guide wire, can then be reinserted.

4. Ensure that the usual nursing protocols are being followed for regular irrigation of the tube.

Polyuria, Frequency, and Incontinence

You will receive many calls at night regarding patients' urinary volume; they may be voiding too much or too little. It is often difficult for a patient to differentiate between problems of polyuria and frequency, and for many elderly patients, either of these problems may manifest as incontinence. Once you clarify which of these three problems is present, treatment is easy.

PHONE CALL

Questions

1. *Which problem is present?*

    Polyuria refers to a urine output of more than 3 L/day. This usually comes to the attention of the nurse when reviewing the fluid balance record or when the urinary drainage bag requires frequent emptying.

    Frequency of urination refers to the frequent passage of urine, whether of large or small volume, and it may occur in concert with polyuria or urinary incontinence.

    Urinary incontinence refers to the involuntary loss of urine.

2. *What are the patient's vital signs?*
3. *Why was the patient admitted?*

Orders

Polyuria, frequency, and incontinence are seldom urgent problems. Urinary incontinence is a common problem in hospitalized elderly patients and is a frequent source of frustration for nurses. Avoid ordering a Foley catheter as the first method of treatment.

Informing the Registered Nurse

Tell the registered nurse (RN), "I will arrive at the bedside in . . . minutes."

If the patient's vital signs are stable and other sick patients require assessment, a patient with polyuria, frequency, or incontinence need not be examined immediately.

ELEVATOR THOUGHTS

What causes polyuria?
1. Diabetes mellitus
2. Diabetes insipidus (central, nephrogenic)
3. Psychogenic polydipsia
4. Large volumes of oral or intravenous (IV) fluids
5. Diuretics (including sodium-glucose cotransporter-2 [SGLT2] inhibitors)
6. Diuretic phase of acute tubular necrosis
7. Postobstructive diuresis
8. Salt-losing nephritis
9. Hypercalcemia

What causes frequency?
1. Urinary tract infection (UTI)
2. Partial bladder outlet obstruction (e.g., prostatism, benign prostatic hypertrophy)
3. Bladder irritation (tumor, stone, infection)

What causes incontinence?
1. Urge incontinence: caused by UTI, diabetes mellitus, urolithiasis, dementia, stroke, normal-pressure hydrocephalus, benign prostatic hypertrophy, pelvic tumor, depression, anxiety
2. Stress incontinence: in multiparous women, caused by lax pelvic bladder support; in men, occurring after prostate surgery
3. Overflow incontinence: caused by bladder outlet obstruction, as in benign prostatic hypertrophy, urethral stricture; spinal cord disease; autonomic neuropathy; fecal impaction
4. Environmental factors: inaccessible call bell, obstacles to the bathroom
5. Iatrogenic factors: diuretics, sedatives, anticholinergics, α-blockers, calcium channel blockers, angiotensin-converting enzyme inhibitors

MAJOR THREAT TO LIFE

- Polyuria: intravascular volume depletion. If polyuria is not caused by fluid excess and continues without adequate fluid replacement, the intravascular volume drops, and the patient may become hypotensive.
- Frequency or incontinence: sepsis. Frequency or incontinence does not pose a major threat to life unless an underlying UTI goes unchecked and progresses to pyelonephritis or sepsis.

BEDSIDE

Quick-Look Test

Does the patient look well (comfortable), sick (uncomfortable or distressed), or critical (about to die)?

Most often, patients with polyuria, frequency, or incontinence look well. If the patient looks sick or critically ill, search for a previously unrecognized problem. For example, if polyuria is caused by previously undetected diabetes mellitus, the patient may be ketoacidotic and appear sick. Similarly, frequency or incontinence may be the presenting manifestation of UTI in a patient who appears sick.

Airway and Vital Signs

Does the patient have postural changes?

A rise in heart rate of more than 15 beats/minute, a fall in systolic blood pressure of more than 5 mm Hg, or any fall in diastolic blood pressure is indicative of significant hypovolemia.

Caution: A resting tachycardia alone may be a sign of decreased intravascular volume.

Does the patient have a fever?

Fever is suggestive of possible UTI.

Selective Physical Examination I

Does the patient have volume depletion?

Cardiovascular system (CVS)	Pulse volume, jugular venous pressure (JVP)
	Skin temperature and color
Neurologic system	Level of consciousness

Management I

What immediate measure must be taken to correct or prevent intravascular volume depletion?

Replace intravascular volume. If the patient has volume depletion, administer IV normal saline or Ringer's lactate, aiming for a JVP of 2 to 3 cm H_2O above the sternal angle and normalization of the vital signs.

Remember that aggressive fluid repletion in a patient with a history of congestive heart failure may compromise cardiac function. Do not overshoot the goal of volume repletion.

Selective History and Chart Review

Identify the specific problem.

Polyuria

Polyuria may be suspected from the history but can be confirmed only through scrutiny of fluid balance sheets that are meticulously kept.

If these are not available, order strict intake-output monitoring. It is worthwhile to document polyuria (>3 L/day) before embarking on an exhaustive workup of a possibly nonexistent problem.

1. Ask about associated symptoms. The presence of both polyuria and polydipsia is suggestive of diabetes mellitus, diabetes insipidus, or compulsive water drinking (psychogenic polydipsia). Of these, diabetes mellitus is the most common.

2. Check the patient's chart for recent laboratory results:
   - Blood glucose level, hemoglobin A1c
   - Potassium level
   - Calcium level

   Hypokalemia and hypercalcemia are important reversible causes of nephrogenic diabetes insipidus. (Refer to Chapter 34 for management of hypokalemia and Chapter 31 for management of hypercalcemia.)

3. Make sure that the patient is not taking any drugs that may cause either nephrogenic diabetes insipidus (lithium carbonate, demeclocycline) or diuresis (diuretics, mannitol).

Frequency

Question the patient about urinary frequency. From the nursing notes or fluid balance sheets, estimate whether the patient is a reliable historian. Ask about associated symptoms. Fever, dysuria, hematuria, and foul-smelling urine are suggestive of UTI. Poor stream, hesitancy, dribbling, or nocturia is suggestive of prostatic hypertrophy.

Incontinence

Incontinence is obvious when it occurs and is often embarrassing to the patient. You need an honest history from the patient to make a proper diagnosis. Address the subject nonjudgmentally. Review the patient's medications to ensure that he or she is not receiving medications that may cause incontinence.

Selective Physical Examination II

Look for specific causes and complications of polyuria, frequency, or incontinence.

Vitals	Fever (UTI)
Head, ears, eyes, nose, throat (HEENT)	Visual fields (pituitary neoplasm)
Respiratory	Kussmaul respiration (diabetic keto-acidosis)
	📖 Kussmaul respiration is characterized by deep, pauseless breathing at a rate of 25-30 breaths/minute.

Abdomen (ABD)	Enlarged bladder (neurogenic bladder, bladder outlet obstruction with overflow incontinence)
	Suprapubic tenderness (cystitis)
Neurologic system	Level of consciousness
	Localizing findings

📖 An alert, conscious patient with polyuria and with free access to fluids and salt will not experience volume depletion. If volume depletion is present, suspect metabolic or structural neurologic abnormalities impairing the normal response to thirst. Perform a complete neurologic examination, looking for evidence of stroke, subdural hemorrhage, or metabolic abnormalities.

Skin	Perineal skin breakdown (a complication of repeated incontinence and a source of infection)
Rectal	Enlarged prostate (bladder outlet obstruction)
	Perineal sensation, resting tone of anal sphincter, lack of anal wink

📖 To elicit an anal wink, gently stroke the skin around the anus. A normal response is manifested by contraction of the external sphincter.

📖 An alternative, albeit more intrusive, sacral reflex test is the bulbocavernosus reflex. To elicit this reflex, the index finger of the examining hand is introduced into the rectum, and the patient is asked to relax the sphincter as much as possible. The glans penis or clitoris is then squeezed with the opposite hand, which normally results in involuntary contraction of the anal sphincter. Innervation of the anus is similar to that of the lower urinary tract; therefore abnormalities in perineal sensation or in the sacral reflexes may be a clue to the presence of a spinal cord lesion that is responsible for the incontinence.

Management II
What more needs to be done tonight?

Polyuria

1. Once intravascular volume is restored, ensure adequate continuing replacement fluid (usually IV) as estimated by urinary losses, insensible losses (400 to 800 mL/day), and other losses (from nasogastric suction, vomiting, or diarrhea). Recheck the volume status periodically to ensure that your mathematical estimates for replacement correlate with an appropriate clinical response.
2. Order that meticulous intake-output records be kept.
3. Order serum or finger-prick blood glucose testing.

   📖 Glucose testing identifies diabetes mellitus before it progresses to ketoacidosis (in type 1 diabetes) or hyperosmolar coma (in type 2 diabetes). The presence of glycosuria on urinalysis provides more rapid evidence of hyperglycemia as a possible cause of polyuria. Random blood glucose levels of 11 mmol/L or lower are seldom accompanied by osmotic diuresis. If hyperglycemia (glucose level >11 mmol/L) exists, refer to Chapter 33, page 394, for further management.
4. It may not be standard practice to measure the serum calcium level as a stat test at night, but if hypercalcemia is strongly suspected (polyuria or lethargy in a patient with malignancy, hyperparathyroidism, or sarcoidosis), contact the laboratory for permission to perform this test on an urgent basis.
5. Maximal urine-concentrating ability measured by the water deprivation test can help differentiate among central diabetes insipidus, nephrogenic diabetes insipidus, and psychogenic polydipsia. This test can be arranged on an elective basis in the morning.

Frequency

1. If other symptoms (urgency, dysuria, low-grade fever, suprapubic tenderness) of UTI (cystitis) are present, empirical treatment with antibiotics may be warranted, pending urine culture and sensitivity results, which usually take 48 hours to complete. The patient's chart may reveal a result of a previous urine culture or previous antibacterial therapy that may affect the selection of empirical treatment.

   Any of the following may be effective therapy in an uncomplicated case of cystitis (i.e., no evidence of upper UTI, no evidence of prostatitis, no renal disease, and no recent urinary tract instrumentation). The usual infecting organisms are *Escherichia coli* and *Staphylococcus saprophyticus*. The condition may resolve spontaneously. Antibiotics are generally used for

3 days in women and for 7 days in men. However, women with diabetes, a structural urinary tract abnormality, or a recently treated UTI should receive a 7-day course.

- Trimethoprim-sulfamethoxazole, 1 tablet (160 mg/800 mg) orally (PO) twice daily
- Nitrofurantoin, 100 mg PO twice daily
- Cephalexin, 500 mg PO every 6 hours
- Fosfomycin 2 to 3 g PO q 2 to 3 days
- Ceftazidime 1 to 2 g IM or IV od if pseudomonas aeruginosa is suspected

2. If the findings of the history and physical examination are suggestive of partial bladder outlet obstruction, examine the abdomen carefully for an enlarged bladder. If the patient has urinary retention, a Foley catheter should be placed. (Refer to Chapter 9 for further investigation and management of urinary retention.)

3. Other causes of frequency, such as bladder irritation by stones or tumors, can be addressed by urologic consultation in the morning. You may be able to expedite the diagnosis of bladder tumor by ordering a collection of urine for cytologic study.

Incontinence

1. Even if incontinence is the only symptom, order a urinalysis and urine culture to check whether a UTI is contributing to the patient's symptoms.

2. Check for hyperglycemia, hypokalemia, and hypercalcemia if polyuria is present. These conditions may manifest as incontinence in an elderly or bedridden patient, and specific treatment may alleviate the incontinence.

3. If findings of the neurologic examination (e.g., abnormal sacral reflexes, diminished perineal sensation, lower limb weakness, or spasticity) are suggestive of the presence of a *spinal cord lesion,* consultation should be arranged with a neurologist.

4. In the case of *overflow incontinence,* you must differentiate between overflow resulting from obstruction of the bladder outlet (e.g., benign prostatic hypertrophy, uterine prolapse) and that resulting from impaired ability of detrusor contraction (e.g., lower motor neuron bladder). This is best done in the morning by assessment of urinary bladder dynamics under the direction of a urologist. If the bladder is palpably enlarged and the patient is in distress, bladder catheterization may be attempted. Forceful attempts at catheterization should be avoided, however, and a urologist should be called for assistance if the catheter does not pass easily (see Chapter 20, pages 246–248). If no correctable obstruction is found, long-term treatment may involve intermittent straight catheterization, which is less likely

to cause infection than is a chronic indwelling Foley catheter. Aim for a urine volume of less than 400 mL every 4 to 6 hours. Greater volumes result in ureterovesical reflux, which promotes ascending UTI. A young, motivated patient with a neurogenic bladder can be taught to self-catheterize. In these cases, a silicone elastomer (Silastic) Foley catheter should be used. This type is less predisposed to calcification and encrustation and may be kept in place for up to 6 weeks at a time.

5. *Urge incontinence* (detrusor instability) is a condition in which the bladder escapes central inhibition, which results in reflex contractions. It is the most common cause of incontinence among elderly persons and is often manifested by involuntary micturition preceded by a warning lasting a few seconds or minutes. Ensure that no physical barriers prevent the patient from reaching the bathroom or commode in time. Does the patient have easy access to the call bell? Are the nurses responding promptly? Are the bed rails kept up or down? Does the patient have a medical condition (e.g., Parkinson's disease, stroke, arthritis) that prevents easy mobilization when the urge to void occurs? If perineal skin breakdown is not evident, *urinary incontinence pads* or *adult diapers with frequent checks* and changes by the nursing staff are adequate. (Urinary incontinence is normal in babies and young children.) If perineal skin breakdown or ulceration is present, placement of a Foley or condom catheter is justified to allow skin healing. Long-term treatment involves (1) regular toileting every 2 to 3 hours while the patient is awake and (2) limiting fluid intake in the evening.

6. Urinary spillage with coughing or straining is suggestive of stress incontinence. Again, if perineal skin breakdown is not evident, urinary incontinence pads or adult diapers are adequate until urologic consultation can be arranged to assess the need for medical versus surgical management.

REMEMBER

Urinary incontinence is an understandable source of frustration for nurses, as well as for patients. Listen to the concerns of the nurses looking after your patients, and discuss with them the reasons for your actions.

Pronouncing Death

One of the duties of medical students and residents on call at night is to pronounce death in recently deceased patients. This includes determining who will inform the family and/or friends of the deceased of the death. This may well be you. The manner in which the information is transmitted will affect their grief process. It must be done with compassion and sensitivity. If you are unsure of the steps that should be taken, the nurse on duty will help you.

You also need to know what must be done to pronounce a patient dead. Unfortunately, the medical and legal definitions of death have long been uncertain.

Traditionally, the determination of death has been solely a medical decision. In the United States, legislation on the criteria for death is within state jurisdiction. Many states have opted to follow the recommendations set forth by the Harvard Medical School Ad Hoc Committee, Capron and Kass (1972), or the Kansas legislation of 1971. It is best to be familiar with the medical and legal criteria accepted for the determination of death in the state in which you work.

The recommended criteria for death issued by the Law Reform Commission of Canada in 1981, and used for all purposes within the jurisdiction of the Parliament of Canada, were as follows:

1. A person is dead when all of a person's brain function has irreversibly ceased.
2. The irreversible cessation of brain function can be determined by the prolonged absence of spontaneous circulatory and respiratory functions.
3. When the prolonged absence of spontaneous circulatory and respiratory functions cannot be determined through the use of artificial means of support, the irreversible cessation of brain function can be determined by any means recognized by the ordinary standards of current medical practice.

Although criterion 1 alone may imply that a complete neurologic examination is required for the pronouncement of death, this is neither practical nor necessary. Criterion 2 accounts for this by assuming that when "prolonged absence of spontaneous circulatory and respiratory functions" exists, the patient's brain function has irreversibly ceased. Therefore in the majority of cases, there is no question that the patients you are asked to pronounce dead are indeed medically and legally dead, because they fulfill criterion 2. Thus in most cases, all that is legally required for you to pronounce a patient dead is to verify that there has been a prolonged absence of spontaneous circulatory and respiratory functions. A slightly more detailed assessment is recommended, however, and takes only a few minutes to complete.

The registered nurse (RN) will page you and inform you of the death of the patient, requesting that you come to the unit and pronounce the patient dead.

1. Identify the patient by the hospital identification tag worn on the wrist.
2. Ascertain that the patient does not rouse to verbal or tactile stimuli.
3. Listen for heart sounds, and feel for the carotid pulse.

   📖 A deceased patient is pulseless and has no heart sounds.
4. Look at and listen to the patient's chest for evidence of spontaneous respirations.

   📖 A deceased patient shows no evidence of breathing movements or of air entry on examination.
5. Record the position of the pupils and their reactions to light.

   📖 A deceased patient shows no evidence of pupillary reaction to light. Although the pupils are usually dilated, this is not invariable.
6. Record the time at which your assessment was completed.

   📖 Although other emergencies take precedence over pronouncing a patient dead, try not to postpone this task too long, since the time of death is legally the time at which you pronounce the patient dead.
7. Document your findings on the chart. A typical chart entry may read as follows: "Called to pronounce Mr. Doe dead. Patient unresponsive to verbal or tactile stimuli. No heart sounds heard; no pulse felt. Not breathing, no air entry heard. Pupils fixed and dilated. Patient pronounced dead at 2030 hours, December 7, 2016."
8. Notify the family physician, attending physician, or both if the nurses have not already done so. Decide, together with the attending physician, whether an autopsy would be useful and appropriate in this patient's case.
9. Notify relatives. Next of kin should be notified as soon as possible. Normally, it is the responsibility of the family physician to notify the relatives once he or she has been told of the patient's death. On occasion, the family physician may have signed over his or her nighttime calls to a partner or to another

physician who does not know the patient or family. In this situation, it is best to inform the physician on call, and if he or she is uncomfortable speaking to the family, a member of the house staff who knows the patient or the family well should notify the next of kin. The family will appreciate hearing the news from a familiar person. If neither the family physician on call nor any member of the house staff knows the patient, spend a few minutes familiarizing yourself with the patient's medical history and mode of death. If you are appointed to deliver the news to the family, the following guidelines may be helpful.

- Identify yourself, "This is Dr. Jones calling from St. Paul's Hospital."
- Ask for the next of kin, "May I speak with Mrs. Doe, please?"
- Deliver the message, "Mrs. Doe, I am sorry to inform you that your husband died at 8:30 this evening."
- You may find that in many instances the news is not unexpected. It is, however, always comforting to know that a relative has died peacefully, "As you know, your husband was suffering from a terminal illness. Although I was not with your husband at the time of his death, the nurses looking after him assure me that he was very comfortable and that he passed away peacefully."
- If an autopsy is desired by one of the medical staff, this question should be broached now: "Your husband had an unusual illness, and if you are agreeable, it would be very useful to us to perform an autopsy. Although it obviously cannot change the course of events in your husband's illness, it may provide some valuable information for other patients suffering from similar problems." If there is any hesitation by the next of kin, emphasize that he or she is under no obligation to grant permission for an autopsy to be performed if it is against the perceived wishes of the patient or the family. If the next of kin refuses, do not argue, no matter how interested you may be in the outcome of the case. Accept the family's decision graciously: "We understand completely, and of course we will respect your wishes."
- Ask the next of kin if he or she would like to come to the hospital to see the patient one last time. Inform the nurses of this decision. Questions pertaining to funeral homes and the patient's personal belongings are best referred to the nurse in charge.

10. The patient may be a potential organ donor. You should inform the medical organ donation team that has the responsibility of initiating the donation process by confirming the deceased as a potential donor, assessing the suitability of

the transplantable organs and initiating discussions with the family. The family has the final say on whether transplantation may be undertaken.

11. You and the attending physician must determine whether the death should be reported to the coroner's service, including sudden or unexplained deaths, accidental deaths, suicides, and homicides.

SPECIAL SITUATIONS

Medical technology has introduced two other scenarios in the pronouncement of a patient's death.

The Mechanically Ventilated Patient Without Circulatory Function

Physicians have a general understanding that in patients being mechanically ventilated, if the heart stops beating, they meet the criteria for legal death through a lack of spontaneous ventilation once the ventilator is turned off. Thus it is reasonable practice to do the following:

1. Ensure that connections are intact and properly attached if the electrocardiogram monitor is attached to the patient. (This ensures that the absence of cardiac electrical activity is not attributable to faulty electrical connections.)
2. Follow the usual procedure for pronouncing death.
3. Discuss your findings with the attending physician and the patient's family before disconnecting the ventilator.
4. After agreement with the attending physician and the patient's family, disconnect the ventilator. Observe the patient for 3 minutes for evidence of spontaneous respiration.
5. Document your findings in the chart: "Called to pronounce Mr. Doe dead. Patient unresponsive to verbal or tactile stimuli. No heart sounds heard; no pulse felt. Pupils fixed and dilated. Patient being mechanically ventilated. Ventilator disconnected at 2030 hours after discussion with attending physician, Dr. Smith. No spontaneous respirations noted for 3 minutes. Patient pronounced dead at 2033 hours, February 7, 2023."

The Mechanically Ventilated Patient With Circulatory Function Intact

This type of patient is usually being cared for in the intensive care unit. A variety of controversial criteria exist for the determination of brain death, and criteria may differ among geographic locations. The task of pronouncing a mechanically ventilated patient dead and the discussion of organ procurement is best left to the staff of the intensive care unit and to associated subspecialists in consultation with the patient's family.

Seizures

A seizure is one of the more dramatic events you may witness while on call. Usually, everyone around is in a panic. The key to controlling the situation is to remain calm.

PHONE CALL

Questions

1. Is the seizure still going on?
2. What type of seizure was witnessed?
   a. Was the seizure partial or generalized?
3. What is the patient's level of consciousness?
4. Has the patient sustained any obvious injury?
5. Why was the patient admitted?
6. Has the patient had previous seizures?

Orders

1. Ask the registered nurse (RN) to make sure that the patient is positioned on his or her side. During both the seizure and the postictal state, the patient should be kept in the lateral decubitus position to prevent him or her from aspirating gastric contents.
2. Ask the RN to have the following available at the patient's bedside:
   a. Oral airway
   b. Intravenous setup with normal saline (flushed through and ready for immediate use)
   c. Two blood tubes (one for chemistry profiles and one for hematologic samples)
   d. **Lorazepam 4 mg for intravenous (IV) use or, if lorazepam is not available, diazepam 20 mg for IV use.**
   e. **Thiamine, 100 mg for IV use**
   f. **Fifty percent dextrose in water (D50W), 50 mL (1 ampule)**
   g. The patient's chart
3. If the patient is in the postictal state (unconscious or semicomatose), ask the RN to remove any dentures, suction the oropharynx, and establish an oral airway.

4. Order a stat finger-prick blood glucose (FPBG) reading if the patient is in the postictal state.

Informing the Registered Nurse

Tell the RN, "I will arrive at the bedside in . . . minutes."

If a patient is having a seizure, you must see the patient immediately.

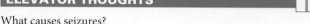

ELEVATOR THOUGHTS

What causes seizures?

An identifiable cause of seizure is found in fewer than half of patients, but it should be searched for diligently, especially in the hospitalized patient with a first-time seizure. You need to know whether the seizure resulted from a central nervous system (CNS) disorder or from a correctable systemic process that, if left undiagnosed, might predispose the patient to further seizures:

1. CNS disorder
   a. Brain tumor
   b. Stroke
   c. Head injury
   d. Meningitis or encephalitis
   e. Idiopathic epilepsy
   f. Post intracranial surgery
   g. Multiple sclerosis
   h. Hemorrhage from arteriovenous malformation
2. Drug-related cause
   a. Drug withdrawal
      i. Antiepileptic medication inadvertently discontinued or reduced to a nontherapeutic level
      ii. Alcohol withdrawal
          Caution: Does the patient have delirium tremens in addition to seizures?
      iii. Benzodiazepine or barbiturate withdrawal
   b. Drug toxicity (does not necessarily imply overdose)
      i. Meperidine overdose (an easily missed diagnosis in an elderly patient after surgery)
      ii. Penicillin at high doses
      iii. Theophylline toxicity
      iv. Lidocaine infusion
      v. Isoniazid
      vi. Lithium carbonate
      vii. Neuroleptic agents (e.g., chlorpromazine)
      viii. Cocaine, amphetamines
3. Endocrine disorder
   a. The four "hypos":
      i. Hypoglycemia

    ii. Hyponatremia

    iii. Hypocalcemia

    iv. Hypomagnesemia

  b. The four "hypers":

    i. Hyperglycemia (nonketotic)

    ii. Hyperthyroidism

    iii. Hypernatremia

    iv. Hyperurea (uremia)

4. Disorders in patients with acquired immunodeficiency syndrome (AIDS)

  a. Mass lesions (toxoplasmosis, CNS lymphoma)

  b. Human immunodeficiency virus (HIV)-related encephalopathy

  c. Meningitis (cryptococcal, herpes zoster, toxoplasmosis, aseptic)

  d. Any of the usual causes of seizures seen in immunocompetent hosts

5. Seizure *mimickers* (some conditions can mimic a seizure and should also be considered when the patient is evaluated)

  a. Syncope

  b. Transient ischemic attack

  c. Migraine

  d. Paroxysmal movement disorders

  e. Psychological disorders (*pseudoseizures*)

6. Miscellaneous

  a. CNS vasculitis

  b. Hypertensive encephalopathy

  c. Hypoxia or hypercapnia

  d. Acute intermittent porphyria

  e. Dialysis disequilibrium syndrome

MAJOR THREAT TO LIFE

- Aspiration
- Hypoxia

The patient should be lying in the lateral decubitus position to prevent the tongue from falling posteriorly and blocking the airway and to minimize the risk of aspirating the gastric contents while in the postictal state. Patients usually keep breathing throughout seizure activity. Most patients can be in status epilepticus as long as 30 minutes with no subsequent neurologic damage.

If the Seizure Has Stopped

In the majority of cases, a seizure will have stopped by the time you arrive at the patient's bedside. The procedures and protocols to follow if the seizure has stopped are discussed as follows. The

procedures and protocols to follow if the seizure persists begin on
page 277.

BEDSIDE

Quick-Look Test

Does the patient look well (comfortable), sick (uncomfortable or distressed), or critical (about to die)?

After a generalized tonic-clonic seizure, most patients are unconscious (the postictal state).

Airway, Vital Signs, and Blood Glucose Results

In what position is the patient lying?

The patient should be positioned in the lateral decubitus position to prevent him or her from aspirating gastric contents (Fig. 23.1).

Remove any dentures and suction the airway. Establish an oral airway if one is not already in place (Fig. 23.2). The patient is not out of danger yet; another seizure might occur, so make sure the airway is protected.

Administer oxygen by facemask or nasal prongs.

What is the (finger stick blood glucose) FPBG result?

Hypoglycemia must be treated immediately to prevent further seizures.

Management I

Draw blood (20 mL) and establish intravenous access. Collect the blood for the following tests:

- Chemistry tube: measurement of *electrolytes, urea, creatinine, random blood glucose, calcium, magnesium, albumin,* and *antiepileptic drug levels* (if the patient is receiving these medications). If the patient is undergoing a 3-day fast for investigation of possible hypoglycemia, order an *insulin level* measurement as well. Screening for *substance abuse* may also be indicated for adolescents and adults with unexplained generalized seizures. A *serum prolactin* level is sometimes helpful in differentiating a true seizure (in which case the level is often elevated when measured 10 to 20 minutes after the seizure and in comparison, with a baseline level measured 6 hours later) from a pseudoseizure, although the finding of a normal prolactin level does not exclude the possibility that a true seizure has occurred.
- Hematology tube: *complete blood cell count (CBC) and manual differential.*

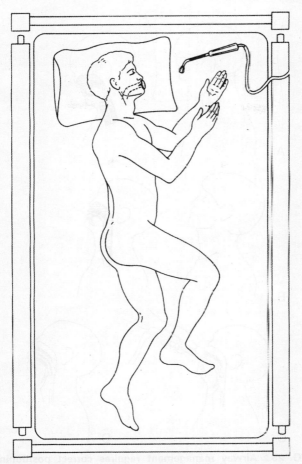

FIG. 23.1 **Lateral decubitus positioning of the patient to prevent him or her from aspirating gastric contents.**

Once intravenous access is established, keep the line open with normal saline. Normal saline is the intravenous fluid of choice because phenytoin is not compatible with dextrose-containing solutions.

If the FPBG reading reveals hypoglycemia, administer **thiamine, 100 mg IV**, by slow, direct injection over 3 to 5 minutes, followed by **D50W 50 mL IV**, by slow, direct injection.

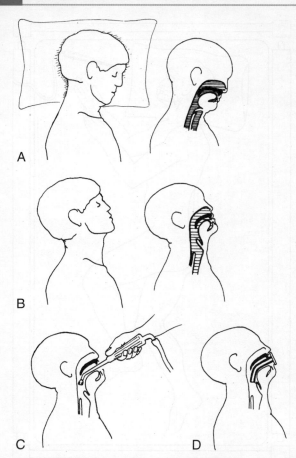

FIG. 23.2 Airway management requires correct positioning of the head, correct suctioning, and correct establishment of an oral airway. *A*, Neck flexion closes the airway. *B*, Neck extension to the sniffing position opens the airway. *C*, Suctioning. *D*, Establishment of the airway.

📖 Thiamine is given before the administration of glucose to prevent an exacerbation of Wernicke encephalopathy.

Check pulse oximetry or measure arterial blood gases if the patient appears cyanotic.

Selective Physical Examination I

Assess the patient's level of consciousness.

Does the patient respond to verbal or painful stimuli? Is the patient in a postictal state (i.e., decreased level of consciousness)?

Remember that if the patient does not regain consciousness between seizures, after 30 minutes the diagnosis becomes *status epilepticus.*

Selective History and Chart Review

1. Ask any witnesses the following details about the seizure:
   a. Duration
   b. Generalized tonic-clonic or partial seizure
   c. Generalized or focal onset of seizure
       📖 A focal onset of a generalized tonic-clonic seizure is suggestive of structural brain disease, which may be old or new.
   d. Any injury observed during the seizure
2. Does the patient have a history of epilepsy, alcohol or sedative withdrawal, head injury (e.g., recent fall while in the hospital), stroke, CNS tumor (primary or secondary), or diabetes mellitus?
3. Is the patient receiving any of the following medications, which may induce seizures?
   a. Penicillin
   b. Meperidine
   c. Insulin
   d. Oral hypoglycemics
   e. Antidepressants, lithium carbonate
   f. Isoniazid
   g. Lidocaine
   h. Neuroleptic agents (e.g., chlorpromazine)
   i. Theophylline
4. Is the patient HIV-positive or otherwise immunosuppressed?
   📖 Seizures are a common manifestation of CNS disease in HIV-positive patients.
5. What are the most recent laboratory results?
   a. Glucose level
   b. Sodium level
   c. Calcium level
   d. Albumin level
   e. Magnesium level
   f. Antiepileptic drug levels
   g. Urea concentration
   h. Creatinine concentration

Review the patient's chart before you conduct a more detailed physical examination because an immediate, treatable cause (e.g., insulin or meperidine overdose, hyponatremia) is more likely to be found in the chart.

Selective Physical Examination II

Vitals	Repeat measurements now
Head, ears, eyes, nose, throat (HEENT)	Tongue or cheek lacerations, nuchal rigidity
Respiratory system	Signs of aspiration
Neurologic system	Complete CNS examination within the limits of level of consciousness.
	Can the patient speak and follow commands?
	Is there any asymmetry of pupils, visual fields, reflexes, or plantar responses?
	Asymmetry in neurologic functioning is suggestive of structural brain disease.
Musculoskeletal system	Palpate skull and face, spine, and ribs.
	Passive range of motion (ROM) of all four limbs
	Are there any lacerations, hematomas, or fractures?

Management II

Establish the *provisional* and *differential diagnoses* of the seizure; they must be causally defined diagnoses (e.g., "generalized tonic-clonic seizure secondary to hypoglycemia").

Are there any complications of the seizure that give rise to a second diagnosis?

For example if a head injury has been sustained, the provisional diagnosis might be forehead hematoma, and the differential diagnosis would include subdural hematoma and frontal bone fracture.

Treat the underlying cause. Seizure is a sign, not a diagnosis.

Maintain intravenous access for 24 hours with a saline lock.

Patients With a Single Seizure

In most patients who have had a single seizure, it is not necessary to administer antiepileptic medications, particularly if a rapidly correctable metabolic cause is found. Exceptions include cases in which patients are already taking antiepileptic medications but have inadequate serum concentrations, patients have suspected structural CNS abnormalities, and patients are HIV-positive (in whom seizures tend to be recurrent). If further seizures are anticipated, a long-acting antiepileptic drug (e.g., phenytoin rather than lorazepam) is recommended (see page 521 for dosage). Although lorazepam is useful as an anticonvulsant to halt seizures, it is not useful as a prophylactic. The antiepileptic medication of choice is phenytoin.

Any patient with an unprovoked first seizure should undergo brain imaging (magnetic resonance imaging [MRI] or computed tomographic [CT] scan of the head) and electroencephalography, which, in most cases, can be arranged in the morning.

Elderly and Other Patients in Whom Structural Central Nervous System Disease Is Suspected to Be a Cause of Seizures

These patients should undergo CT scanning of the head.

Human Immunodeficiency Virus–Positive Patients

HIV-positive patients should undergo MRI or CT scanning of the head (because of the high incidence of CNS mass lesions) and, if there is no risk of herniation, a lumbar puncture. On occasion, cryptococcal meningitis may coexist in an HIV-positive patient in whom a mass lesion is evident on brain imaging.

Seizure precautions should be instituted for the next 48 hours and then reviewed (Box 23.1).

If the Seizure Persists

Do not panic (almost everybody else will). Most seizures resolve without treatment within 2 minutes.

BEDSIDE

Quick-Look Test

Does the patient look well (comfortable), sick (uncomfortable or distressed), or critical (about to die)?

BOX 23.1	Seizure Precautions

1. Place the patient's bed in the lowest position.
2. At the head of the bed, provide equipment for establishing an oral airway.
3. Keep the side rails up when the patient is in bed. In the case of generalized tonic-clonic seizures, pad the side rails.
4. Provide the patient with a firm pillow.
5. Provide suction at the patient's bedside.
6. Provide oxygen at the patient's bedside.
7. Allow the patient to use the bathroom only with supervision.
8. Allow the patient to take baths or showers only with a nurse in attendance.
9. To measure temperature, use only an axillary or forehead thermometer.
10. Provide direct supervision when the patient uses sharp objects such as a straight razor or nail scissors.

A generalized tonic-clonic seizure often engenders anxiety in observers. Remember that if the patient is having a seizure, you must ensure that he or she has both a blood pressure (BP) and a pulse.

Ask the RN to notify your resident of the situation—a seizure is a medical emergency.

Airway, Vital Signs, and Blood Glucose Value

In what position is the patient lying?

The patient should be positioned and maintained in the lateral decubitus position to prevent him or her from aspirating gastric contents. One or two assistants may be needed to hold the patient in this position if the seizure is violent.

Suction the patient's airway. Do not establish an oral airway or attempt to remove dentures if force is required; you might break the patient's teeth.

Administer oxygen by facemask or nasal prongs.

What is the patient's BP?

It is virtually impossible to measure BP during a generalized tonic-clonic seizure; therefore palpate the femoral pulse instead. (You may need an assistant to hold the patient's knee against the bed.) A palpable femoral pulse usually indicates a systolic BP of higher than 60 mm Hg.

What is the FPBG result?

Hypoglycemia, if present, must be treated immediately.

Management I

How long has the seizure lasted?

If the seizure has stopped, refer to page 272.

If the seizure has lasted less than 3 minutes:

- Do not administer lorazepam yet.
- Recheck the patient's airway.
- Observe the seizure activity.
- Do not attempt to start an intravenous line yet; it will be much easier in 1 or 2 minutes, after the seizure has stopped.
- Ensure that intravenous tubing is flushed through with normal saline and that thiamine, D50W, lorazepam, and two blood tubes are available at the bedside.

  If the seizure has lasted 3 minutes or longer and continues:
- Draw blood (20 mL) and establish intravenous access.

Tips on Starting the Intravenous Line

If the seizure is persisting, establishing an IV line is very difficult. Because a seizure is an emergency, it is not the appropriate time for a novice to practice starting an IV line. Appoint the most experienced person present to obtain IV access. The patient's arm should be held firmly by one or two assistants while the patient is held on his or her side. Try for the largest vein available, but avoid using the antecubital vein unless necessary, because the elbow will then have to be splinted to avoid losing IV access.

Medications

Order the following medications to be administered immediately:

1. **Thiamine, 100 mg IV**, by slow, direct injection over 3 to 5 minutes.
2. **D50W, 50 mL IV**, by slow, direct injection. If the patient is hypoglycemic, he or she will abruptly regain consciousness while receiving the first 30 mL of D50W. Do not proceed with any further medication; change the IV fluid to D5W. Thiamine is given before the administration of glucose to protect against an exacerbation of Wernicke encephalopathy.
3. **Lorazepam 0.1 mg/kg (maximum 4 mg) over a few minutes IV.** If injected into the IV tubing, do so as close to the vein insertion as possible to avoid interactions. If lorazepam is not available, a good alternative is **diazepam 2 mg IV over 3 to 5 minutes.** Alternatively, if IV access is unobtainable, **intranasal diazepam may be given at a dose of 0.2 mg/kg.**
4. If no response, ask an assistant to do the following:
    - Establish a second intravenous line with normal saline in preparation for administering phenytoin (Fig. 23.3).
      📖 Phenytoin should only be administered in normal saline.
    - Administer **phenytoin, loading dose of 15 mg/kg (1050 mg for a 70-kg patient).** The phenytoin loading dose can be injected directly through the normal saline intravenous line at a rate no faster than 25 to 50 mg/minute, or it can be

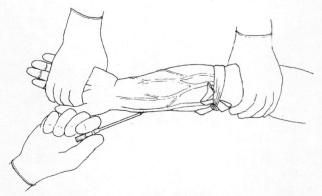

FIG. 23.3 Two intravenous lines are needed if both lorazepam and phenytoin are to be administered.

administered as an infusion (add the loading dose to 100 mL of normal saline) at a rate no faster than 25 to 50 mg/minute. After phenytoin administration, the IV line should be flushed through with normal saline to avoid local venous irritation caused by the drug's alkalinity.

📖 Phenytoin may cause hypotension and cardiac dysrhythmias. The heart rhythm and BP should be monitored frequently until the patient can be transferred to the intensive care unit or a telemetry unit. If hypotension or dysrhythmias occur, slow the phenytoin infusion rate.

If the seizure stops, stop administering lorazepam but administer the full loading dose of phenytoin. It is now practical to arrange for continuous electrocardiographic monitoring and repeated measurements of BP, which are important while the remainder of the phenytoin is being infused. See page 280 for further instructions. Most seizures can be controlled with diazepam and phenytoin. If not, CNS infection or structural brain disease may be present.

If the seizure has persisted for more than 5 to 10 minutes, the patient is now in status epilepticus. *This is an emergency.* A neurologist, intensivist, or anesthesiologist should be consulted immediately. The patient should be transferred to the intensive care unit/cardiac care unit (ICU/CCU) for management of the airway and probable intubation.

Status epilepticus is rare. It is defined as a single seizure lasting more than 5 to 10 minutes or repetitive seizures without intervening periods of normal consciousness.

Additional treatment in the ICU/CCU may include intravenous infusions of benzodiazepine, phenobarbital, levetiracetam, pentobarbital, or propofol.

Shortness of Breath

Calls at night to assess a patient's breathing are common. Do not become overwhelmed by the myriad causes of shortness of breath that you learned in medical school. In hospitalized patients, shortness of breath is commonly caused by only four entities: congestive heart failure (CHF), pulmonary embolism, pneumonia, and bronchospasm.

PHONE CALL

Questions

1. How long has the patient had shortness of breath? The sudden onset of shortness of breath is suggestive of pulmonary embolus, pneumothorax, or anaphylaxis.
2. Is the patient choking or wheezing? Immediate attention to ensuring an adequate airway is essential. Wheezing may signal an anaphylactic reaction.
3. Is the patient cyanotic? Clinical cyanosis is indicative of significant hypoxia, and you must see the patient immediately.
4. What are the patient's vital signs?
5. Why was the patient admitted?
6. What is the pulse oximetry reading? A normal oxygen saturation is greater than 94%. A pulse oximetry reading less than 93% suggests significant hypoxia, in which case you must see the patient immediately.
7. Does the patient have chronic obstructive pulmonary disease (COPD)? What you need to know is whether the patient retains CO_2. In most cases, this condition is present in patients with COPD or with a history of heavy smoking.

Orders

Airway Management

1. *Oxygen.* If you are certain that the patient does not retain CO_2, you can safely order any concentration of O_2 in the short-term situation. If you are not certain, order O_2, 28% by Venturi mask, and

reassess the patient on arrival at the patient's bedside. For most patients the concentration of oxygen delivered can be adjusted to maintain a pulse oximetry reading of greater than 94%.

2. If the admitting diagnosis is asthma and the patient has not received an inhaled bronchodilator within the past 2 hours, order nebulized **salbutamol, 2.5 to 5 mg,** in 3 mL of normal saline (NS) or **180 mcg (2 puffs)** by metered-dose inhaler, immediately.

Informing the Registered Nurse

Tell the registered nurse (RN), "I will arrive at the bedside in . . . minutes."

If a patient has shortness of breath, you must see the patient immediately.

ELEVATOR THOUGHTS

What causes shortness of breath?

1. Common cardiovascular causes
   a. CHF
   b. Pulmonary embolism
2. Common pulmonary causes
   a. Pneumonia
   b. Bronchospasm (asthma, COPD)
3. Miscellaneous causes
   a. Upper airway obstruction
   b. Anxiety
   c. Pneumothorax
   d. Massive pleural effusions
   e. Massive ascites
   f. Postoperative atelectasis
   g. Cardiac tamponade
   h. Aspiration of gastric contents
   i. Anxiety

MAJOR THREAT TO LIFE

- Upper airway obstruction

  Most causes of upper airway obstruction due to foreign bodies (e.g., aspiration) are immediately evident to the RN and manifested as choking, anxiety, and an inability to speak. Upper airway obstruction due to anaphylaxis may occur suddenly, progress rapidly, and end in death. Therefore your initial approach must be to determine whether there is evidence of present or impending upper airway obstruction.

- Hypoxia

  Inadequate tissue oxygenation is the most worrisome end result of any process causing shortness of breath. A second, simultaneous determination must be whether *hypoxia* is present.

BEDSIDE

Quick-Look Test

Does the patient look well (comfortable), sick (uncomfortable or distressed), or critical (about to die)?

This simple observation helps determine the necessity of immediate intervention. If the patient looks sick, ask the RN to bring the cardiac arrest cart to the bedside, attach the patient to the electrocardiographic (ECG) monitor, and prepare for possible intubation. Consult the intensive care unit (ICU) immediately. **Order arterial blood gas (ABG) measurements, O_2, and an intravenous line to keep the vein open.**

Airway and Vital Signs

Is the patient ventilating adequately?

To ventilate adequately, a patient must do two things: make adequate breathing efforts and have an open airway.

Is the patient making adequate breathing efforts?

If the patient is no longer breathing or is making inadequate breathing efforts, you must perform a head tilt–chin lift or a jaw-thrust maneuver to open the airway and begin ventilation with a bag-mask device.

Is the patient's airway open?

If the patient is making adequate breathing efforts (looks tachypneic, is agitated, and is struggling to breathe) but is not ventilating, suspect an upper airway obstruction. In the conscious patient there may be evidence of stridor, suggesting an obstruction to air inflow. In the hospitalized patient this may be a sign of anaphylaxis, even in the absence of hypotension, urticaria, or facial swelling. In an unconscious patient, such obstruction is more commonly due to prolapse of the tongue into the posterior pharynx, a situation that can be corrected with the head tilt–chin lift or jaw-thrust maneuver. Other causes of upper airway obstruction include a food bolus in the posterior pharynx, tracheal collapse resulting from loss of tone in the supporting muscles, and laryngospasm resulting from aspiration of oral secretions. These situations may necessitate a *finger sweep*, to clear the airway of foreign material; positive pressure ventilation with a bag-mask device; or endotracheal intubation.

What is the patient's respiratory rate?

Rates slower than 12 per minute are suggestive of a central nervous system depression of ventilation, which is usually caused by a stroke, narcotic overdose, or some other drug overdose. Rates faster than 20 per minute are suggestive of hypoxia, pain, or anxiety. Look also for thoracoabdominal dissociation, which may be a sign of impending respiratory failure. Remember that the chest cage and abdominal wall normally move in the same direction.

What is the patient's heart rate?

Sinus tachycardia is expected to accompany hypoxia. This is because vascular beds supplying hypoxic tissue dilate, and a compensatory sinus tachycardia occurs in an effort to increase cardiac output and thereby improve oxygen delivery.

What is the patient's temperature?

An elevated temperature is suggestive of infection (pneumonia, pyothorax, or bronchitis) but is also consistent with pulmonary embolism.

What is the patient's blood pressure (BP)?

Hypotension may be indicative of anaphylaxis, CHF, septic shock, massive pulmonary embolism, cardiac tamponade, or tension pneumothorax (see Chapter 18). If you suspect any of these conditions, call your resident for help. Also, measure the amount of pulsus paradoxus, which, in asthmatic patients, correlates approximately with the degree of airflow obstruction. Pulsus paradoxus also may be a clue to the presence of cardiac tamponade.

📖 Pulsus paradoxus is an inspiratory fall in systolic BP of more than 10 mm Hg. To determine whether a pulsus paradoxus is present, inflate the BP cuff 20 to 30 mm Hg above the palpable systolic BP. Deflate the cuff slowly. Initially, Korotkoff sounds are heard only in expiration. At some point during cuff deflation, Korotkoff sounds appear in inspiration as well. The number of millimeters of mercury between the initial appearance of Korotkoff sounds and their appearance throughout the respiratory cycle represents the degree of pulsus paradoxus (Fig. 24.1).

Selective Physical Examination

Is there evidence of present or impending upper airway obstruction?
   Is the patient hypoxic?

Vitals	Repeat measurements now; again, ensure airway patency.
Head, ears, eyes, nose, throat (HEENT)	Check for swelling of the face, lips, tongue, uvula, and neck and for urticaria (suggests possible anaphylaxis).
	Check for central cyanosis (blue tongue and mucous membranes).
	📖 Cyanosis often does not occur until hemoglobin desaturation is severe, and it may not occur at all in an anemic patient. If hypoxia is suspected, confirm by ABG measurement. Remember that cyanosis is a helpful sign only if it is present; its absence does not mean that the partial pressure of oxygen (Po_2) is adequate.
	Check that the trachea is in the midline.

Respiratory system	Are breath sounds present and of normal intensity?
	Check for stridor, wheezing, crackles, consolidation, or pleural effusion.
Neurologic system	Check the level of sensorium: is the patient alert, confused, drowsy, or unresponsive?

Management

What measure needs to be taken immediately to correct the upper airway obstruction?

If there is evidence of a foreign body, institute basic life support measures, including the Heimlich maneuver if appropriate.

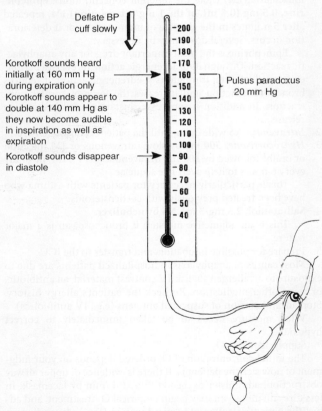

FIG. 24.1 **Determination of pulsus paradoxus.** *BP,* Blood pressure.

If there is no evidence of a foreign body, but air *entry* appears compromised, consider anaphylaxis. Call your resident and an anesthetist for help immediately. Treat rapidly, as follows:

1. Epinephrine

    Two strengths of epinephrine are available for injection. Make sure that you are using the correct strength.

    For profound anaphylaxis that is immediately life-threatening, use the intravenous route: **epinephrine, 1 mg (10 mL of the 0.1 mg/mL solution)**, administered every 3 to 5 minutes. Follow each dose with a 20-mL flush of NS, and elevate the arm for 10 to 20 seconds after each dose. See page 426 for alternative doses and routes.

    For less severe situations, epinephrine can be given intramuscularly (IM) (note the different concentration): **epinephrine, 0.5 mg (0.5 mL of the 1 mg/mL solution) IM**, repeated after 5 minutes in the absence of improvement or if deterioration occurs. Several doses may be necessary.

    Epinephrine is the most important drug for any anaphylactic reaction. Through its α-adrenergic action, it reverses peripheral vasodilatation; through its β-adrenergic action, it reduces bronchoconstriction and increases the force of cardiac contraction. In addition it suppresses histamine and leukotriene release.

2. *Intravenous NS* wide open until the patient is normotensive.

3. *Hydrocortisone, 500 mg* by slow intravenous or IM injection or orally, followed by 100 mg intravenously (IV), IM, or orally every 6 hours to help avert late sequelae.

    This is particularly necessary for patients with asthma who have been treated previously with corticosteroids.

4. **Salbutamol, 2.5 mg/3 mL NS by nebulizer**

    This is an adjunctive measure if bronchospasm is a major feature.

5. Prepare for possible intubation, and transfer to the ICU.

Most causes of anaphylaxis in hospitalized patients are due to exposure to an allergen such as IV contrast material, an antibiotic, or some other medication. Recheck the patient's allergy history. Stop administration of suspected antigens (e.g., IV antibiotics).

What measure needs to be taken immediately to correct hypoxia?

Supply adequate O_2.

The initial concentration of O_2 ordered depends on your judgment of how sick the patient is. If there is evidence of upper airway obstruction, administer oxygen at 8 to 10 L/min by facemask. In less dire situations you may begin empirical O_2 treatment, and adjust the patient's fraction of inspired oxygen (Fio_2), depending on the results of subsequent ABG measurements or pulse oximetry.

If pulse oximetry is available, gradually increase the FiO_2 until the O_2 saturation is higher than 94%; then recheck the ABG measurements. Remember that pulse oximetry tells you nothing about partial pressure of carbon dioxide (Pco_2), hydrogen ion concentration (pH), or alveolar-arterial oxygen ($A-aO_2$) gradient. In most cases, a Po_2 higher than 60 mm Hg or an O_2 saturation of 94% is adequate. Some patients with COPD chronically run O_2 saturations of 88% to 92%, and in these patients maintaining the O_2 saturation in the 90% to 92% range is sufficient.

What harm can your treatment cause?

Some patients with COPD retain CO_2 and are dependent on mild hypoxia to stimulate the respiratory center. An FiO_2 higher than 0.28 may remove this hypoxic drive to breathe. Unless the patient has ever had hypercarbia (check the patient's old chart), it is difficult to predict which patients with COPD retain CO_2. It is therefore prudent to assume that all patients with COPD and a history of heavy smoking retain CO_2 until proved otherwise.

📖 Administration of 100% O_2 can cause atelectasis or O_2 toxicity if continued over a period of days. This is of greater concern in a mechanically ventilated patient, because such FiO_2 levels are impossible to attain unless the patient is intubated.

Why is the patient short of breath or hypoxic?

Upper airway obstruction is not the most common cause of dyspnea in hospitalized patients, but if unrecognized, it may be the most rapidly fatal. Once this condition has been ruled out, direct your attention to the more common causes of shortness of breath encountered in hospitalized patients, of which there are primarily four:

- CHF (cardiovascular cause)
- Pulmonary embolism (cardiovascular cause)
- Pneumonia (pulmonary cause)
- Bronchospasm, as in asthma or COPD (pulmonary cause)

In most cases, it is easy to distinguish among these four conditions. Look for specific associated signs and symptoms (Table 24.1) to help you identify the cause of your patient's shortness of breath, and then treat the condition accordingly. Once you establish the cause, obtain a more thorough selective history and physical examination.

Cardiovascular Causes

CONGESTIVE HEART FAILURE

CHF refers to a clinical syndrome in which shortness of breath is caused by fluid in the pulmonary interstitium and alveolar spaces as a result of elevated left ventricular filling pressures. It is most often caused by left ventricular systolic dysfunction

TABLE 24.1	Discriminating Features in the History and Physical Examination of a Patient With Shortness of Breath

		Characterization		
Feature	CHF	Pulmonary Embolism and Infarction	Pneumonia	Asthma or COPD
History				
Onset	Gradual	Sudden	Gradual	Gradual
Other	Orthopnea	Risk factors (see page 293)	Cough Fever Sputum production	Previous history
Physical Examination				
Temperature	Normal	Normal or slightly elevated	High	Normal
Pulsus paradoxus	None	None	None	Yes
JVP	Elevated	Elevated or normal	Normal	Normal
S_3	Present	Occasional right ventricular S_3 present	Absent	Absent
Respiratory				
Crackles	Bibasal	Unilateral	Unilateral	None
Wheezes	May or may not be present	May or may not be present	May or may not be present	Present
Friction rub	None	May or may not be present	May or may not be present Consolidation	None
Other	—	Pleural effusions	Bronchial breath sounds Whispering pectoriloquy	—

CHF, Congestive heart failure; *COPD,* chronic obstructive pulmonary disease; *JVP,* jugulovenous pressure; *S_3,* third heart sound.

(so-called heart failure with reduced ejection fraction or HFrEF) or left ventricular diastolic dysfunction (so-called heart failure with preserved ejection fraction or HFpEF), but may also be seen with administration of excess IV fluids, severe hypertension, and renal failure. HFrEF and HFpEF can be differentiated by measurement of the left ventricular ejection fraction by echocardiography. However, treatment should not be delayed while awaiting an echocardiogram, as the initial steps are the same, that is, shifting the excess intravascular volume from the central veins.

Selective History

Does the patient have a history of CHF or cardiac disorder?
Does the patient have orthopnea?
Does the patient have paroxysmal nocturnal dyspnea?
Does the patient exhibit trends in daily weight or fluid balance records that heighten your suspicion of fluid retention and hence CHF?

Selective Physical Examination

Assess the patient's volume status. Does the patient have volume overload?

Vital signs	Tachycardia, tachypnea
HEENT	Elevated jugular venous pressure (JVP)
Respiratory system	Inspiratory crackles with or without pleural effusions (more often on the right side)
Cardiovascular system (CVS)	Cardiac apex displaced laterally
	S_3
	Systolic murmurs (aortic stenosis, mitral regurgitation, ventricular septal defect, tricuspid regurgitation)
	Diastolic murmur (aortic regurgitation)
Abdomen	Hepatomegaly with positive hepatojugular reflex (HJR)
Extremities	Presacral or ankle edema

Crackles and S_3 are the most reliable indication of left-sided heart failure, whereas elevated JVP, enlarged liver, positive HJR,

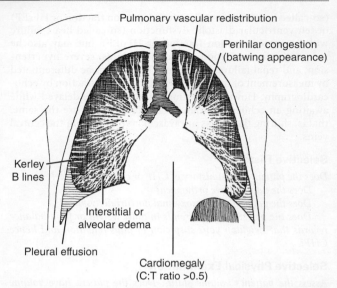

FIG. 24.2 **Diagram of radiographic features of congestive heart failure.** *C:T,* Chest-to-thorax.

and peripheral edema are indicative of right-sided heart failure. Although right-sided heart failure alone does not necessarily cause shortness of breath, it commonly accompanies left-sided heart failure and pulmonary disorders (cor pulmonale).

Other Investigations

Chest Radiography

A chest radiograph (Fig. 24.2) can reveal the following conditions:
- Cardiomegaly
- Perihilar congestion
- Bilateral interstitial infiltrates (early) or alveolar infiltrates (more advanced)
- Redistribution of pulmonary vascular markings
- Kerley B lines
- Pleural effusions

Bloodwork

Order CBC, electrolytes, and Mg levels. A brain natriuretic peptide (BNP) or N-terminal pro B-type natriuretic peptide (NT-proBNP) level is helpful if the diagnosis is uncertain.

Treatment

General Measures

- Insert an IV

    📖 Intravenous access is needed to deliver medications. Switch to saline lock when the acute episode has resolved.

- O_2
- Restricted-sodium (<2 to 3 g/day) and fluid (1.5 to 2 L/day) diet
- Bed rest
- **Low-molecular-weight heparin, Dalteparin 5000 U subcutaneous (SC) injection daily or unfractionated heparin (5000 U SC every 8 hours).**

    Patients with CHF are predisposed to venous thrombosis and pulmonary emboli and should receive prophylactic subcutaneous heparin while on bed rest.

- Fluid balance charting
- Daily weight

Specific Measures

POSITION

Ensure the patient is sitting up. This position pools blood in the legs.

DIURESIS

- Administer **furosemide, 40 mg IV over 2 to 5 minutes.** If no response (e.g., lessening of the symptoms and signs of CHF, diuresis) is achieved, double the dose every 1 to 2 hours (i.e., 40, 80, and then 160 mg) up to a total dose of about 400 mg. Larger initial doses (e.g., 80 to 120 mg) may be required if the patient has renal insufficiency, has severe CHF, or is already receiving furosemide for maintenance. Doses of furosemide that exceed 100 mg should be infused at a rate not exceeding 4 mg per minute, to avoid ototoxicity. Smaller initial doses (e.g., 10 mg) may suffice for frail elderly patients (aged 80 years and older). Alternative loop diuretics such as bumetanide (1 mg equivalent to 40 mg of furosemide) or torsemide (20 mg equivalent to 40 mg of furosemide) may be available in your institution but have no clear advantage over IV furosemide.
- The addition of a diuretic with a different site of action (e.g., a thiazide) may result in diuresis in patients who are resistant to furosemide alone.

    📖 The diuretics mentioned may cause hypokalemia, which is of particular concern in a patient receiving digitalis. Monitor the serum potassium level once or twice daily in the acute situation. High doses of these diuretics may also lead to serious sensorineural hearing loss, especially if the patient is also receiving other ototoxic agents, such as aminoglycoside antibiotics.

If diuretics are ineffective, it is unlikely that the patient will produce urine. Other methods of removing intravascular volume, such as phlebotomy (200 to 300 mL) and *rotating tourniquets,* are seldom required in the hospital setting. If bronchospasm persists (cardiac asthma), an inhaled β-agonist may improve oxygenation.

Digoxin is not of benefit acutely unless the CHF was precipitated by a bout of supraventricular tachycardia (e.g., atrial fibrillation or atrial flutter with rapid ventricular response rates), which can be slowed by digoxin. (Refer to Chapter 15 for the management of tachydysrhythmias.)

VASODILATORS

- Nitroglycerin, which is more of a venous than arterial dilator, may be used in patients with inadequate response to diuretics. Often IV nitroglycerin is required in a monitored setting. However as a temporary measure, you may administer **nitroglycerin ointment, 2.5 to 5 cm (1–2 inches) topically every 6 hours, or place a transdermal nitroglycerin patch**. If nitroglycerin ointment is not readily available, you can administer nitroglycerin tablets, 0.3 to 0.6 mg sublingually, or **nitroglycerin spray, 1 puff sublingually every 5 minutes,** until the patient feels less short of breath, as long as the systolic BP remains higher than 90 mm Hg. All nitroglycerin preparations cause blood to pool in the peripheral circulation. Nitroglycerin preparations commonly cause headaches, which can be treated with acetaminophen, 325 to 650 mg orally (PO) every 4 hours as needed. Nitrates are contraindicated if there has been recent ingestion of phosphodiesterase type-5 inhibitors (e.g., sildenafil, tadalafil, vardenafil, avanafil).
- Nitroprusside, a balanced venous and arterial dilator, should be considered in patients with CHF due to severe hypertension or acute mitral or aortic insufficiency. These patients must be monitored in an ICU setting.

DETERMINING THE CAUSE

After you have initiated treatment measures, determine why the patient developed CHF. If the patient has a history of CHF, the etiologic factor may already be identified in the patient's chart. Otherwise, an echocardiogram will help differentiate HFrEF from HFpEF and also provide specific clues to the etiology. Common causes of HFrEF include coronary artery disease, hypertension, viruses, alcohol, and rate-related cardiomyopathies due to atrial fibrillation or flutter. Common causes of HFpEF include coronary artery disease, hypertension, diabetes, hypertrophic obstructive cardiomyopathy, and restrictive cardiomyopathy.

Regardless of the underlying etiology of CHF, there is often a precipitating factor, of which the following 10 are most common:

1. Myocardial infarction or ischemia
2. Infection with fever
3. Dysrhythmia (commonly atrial fibrillation)
4. Pulmonary embolism
5. Increased sodium load (dietary, medicinal, parenteral)
6. Cardiac depressant drugs (e.g., β-blockers, disopyramide, calcium entry blockers)
7. Sodium-retaining agents (e.g., nonsteroidal anti-inflammatory drugs [NSAIDs])
8. Noncompliance with diet or medication regimen
9. Renal disease
10. Anemia

Document the suspected etiologic and precipitating factors in the patient's chart.

PULMONARY EMBOLISM

Positive findings on radiography depend on the presence of pulmonary infarction. An entirely normal chest radiograph in the setting of severe shortness of breath, however, is very suggestive of a pulmonary embolism.

The classic triad of shortness of breath, hemoptysis, and chest pain actually occurs in only a minority of cases. The best way to avoid missing this diagnosis is to consider it in every patient with shortness of breath.

Selective History

Look for predisposing causes.

Stasis

- Prolonged bed rest or hospitalization
- Immobilized limb (e.g., stroke)
- CHF
- Pregnancy (particularly during the postpartum period)

Vein Injury

- Lower extremity trauma
- Recent surgery (especially abdominal, pelvic, and orthopedic procedures)

Hypercoagulability

- Congenital or inherited (factor V Leiden, protein C or S deficiency, antithrombin III deficiency, G20210A prothrombin gene mutation, dysfibrinogenemia, hyperhomocysteinemia)
- Acquired (after orthopedic surgery; antiphospholipid antibody; from drugs, such as oral contraceptive or hormone replacement therapy, tamoxifen, raloxifene)
- Associated with systemic disease (malignancy, inflammatory bowel disease, nephrotic syndrome, polycythemia vera)
- Older age (>50 years)
- Obesity
- Prior episode of venous thromboembolism

Selective Physical Examination
Features suggestive of pulmonary embolism include the following:

- Pleural friction rub
- Pulmonary consolidation
- Unilateral or bilateral pleural effusion
- Sudden-onset cor pulmonale
- New-onset tachydysrhythmia
- Simultaneous deep vein thrombosis (DVT)

Determine the Pretest Probability

Most pulmonary emboli are due to venous thromboembolism arising in the deep veins of the pelvis or legs. Therefore, determining the pretest probability for a deep vein thrombosis can help identify which patients with shortness of breath may have suffered a pulmonary embolism. Several tools are available to determine the pretest probability. One is the Wells' Criteria for Pulmonary Embolism, which can be found online at mdcalc.com/calc/115/wells-criteria-pulmonary-embolism.

Other Investigations
Chest Radiography

If the patient is clinically stable, obtain upright posteroanterior and lateral chest radiographs (Fig. 24.3), rather than a portable chest radiograph, to ensure optimal imaging and prevent the masking of pleural fluid, which can occur when images are taken with the patient in the supine position. A chest radiograph may reveal the following abnormalities:

- Atelectasis (loss of volume)
- Unilateral wedge-shaped pulmonary infiltrate

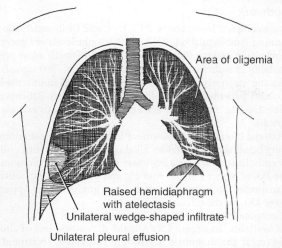

FIG. 24.3 **Diagram of variable radiographic features of pulmonary embolism.**

- Unilateral pleural effusion
- Raised hemidiaphragm
- Areas of oligemia
  A chest radiograph may also yield normal findings.

Electrocardiography

Only a massive pulmonary embolism causes the classic right ventricular strain pattern of S1, Q3, right-axis deviation, and right bundle branch block. The most common ECG finding is a *sinus tachycardia,* but other supraventricular tachycardias also may occur.

Ultrasound Studies

An echocardiogram may give important clues to the diagnosis if an urgent computed tomography pulmonary angiogram (CTPA) is unavailable. Findings suggestive of a pulmonary embolism include right ventricular dilatation and hypokinesis and an elevated pulmonary artery systolic pressure, although absence of these findings does not exclude the diagnosis. Similarly, positive findings of a deep venous thrombosis on lower limb ultrasonography makes the diagnosis of pulmonary embolism more likely, but a negative leg ultrasound does not exclude the diagnosis.

Bloodwork

Order a complete blood count, PTT, INR, and Cr in anticipation of beginning anticoagulation. BNP and troponin levels are generally not helpful in making the diagnosis. In patients with a low pretest probability of pulmonary embolism, a D-dimer <500 ng/mL excludes the diagnosis of pulmonary embolism, and in intermediate probability patients makes the diagnosis very unlikely. Patients with a value ≥500 ng/mL should have a CTPA to confirm or exclude the diagnosis.

Arterial blood gas measurement is helpful, the most common finding being acute respiratory alkalosis. Of patients with pulmonary embolism, 85% have a Po_2 lower than 80 mm Hg on room air. If the Po_2 is higher than 80 mm Hg and pulmonary embolism is still suspected, look for an elevated $A-Ao_2$ gradient. (See Appendix C, page 430, for the calculation.)

Computed tomography pulmonary angiogram

If available, an urgent CTPA is the diagnostic test of choice. However, if the diagnosis is strongly suspected, treatment for presumed pulmonary embolism should not be delayed while awaiting this test. A ventilation/perfusion (V/Q) scan may be helpful if the CTPA is unavailable, contraindicated, or inconclusive.

Management

Fibrinolytic Therapy

If you strongly suspect pulmonary embolism and the patient is persistently hypotensive, you should consider fibrinolytic therapy. In this case, call your resident immediately. The aim of fibrinolytic therapy is to dissolve the pulmonary embolism; **tissue plasminogen activator, 100 mg IV over 2 hours** is preferable to streptokinase because of its relatively rapid administration time. Pulmonary arteriotomy with embolectomy, when immediately available, may also be lifesaving.

Anticoagulation Therapy

If you strongly suspect pulmonary embolism and the patient is hemodynamically stable, you must begin anticoagulation therapy without further confirmation of the diagnosis. The aim of anticoagulation is not to dissolve the pulmonary embolism but rather to prevent further embolization from the site of venous thrombosis, which may prove fatal.

Before you order an anticoagulant, however, ensure that the patient has no active bleeding, no severe bleeding diathesis, a platelet count higher than 20,000/mm³, hasn't had an acute intracranial hemorrhage, recent major trauma, and hasn't had high-bleeding-risk surgery or is about to undergo emergency high-bleeding-risk surgery—these conditions are absolute contraindications to anticoagulation. Relative contraindications include brain or spinal tumors, large abdominal aortic aneurysms in the context of severe hypertension, stable aortic dissection, recurrent bleeding from gastrointestinal telangiectasias, and recent or planned emergency low-bleeding-risk surgery.

In patients with these relative contraindications, pulmonary embolism must be confirmed with CTPA or V/Q scan, or pulmonary angiography; if an embolism is documented, obtain consultation to consider interruption of the inferior vena cava by inserting a transvenous intracaval device.

If there are no contraindications, administer low-molecular-weight heparin (LMWH), e.g., Dalteparin 200 U/kg by deep SC injection once daily. Alternatively, **unfractionated heparin (UFH) at a dose of 80 U/kg by intravenous bolus (usual dose, 5000 to 10,000 U IV), followed by a maintenance infusion of 18 U/kg/ hour (maximum dose 2000 U/hour) may be used.**

📖 If used, **unfractionated heparin** should be delivered by infusion pump, as maintenance dosing: **for example 25,000 U/500 mL 5% dextrose in water (D5W) to run at 20 mL/hour, which is 1000 U/hour.** It is dangerous to put large doses of heparin in small-volume intravenous bags, because runaway intravenous bags filled with heparin can result in serious overdose.

📖 Anticoagulants are dangerous drugs because of their potential for causing bleeding disorders. Write and double-check your heparin orders carefully. Also, measure platelet counts once or twice a week to detect reversible heparin-induced thrombocytopenia, which may occur at any time while a patient is receiving heparin.

LMWH is a safe and effective alternative to intravenous unfractionated heparin in the treatment of patients with pulmonary embolism. The onset of action of IV UFH is immediate whereas that of LMWH SC is between 3 to 5 hours. Several formulations of LMWH exist, with different distributions of molecular weight, which result in differences in inhibitory activities against factor Xa and thrombin, the extent of plasma protein binding, and plasma half-lives. Familiarize yourself with the LMWH formulation used in your hospital. Also, be careful to note that the dose of LMWH used in the *treatment* of pulmonary embolism is considerably higher than that used for *prophylaxis* of DVT.

After heparin is started, obtain a CTPA as soon as possible to confirm the diagnosis of pulmonary embolism.

In patients receiving intravenous unfractionated heparin, monitor the aPTT every 4 to 6 hours, and adjust the heparin maintenance dose until the aPTT is in the therapeutic range (1.5 to

2.5 × normal level). After this, daily aPTT measurements are sufficient. Initial measurements of aPTT are made only to ensure adequate anticoagulation. Because of the more predictable anticoagulant response to LMWH, patients receiving this medication do not require monitoring of the aPTT.

If transitioning from unfractionated heparin to warfarin (Coumadin), add it on the first day, beginning at 10 mg PO and titrating the dose to achieve a prothrombin time with an international normalized ratio (INR) of 2.0 to 3.0 (this corresponds to a prothrombin time of 1.3 to 1.5 × control value, with rabbit brain thromboplastin; if you are unsure of the method used by your laboratory, call and ask). Attainment of a therapeutic INR usually takes 5 days, at which time heparin can be discontinued.

If transitioning from unfractionated heparin to LMWH, stop the UFH IV infusion and within 1 hour initiate LMWH SC.

If transitioning from UFH to a DOAC, stop the UFH heparin as soon as the first dose of DOAC is administered.

If transitioning from LMWH to warfarin, start warfarin and continue LMWH until INR is 2 to 3 on 2 consecutive days.

If transitioning from LMWH to a DOAC, begin the DOAC within 2 hours of the next scheduled dose of LMWH.

📖 Numerous drugs interfere with warfarin metabolism to increase or decrease the prothrombin time. Before you prescribe any drug to a patient receiving warfarin, ascertain its effect on warfarin metabolism, and monitor prothrombin time carefully if an interaction is anticipated. Metabolism of the DOACs is also influenced by many unrelated drugs; before prescribing a DOAC, review the patient's medication list to ensure that there are no potential interactions that might result in more or less anticoagulation than is desired.

📖 Except in unusual circumstances, a patient receiving heparin should receive no platelet inhibitors (e.g., aspirin, clopidogrel) or fibrinolytic agents and no intramuscular injections.

Ask your patient daily about signs of bleeding or bruising. Instruct your patient that prolonged pressure is required after venipuncture to prevent local bruising while the patient undergoes anticoagulation.

Pulmonary Causes

PNEUMONIA

Selective History and Physical Examination

Check for the presence of the following signs and symptoms:

- Cough: a cough productive of purulent sputum is typical; however, the cough may be dry in the early stages of pneumonia
- Fever, chills

- Pleuritic chest pain
- Pulmonary consolidation with or without pleural effusion

Other important information to check is whether the patient is immunocompromised.

Other Investigations
Complete Blood Count

A white blood cell count higher than 15,000/mm^3 is suggestive of a bacterial infection. Lower counts, however, do not preclude a bacterial cause of pneumonia. Lymphopenia (absolute lymphocyte count <1000/mm^3) or a low CD4 cell count (<200/mm^3) is suggestive of pneumonia in a patient infected with the human immunodeficiency virus (HIV).

Chest Radiography

Findings are variable, from patchy diffuse infiltrates to consolidation (pleural effusion). Remember that a patient with volume depletion may not manifest the typical findings of pneumonia on chest radiographs until the intravascular volume is restored to normal. Trust the findings of your clinical examination.

Identification of the Organism

1. Gram stain and culture of sputum. If the patient is unable to spontaneously cough up sputum, you can induce it with ultrasonic nebulization or chest physical therapy. Send a sputum sample to the laboratory for Gram stain. Confirm that the sputum is from the lower respiratory tract (<25 squamous epithelial cells per low-power field). (See Appendix C, page 431, for interpretation of the Gram stain.)
2. Special cultures if *Mycobacterium tuberculosis*, *Legionella* species, or fungi such as *Blastomyces dermatitidis* are suspected.
3. Nucleic acid amplification tests (polymerase chain reaction [PCR]) to determine the deoxyribonucleic acid (DNA) of *Legionella* species, *Mycoplasma pneumoniae*, influenza A and B, and other viruses, if they are available in your laboratory.
4. Urine test for *Legionella* antigen if Legionnaires' disease is strongly suspected.
5. Blood culture (× 2)
6. Blood for measurement of *Mycoplasma* immunoglobulin M
7. Thoracentesis: moderate-sized to large pleural effusions should be tapped to confirm or rule out empyema; pleural biopsy is necessary if tuberculosis is a consideration. Pleural fluid should be sent to the laboratory for the following:
   - Gram stain and aerobic and anaerobic cultures
   - Ziehl-Neelsen stain and tuberculosis cultures
   - Cell count and differential

- Lactate dehydrogenase level
- Protein level
- Glucose level
8. If the following studies are appropriate, request them:
   - Fungal cultures
   - pH measurement
   - Cytologic profile
   - Amylase measurement
   - Triglyceride measurements

Immediately after the pleural tap has been completed, a sample should be drawn to measure simultaneous serum glucose, protein, and lactate dehydrogenase levels. These serum determinations are necessary to compare with pleural fluid values in assessing whether the fluid is a transudate or exudate.

Always consider tuberculosis in your differential diagnosis. Order Ziehl-Neelsen stains and sputum for culture if tuberculosis is suspected.

Pneumocystis carinii is the most common cause of pneumonia in patients who are HIV-positive. This organism can occasionally be demonstrated by immunofluorescent staining of a sputum sample obtained by inducing sputum production, although bronchoalveolar lavage is the best method of confirming the diagnosis.

Management

General Measures

- O_2
- Chest physical therapy
- Antimicrobial agents

Your choice of treatment depends on the results of Gram stain or other available stains. However, in the absence of a definitive smear, the choice of antimicrobial agent should be based on the rapidity of progression, the severity of pneumonia, the presence of comorbid conditions, and your knowledge of local etiologic organisms and resistance patterns.

COMMUNITY-ACQUIRED PNEUMONIA

For community-acquired pneumonia in immunocompetent individuals that is severe enough to necessitate hospitalization, the probable causative bacteria include the following:

- *Streptococcus pneumoniae*
- Atypical agents (*M. pneumoniae, Chlamydia pneumoniae, Enterobacteriaceae, Legionella* species)
- *Hemophilus influenzae*

The sensitivities of respiratory pathogens to antibiotics vary partly in relation to the use of antibiotics. Knowledge of the local sensitivity patterns should aid in determining the drug selection. For a patient who has acquired pneumonia outside of the hospital, has no premorbid conditions, and is younger than 65 years, a useful choice is either of the following:

- **Amoxicillin 750 mg to 2 g PO or IV q8h**

  or

- **Doxycycline, 100 mg PO every 12 hours or 100 to 200 mg IV daily in one or two infusions**

📖 Because of the greater risk of resistant *S. pneumoniae*, a useful choice for individuals older than 65 years is **levofloxacin, 250 to 500 mg PO or IV daily.**

Viral causes are not uncommon (including human rhinovirus, influenza A and B, human metapneumonia virus, respiratory syncytial virus, parainfluenza virus, and adenovirus). Symptoms suggestive of this diagnosis include fever (usually high), extreme fatigue, headache, muscle aches, dry cough, and runny or stuffed nose.

Severely ill patients should be treated as soon as possible since the spread of the virus is rapid and the drugs lose their effectiveness. Timely treatment also helps curtail spread to others. Empiric treatment is recommended and should not be delayed until the results of diagnostic testing are available.

Current *influenza A and B* antivirals are listed in the Formulary.

COMPLEX PNEUMONIAS

For complex pneumonias (pneumonia complicating COPD, pneumonia acquired in hospitals or nursing homes, pneumonia in patients with previous antibiotic exposure), the following additional organisms may be present:

- Oral anaerobes
- Gram-negative bacilli
- *Staphylococcus aureus*

  A useful antibiotic choice in these situations is the following:

- **Ceftriaxone, 1 to 2 g IV daily, plus**
- **Levofloxacin, 250 to 500 mg PO or IV daily**

  If infection with multiple resistant gram-negative organisms or *Pseudomonas aeruginosa* is a consideration

- **Ceftaroline 600 mg IV q12h plus**
- **Levofloxacin, 250 to 500 mg PO or IV daily**

  If methicillin-resistant *S. aureus* is a risk, vancomycin or rifampin may be necessary.

ASPIRATION PNEUMONIA

Aspiration pneumonia should be considered in any situation in which the level of consciousness is decreased or the cough reflex is hampered (e.g., alcoholism, stroke, seizure, after surgery). Episodes of aspiration do not necessitate antibiotic treatment unless the patient has clinical signs of bacterial infection (e.g., fever, sputum production, leukocytosis).

PNEUMONIA IN ALCOHOLIC PATIENTS

Alcoholic patients, like patients with aspiration pneumonia, have a high frequency of *Klebsiella pneumoniae* infection. This should be treated with two drugs—usually a cephalosporin, such as **ceftazidime, 1 to 2 g IV every 8 hours**, and an aminoglycoside, such as **gentamicin, 5 to 7 mg/kg IV daily**—if renal function is normal. See Appendix for alternative antibiotics for pneumonia.

📖 Aminoglycosides can cause nephrotoxicity and ototoxicity. Avoid these side effects by monitoring serum aminoglycoside levels, usually after the third or fourth maintenance dose, and by monitoring serum creatinine levels. If the patient already has renal insufficiency, administer the same initial dose, but adjust the maintenance dose or interval according to the creatinine clearance (see Appendix C, page 430).

PNEUMONIA IN IMMUNOCOMPROMISED PATIENTS

In addition to the usual infecting organisms, uncommon infections should be considered in the immunocompromised patient with pneumonia. Conditions associated with neutropenia (e.g., chemotherapy, HIV/AIDS) predispose patients to infection with Gram-negative bacilli, *Staphylococcus aureus*, coagulase-negative staphylococcus, streptococci, and fungi. In patients with T-lymphocyte deficiency (e.g., HIV/AIDS, transplant recipients, glucocorticoids), organisms such as viruses, mycobacteria, fungi (e.g., Pneumocystis, Cryptococcus), and parasites (e.g., Strongyloides, Toxoplasma) should be considered. Patients with B-lymphocyte deficiency (e.g., multiple myeloma, leukemia, burns, glucocorticoids) are prone to infection with Salmonella, Campylobacter, and Giardia.

BRONCHOSPASM (ASTHMA AND CHRONIC OBSTRUCTIVE PULMONARY DISEASE)

Asthma is a condition characterized by airflow obstruction that varies significantly over time.

COPD may take the form of chronic bronchitis, which is a clinical diagnosis (production of mucoid sputum on most days for 3 months of the year in 2 consecutive years), or of emphysema, which is a pathologic diagnosis (enlargement of airways distal to the terminal bronchioles). Most patients with COPD have features of both.

Selective History

Does the patient smoke cigarettes?

Is the patient taking theophylline or steroids?

Has the patient ever required intubation?

Can precipitating factors (e.g., specific allergies, nonspecific irritants, upper respiratory tract infection, pneumonia, β-blocker administration) be identified?

Is the patient having an anaphylactic reaction?

Look for evidence of systemic autocoid (e.g., histamine) release: wheezing, itch (urticaria), and hypotension. Anaphylactic reactions in hospitalized patients occur most commonly after the administration of intravenous dye, penicillin, or aspirin. If anaphylaxis is suspected, refer immediately to Chapter 18, page 196, for appropriate management. This is an emergency!

Selective Physical Examination

Does the patient exhibit evidence of obstructive airway disease?

Vital Signs	Pulsus Paradoxus
HEENT	Cyanosis
	Elevated JVP (cor pulmonale):
	Cor pulmonale is defined as right-sided heart failure secondary to pulmonary disease.
	Position of trachea
	Pneumothorax may be a complication of asthma or COPD and results in a shift of the trachea away from the affected side.
Respiratory system	Intercostal indrawing
	Use of accessory muscles of respiration
	Increased anteroposterior diameter
	Hyperinflated lungs with depressed hemidiaphragms
	Wheezing
	Diffuse wheezing is most often a manifestation of asthma or COPD but may also be seen in CHF (cardiac asthma), pulmonary embolism, pneumonia, or anaphylactic reactions. Ensure that the patient has not undergone intravenous dye studies within the past 12 hours.
	Prolonged expiratory phase
CVS	Loud P_2
	Right ventricular heave, right ventricular S_3 (pulmonary hypertension, cor pulmonale)

Other Investigations

Chest Radiography

A chest radiograph may reveal the following:

- Hyperinflation of lung fields
- Flattened diaphragms
- Increased anteroposterior diameter
- Infiltrates (suggestive of concomitant pneumonia), atelectasis (suggestive of mucous plugging), pneumothorax, or pneumomediastinum

Spirometry

Spirometry provides an objective measurement of the severity of airflow limitation and is helpful in evaluating the efficacy of therapy in patients with mild to moderate asthma. Some patients with severe asthma are too unwell to be evaluated by spirometry. The common parameters followed are the forced expiratory volume in 1 second (FEV_1) and the peak expiratory flow rate. The results from the best of three attempts should be recorded.

Management

General Measures

- O_2
- Hydration
- Pulse oximetry monitoring

Specific Measures

STEP 1

Administer inhaled β_2 adrenergic agonists, such as **salbutamol, 2.5 to 5 mg, in 3 mL of NS by nebulizer or 180 mcg (2 puffs) by metered-dose inhaler every 4 hours**.

📖 When delivered properly (Box 24.1) under supervision, therapy delivered by a metered-dose inhaler is as effective as, and less expensive than, nebulizer treatments. If a patient is too dyspneic and distressed to coordinate the efforts necessary to allow effective delivery of a β_2 adrenergic agonist by metered-dose inhaler, nebulization of the drug may be preferable.

An anticholinergic agent, such as **ipratropium bromide, 250 to 500 mcg (1 to 2 mL) in 3 mL of NS by nebulizer**, may also improve oxygenation, but its ingestion should always be preceded or followed by an inhaled β-agonist because it occasionally worsens bronchoconstriction.

BOX 24.1	Technique for Inhalation of β_2 Agonists From Metered-Dose Inhalers

1. Shake the canister thoroughly.
2. Hold the mouthpiece of the inhaler 4 cm in front of the open mouth, or use a spacer between the inhaler and the mouth.
3. Breathe out slowly and completely.
4. Discharge the inhaler while taking a slow, deep breath (5–6 s).
5. Hold the breath at full inspiration for 10 s.

From Nelson, H. S. (1995). β-Adrenergic bronchodilators. *New England Journal of Medicine, 333,* 501.

Although standard dosing intervals for β-agonists are every 4 to 6 hours, they may be administered almost continuously in severe bronchospasm, as long as you watch closely for potential side effects (supraventricular tachycardias, premature ventricular contractions, muscle tremors).

STEP 2

Administer steroids (most useful in patients with pure asthma). In hospitalized patients, intravenous steroids have no advantage over oral steroids in hastening the resolution of bronchospasm. The optimal steroid preparation and dosage are controversial. However, because pure asthma is predominantly a response to airway inflammation, steroids should be used early in the management of exacerbations. In addition, steroids may take 6 hours to work, and so they must be administered immediately if persistent wheezing is anticipated in the next 6 to 24 hours. **Prednisone, 40 to 60 mg PO daily,** is recommended. If the patient is unable to swallow or absorb oral medications, **methylprednisolone, 125 mg IV, followed by 40 to 60 mg IV every 6 hours,** or **hydrocortisone, 500 mg as an intravenous bolus, followed by a maintenance dose of 100 mg IV every 6 hours,** may be administered. Beclomethasone dipropionate (Beclovent) is not useful in acute bronchospasm.

Steroids have few side effects in the short-term situation. Sodium retention is of concern in a patient with CHF or hypertension; hyperglycemia may occur in diabetic patients.

Tapering steroids too rapidly has been a concern. A person who has taken steroids for less than 2 weeks, however, can discontinue taking the steroids abruptly without fear of steroid withdrawal. Of more concern is exacerbation of wheezing as steroids are tapered. This may limit the rate at which steroids can be withdrawn.

STEP 3

In patients whose asthma remains severe after an hour of intensive step 1 and 2 therapy, a single dose of **magnesium sulfate 2 g IV** given over 20 minutes may be helpful.

IV magnesium acts as a bronchodilator in acute asthma. Its use is contraindicated in the presence of renal insufficiency, because of the risk of hypermagnesemia.

When a patient develops an exacerbation of bronchospasm, a general rule is to administer medications *beyond* what is usually required for an outpatient. For example, a patient in whom asthma is normally controlled with a salbutamol inhaler at home probably requires more frequent inhaled β-agonist with or without ipratropium, as well as steroids, during an exacerbation. If a patient with COPD is wheezing despite outpatient treatment with a β-agonist and a theophylline preparation, or if the patient is already taking a small dose of prednisone, he or she should be given higher doses of prednisone during the acute attack. Theophylline preparations do not produce more bronchodilation than that achieved by β_2 adrenergic agonists in patients with acute severe asthma and are no longer recommended.

Look for evidence of bronchitis or pneumonia as the precipitant of bronchospasm. In patients so affected, bronchospasm may persist until appropriate antibiotics are administered.

Five Warnings in Asthma

1. Sudden acute deterioration in an asthmatic patient may represent a *pneumothorax*.
2. Patients with an acute attack of asthma hyperventilate, and the Pco_2 rises. A *normal Pco_2* of 40 mm Hg in the acute situation may signify impending respiratory failure.
3. *Disappearance of wheezing* in the acute situation is an ominous sign, indicating that the patient is not moving sufficient air in and out to generate a wheeze.
4. *Sedatives are contraindicated in asthma and COPD.* The RN may not be aware of this and may unknowingly request a sleeping aid for such patients while you are off duty. To avoid this pitfall, write clearly in your orders, "No sedatives or sleeping pills."
5. Some asthmatic patients have a triad of asthma, nasal polyps, and aspirin sensitivity. When you prescribe analgesics for asthmatic patients, it is best to *avoid NSAIDs,* including aspirin, because fatal anaphylactoid reactions have occurred in some patients who are given these medications.

Respiratory Failure

Any of the four conditions causing shortness of breath may lead to respiratory failure, as may various other conditions. Suspect that this is occurring if the respiratory rate is lower than 12 per minute or if thoracoabdominal dissociation is present. Confirm the diagnosis of acute respiratory failure by ABG determination. A Po_2 lower than 60 mm Hg or a Pco_2 higher than 50 mm Hg with a pH lower than 7.30 while the patient is breathing room air is an indication of *acute respiratory failure*.

1. Ensure that the patient has not received narcotic analgesics in the past 24 hours, which may depress the respiratory rate. Pupillary constriction may provide a clue that a narcotic is the culprit. If a narcotic has been administered or if you are uncertain, order **naloxone hydrochloride, 0.2 to 2 mg IV**, immediately. Naloxone is also available by nasal spray as Narcan 2 mg or 4 mg or higher dose Kloxxado 8 mg.

2. If the patient does not respond to naloxone, arrange for the patient's transfer to the ICU/cardiac care unit. Acute respiratory acidosis with a pH lower than 7.30 may respond to aggressive treatment of the underlying respiratory or neuromuscular disorder. Noninvasive pressure support ventilation delivered by facemask may be useful for acute exacerbations of COPD (if the respiratory rate >30/minute and the pH <7.35) and may prevent the need for intubation. However, if improvement is not rapid, make arrangements for possible endotracheal intubation. Acute respiratory acidosis with a pH lower than 7.20 usually necessitates mechanical ventilation until the precipitating cause of respiratory deterioration can be reversed.

REMEMBER

1. Abdominal problems can masquerade as shortness of breath. (In one of our cases, a patient's shortness of breath resolved as soon as urinary retention was relieved by placement of a Foley catheter; 1300 mL of urine was drained.) Massive ascites and obesity may also compromise respiratory function.

2. Do not worry about your inexperience with endotracheal intubation. A patient in respiratory failure can be bagged and masked effectively until someone with intubation experience is available to assist you.

3. Notice that *epinephrine* does not appear in the protocol for the treatment of asthma. There is no need to use epinephrine in an adult with an attack of asthma or COPD unless bronchospasm is a component of an anaphylactic reaction.

Epinephrine administered inadvertently in cases of cardiac asthma has resulted in fatal myocardial infarction.

4. An occasional patient has shortness of breath as a manifestation of anxiety. In this instance, shortness of breath is often qualitatively unique, in that the patient describes "shortness of the *deep* breath," with the sensation that he or she cannot get a satisfactory deep breath. Sighing and yawning are common accompaniments.

Skin Rashes and Urticaria

Reading this chapter will not transform you into a dermatologist, able to diagnose any rash with one quick glance. It will, however, help you accurately describe rashes you are asked to examine while you are on call at night. This ability will facilitate confirmation of the diagnosis in the morning by more experienced physicians. You may be called because a rash has appeared abruptly (e.g., drug reaction) or because a patient has been admitted with a rash and the nursing staff is concerned that it may be infectious (e.g., scabies or lice). Urticarial rashes are rare in hospitalized patients; however, they are important to recognize because they may be the prodrome of anaphylactic shock.

PHONE CALL

Questions

1. How long has the patient had the rash?

   If the rash appeared abruptly, a drug reaction is the most likely cause.

2. Is any urticaria (hives) present?

   Urticaria is often the first sign of an impending anaphylactic reaction. Urticaria of the central part of the face is a common manifestation of angioedema.

3. Does the patient have any facial swelling, audible wheezing, or shortness of breath?

   These features are suggestive of impending airway obstruction.

4. What are the patient's vital signs?

5. What drugs has the patient received within the past 12 hours? Has the patient received blood products or intravenous (IV) contrast material within the past 12 hours?

   Remember that patients undergoing computed tomography (CT) and magnetic resonance imaging (MRI) scans are often given IV contrast material.

6. Does the patient have any known allergies?
7. Why was the patient admitted?

Orders

If the patient has evidence of anaphylaxis or angioedema (urticaria, wheezing, shortness of breath, or hypotension), ask the registered nurse (RN) to bring the following to the patient's bedside:
1. IV line, to be started immediately with normal saline
2. **Epinephrine, 1 mg (10 mL of the 0.1 mg/mL solution) for IV administration**. For less severe situations, **epinephrine, 0.5 mg intramuscularly (0.5 mL of the 1 mg/mL solution)**, can be given. Note the different concentrations and different routes of administration.

Informing the Registered Nurse

Tell the RN, "I will arrive at the bedside in . . . minutes."

If a patient exhibits evidence of facial urticaria (which may be the first manifestation of angioedema) or of anaphylaxis (urticaria, wheezing, shortness of breath, or hypotension), you must see the patient immediately. Also, if the rash is acute and the patient has been or is receiving systemic medication, blood, or IV contrast material, you must see the patient immediately. Assessment of a rash with no associated symptoms of anaphylaxis can wait an hour or two if you have patients with higher priority problems.

ELEVATOR THOUGHTS

What causes skin rashes?

The majority of calls at night regarding acute-onset skin rashes involve drug reactions. The lesions may be urticarial and are occasionally associated with life-threatening anaphylaxis. Other drug reactions can have widely varied morphologic features but are usually symmetric and often start on the buttocks. Early drug reactions are often localized.
1. Urticaria (rare but life-threatening)
   a. Drugs
      i. IV contrast material
      ii. Opiates (codeine, morphine, meperidine)
      iii. Antibiotics (penicillins, cephalosporins, sulfonamides, tetracycline, quinine, polymyxin, isoniazid)
      iv. Anesthetic agents (curare)
      v. Angiotensin-converting enzyme (ACE) inhibitors (captopril, enalapril, lisinopril, fosinopril)
      vi. Aspirin and other nonsteroidal anti-inflammatory drugs (NSAIDs)
   b. Blood transfusion reaction

    c. Food allergies, especially to nuts, fruits, tomatoes, lobster, shrimp

    d. Physical urticaria: cold, heat, pressure, vibration

2. Erythematous maculopapular (morbilliform) rashes

    a. Antibiotics (penicillin, ampicillin, sulfonamides, chloramphenicol)

        📖 Ampicillin commonly causes a generalized maculopapular eruption 2 to 4 weeks after administration of the first dose; thus, it is important to check not only the current drugs the patient is receiving but also all recently discontinued drugs, because the eruption may appear several weeks after the patient has stopped taking the drug. A rash associated with β-lactam antibiotics often has a raised papular component.

    b. Antiretroviral agents (nelfinavir, abacavir, didanosine, stavudine)

        📖 Severe allergic reactions consisting of fever, rash, nausea, vomiting, diarrhea, and abdominal pain have been reported in 3% to 5% of people who take abacavir.

    c. Antihistamines

    d. Antidepressants (amitriptyline)

    e. Diuretics (thiazides)

    f. Oral hypoglycemic agents

    g. Anti-inflammatory agents (gold, phenylbutazone)

    h. Sedatives (barbiturates)

    i. Sulfonamides (usually morbilliform)

    j. Delavirdine, nevirapine, efavirenz

    k. Scabies and lice

        📖 Lice and mites (the organisms that cause scabies) commonly produce excoriated papules. The lesions of scabies are usually present on the finger webs, wrists, waist, axillae, areolae, genitals, and feet. Lesions from lice may occur anywhere on the body but are common on the scalp, pubic area, neck, flanks, waistline, and axillae. Infestation with both organisms is associated with intense itching.

    l. Drug reaction with eosinophilia and systemic symptoms (DRESS)

A rare condition that that can be life-threatening. The diffuse erythematous rash is accompanied by systemic involvement including fever, lymphadenopathy, flu-like symptoms, and liver and kidney damage (anticonvulsants, allopurinol, abavir, minocycline, sulfasalazine, proton pump inhibitors).

Viral infections—for example, monkeypox

3. Vesicobullous rashes

    a. Antibiotics (sulfonamides, dapsone)

    b. Anti-inflammatory drugs (penicillamine)

   c. Sedatives (barbiturates)

   d. Halogens (iodides, bromides)

   e. Herpes zoster

   f. Toxic epidermal necrolysis and Stevens-Johnson syndrome (sulfonamides, allopurinol)

   g. Viral infections—for example, monkeypox

4. Purpura

📖 Drug-induced thrombocytopenia causes nonpalpable purpura, whereas vasculitis causes palpable purpura.

   a. Antibiotics (sulfonamides, chloramphenicol)

   b. Diuretics (thiazides)

   c. Anti-inflammatory drugs (phenylbutazone, indomethacin, salicylates)

   d. Coronavirus vaccine (Johnson and Johnson)

5. Exfoliative (skin shedding) rashes = erythroderma

📖 If a drug eruption is not recognized early and the drug is not discontinued, the patient may develop mucosal erosions and profound skin injury, with blistering and extensive loss of epidermis (Stevens-Johnson syndrome or toxic epidermal necrolysis).

   a. Antibiotics (sulfa derivatives, co-trimoxazole, penicillins, streptomycin, isoniazid)

   b. Anti-inflammatory drugs (phenylbutazone, piroxicam)

   c. Antiseizure medication (carbamazepine, phenytoin)

   d. Sedatives or anxiolytics (barbiturates, chlormezanone)

   e. Miscellaneous (allopurinol, chloroquine)

6. Fixed drug eruption

📖 Certain drugs may produce a skin lesion in a specific area. Repeated administration of the drug causes the skin lesion to reappear in the same location. The lesion is usually composed of dusky red patches distributed over the trunk or proximal limbs.

   a. Antibiotics (sulfonamides, metronidazole)

   b. Anti-inflammatory drugs (phenylbutazone)

   c. Analgesics (phenacetin)

   d. Sedatives (barbiturates, chlordiazepoxide)

   e. Laxatives (phenolphthalein)

   f. Viral infections—for example, monkeypox

MAJOR THREAT TO LIFE

- Upper airway obstruction as a result of angioedema
- Anaphylactic shock
- (Drug reaction with eosinophilia and systemic symptoms—DRESS)
- Toxic epidermal necrolysis

Urticarial skin rash may be a prodrome of *angioedema* or *anaphylaxis,* whereas other types of skin rashes are not. Drugs and IV contrast material are the usual causes of anaphylactic shock in hospitalized patients, except in cases of wasp stings or eating shrimp.

DRESS syndrome is characterized by a maculopapular eruption that may coalesce, along with fever, lymphadenopathy, eosinophilia, neutrophilia, and atypical lymphocytosis, along with internal organ involvement including liver involvement, interstitial nephritis, interstitial pneumonia, and myocarditis.

The skin of a patient with toxic *epidermal necrolysis* looks scalded, with peeling of the outer surface. Frequently, fever is difficult to control. If you suspect DRESS syndrome or toxic epidermal necrolysis, call for a dermatologic consultation immediately. Drugs commonly involved in the DRESS syndrome and toxic epidermal necrolysis include allopurinol, sulfonamides, and anticonvulsants. With *toxic shock syndrome* (see page 199) and *necrotizing fasciitis* (see page 210), the patient is more ill or complains of more local pain than you would expect from objective signs. Obtain a dermatologic or infectious disease consultation immediately.

BEDSIDE

Quick-Look Test

Does the patient look well (comfortable), sick (uncomfortable or distressed), or critical (about to die)?

Patients with upper airway obstruction as a result of angioedema and those with anaphylactic reactions look apprehensive, usually have shortness of breath, and are sitting upright in bed.

Airway and Vital Signs

What is the patient's respiratory rate?

Tachypnea, particularly if associated with audible stridor or wheezing, is an ominous sign. Inspiratory stridor is suggestive of impending obstruction of the upper airway. Notify your resident and an anesthetist immediately.

What is the patient's blood pressure?

Hypotension is a sign of impending or established anaphylactic shock, and the patient requires immediate treatment. If anaphylaxis is suspected, insert a large-bore IV line (size 16 if possible), if this has not already been done, and run normal saline in as fast as possible.

What is the patient's temperature?

Skin rashes are often more prominent when the patient is febrile.

Selective Physical Examination

Does the patient show evidence of an impending anaphylactic reaction?

Head, ears, eyes, nose, throat (HEENT)	Tongue, pharyngeal, or facial edema (angioedema)
Respiratory system	Wheezing (anaphylaxis)
	If evidence of an impending anaphylactic reaction exists, refer to page 310 for immediate treatment.
Skin	If an urticarial rash resulting from angioedema or anaphylaxis has been ruled out, provide an accurate description of the rash to establish the diagnosis or to help someone else make a diagnosis if the rash disappears or changes by morning; with the patient's consent, a photograph of the rash using a smartphone may also be helpful.

Where is the rash located?

Is it generalized, acral (hands, feet), or localized? Remember to examine the patient's buttocks, a common site for the onset of drug eruptions.

What color is the rash?

It may be red, pink, brown, or white.

What does the primary lesion look like?

See Fig. 25.1.

- *Macule:* flat (noticeable from the surrounding skin because of the color difference)
- *Patch:* a large macule
- *Papule:* solid, elevated, smaller than 1 cm
- *Plaque:* solid, elevated, larger than 1 cm
- *Vesicle:* elevated, well circumscribed, smaller than 1 cm
- *Bulla:* elevated, well circumscribed, larger than 1 cm
- *Nodule:* deep-seated mass, indistinct borders, smaller than 0.5 cm in both width and depth
- *Cyst:* nodule filled with expressible fluid or semisolid material
- *Wheal (hives):* well-circumscribed, flat-topped, firm elevation (papule, plaque, or dermal edema) with or without central pallor and irregular borders
- *Petechia:* red or purple nonblanchable macule, smaller than 3 mm
- *Purpura:* red or purple nonblanchable macule or papule, larger than 3 mm

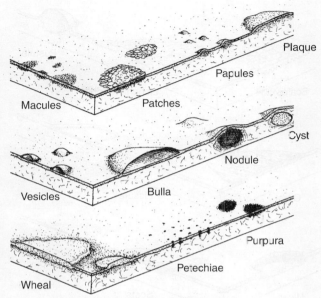

FIG. 25.1 **Primary skin lesions.**

What does the secondary lesion look like? (Fig. 25.2)
- *Scale:* dry, thin plate of thickened keratin layers (white color differentiates it from crust)
- *Lichenification:* dry, leathery thickening; shiny surface; accentuated skin markings
- *Pustule:* vesicle containing purulent exudate
- *Crust:* dried, yellow exudate of plasma (result of broken vesicle, bulla, or pustule)
- *Fissure:* linear, epidermal tear
- *Erosion:* wide, epidermal fissure; moist and well circumscribed
- *Ulcer:* erosion into the dermis
- *Scar:* flat, raised, or depressed area of fibrosis
- *Atrophy:* depression secondary to thinning of the skin
  What is the configuration of the rash?
- *Annular:* circular
- *Linear:* in lines
- *Grouped:* in clusters, such as the vesicular lesions of herpes zoster or herpes simplex

Selective History and Chart Review
- How long has the rash been present?
- Does it itch?

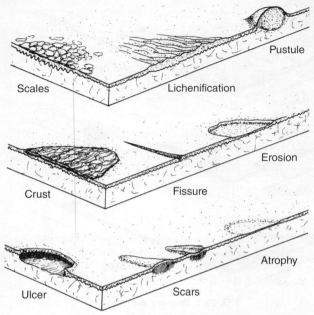

FIG. 25.2 **Secondary skin lesions.**

- How has it been treated?
- Is it a new or a recurrent problem?
- Which drugs was the patient receiving before the rash started?

Management

1. In patients with DRESS or toxic epidermal necrolysis, the suspected offending drug should be discontinued. In severe DRESS involving the lungs or kidneys, management with oral glucocorticoids – prednisone 0.5 to 1.0 mg/kg/day – may be helpful. Glucocorticoids are not helpful in patients with toxic epidermal necrolysis.
2. If the rash is associated with urticaria and is thought to be secondary to a drug reaction, the drug should be withheld until the diagnosis is confirmed in the morning.
3. Seemingly minor nonurticarial maculopapular rashes are occasionally the initial manifestation of a more serious reaction, such as toxic epidermal necrolysis. Ideally, if the rash is thought to be a drug reaction, the offending drug should be stopped. If the offending medication is essential to the patient's

management overnight, a suitable alternative may be chosen. If no suitable alternative exists, the decision to stop or continue the offending medication must be made with the help of your resident or attending physician.

4. When the skin rash is not a drug eruption and the diagnosis is clear, the standard recommended treatment can be instituted. (Refer to a dermatology text for specific treatment.)

5. Often, house staff have difficulty diagnosing skin rashes with confidence. If you are uncertain, it is often sufficient to describe the lesion accurately and refer the patient to a dermatologist in the morning. Several important exceptions exist:

   a. A *petechial rash* is suggestive of a disorder of platelet number or function; a *purpuric rash* may be indicative of a coagulation disorder. Measurements of activated partial thromboplastin time and prothrombin time and platelet studies should be ordered when appropriate.

   b. *Herpes zoster* in an immunocompromised patient (e.g., one with AIDS) may necessitate urgent treatment because of the risk of systemic dissemination, especially to the central nervous system. If you suspect herpes zoster (manifesting initially as erythematous macules and papules in a dermatomal distribution and progressing to grouped vesicles and hemorrhagic crusts) in an immunocompromised patient, consult your resident or attending physician for possible treatment with IV acyclovir.

   c. Patients with hereditary *deficiency of protein* C may develop skin necrosis, typically 3 to 5 days after beginning warfarin therapy. The skin lesions usually begin as painful red plaques overlying areas of fat. In these cases, warfarin must be stopped immediately, its effect reversed with vitamin K, and heparin substituted as an anticoagulant.

Stroke

As patients age, they accumulate *morbid conditions,* some of which may not be evident at the time of admission. The most common of these is atherosclerosis, which often manifests in the coronary and cerebrovascular circulations. Stroke is a common reason for hospital admission, but a stroke may also occur as an unexpected event in a hospitalized patient whose reason for admission may not be remotely neurologic. With the more prevalent use of fibrinolytic agents and endovascular thrombectomy for acute stroke, the physician on call must be familiar with the pathophysiologic features and treatment of acute stroke. You might receive information such as "I think Mr. Jones has had a stroke," but you are more likely to be given information such as "Mr. Jones is less responsive than usual"; "Mr. Jones is not moving his right side"; or "Mr. Jones' speech is slurred."

PHONE CALL

Questions

1. What are the patient's symptoms?
2. For how long has the patient had symptoms?

    The time of stroke onset is defined as when the patient was last symptom free. For patients who are unable to provide this information or who awaken with stroke symptoms, the time of onset is defined as when the patient was last awake and symptom free.

    A stroke onset of more than 4.5 hours ago is a contraindication to fibrinolytic therapy.

3. What are the patient's vital signs?
4. What is the patient's blood glucose level?

    A finger-prick blood glucose test should be performed immediately, because hypoglycemic symptoms may mimic stroke, and hypoglycemia is a readily reversible disorder.

5. Is the patient taking anticoagulants?

    An intracerebral hemorrhage should be considered in any patient receiving anticoagulants.

6. Why was the patient admitted?

Orders

1. Intravenous line in place
2. Complete blood cell count, platelet count, and measurements of partial thromboplastin time, international normalized ratio (INR), glucose level, electrolyte levels, creatinine level, troponin level, and creatine phosphokinase level
3. Electrocardiography
4. Pulse oximetry

Informing the Registered Nurse

Tell the registered nurse (RN), "I will arrive at the bedside in … minutes."

Stroke is a medical emergency, and recombinant tissue plasminogen activator (rt-PA) (tenecteplase or alteplase), when administered within 3 hours after the onset of symptoms, has beneficial effects against acute ischemic stroke and may be of some benefit in selected patients up to 4.5 hours after the onset of symptoms. As is the case with thrombolytic therapy for myocardial infarction, the sooner the agent can be given, the more potential benefit. Accordingly, a patient with a disabling stroke must be examined immediately to determine eligibility for treatment with intravenous rt-PA.

ELEVATOR THOUGHTS

You should consider five questions on your way to the patient's bedside:
1. Is the patient receiving oxygen therapy properly, and is the patient hemodynamically stable?
2. Is the event a stroke? (Is the patient truly having a stroke, or are the patient's symptoms caused by a stroke mimicker?)
3. If the event is a stroke, is it an *acute ischemic stroke?*
4. If the event is an acute ischemic stroke, is the patient *eligible for fibrinolytic therapy?*
5. If the patient is eligible for fibrinolytic therapy, how is this most safely accomplished?

These five questions help organize and direct your approach to evaluating and managing a possible stroke.

MAJOR THREAT TO LIFE

Stroke may result in compromise of the airway and abnormalities in heart rate, heart rhythm, and blood pressure (BP). The predominant threat to the patient, however, is a potentially devastating loss of quality of life if neurologic deterioration continues untreated.

BEDSIDE

Is the patient oxygenating properly, and hemodynamically stable?

Vital Signs

Blood pressure (BP)	High BP is common in the first hours after a stroke; causes include preexisting hypertension, stress, a full bladder, nausea, pain, hypoxia, and increased intracranial pressure.
Heart rate (HR)	Atrial fibrillation is the most common arrhythmia seen in the setting of stroke and may be either a cause or a complication of stroke.
Respiratory system and pulse oximetry	The most common causes of hypoxia are airway obstruction, hypoventilation, aspiration pneumonia, and atelectasis.
Temperature	Fever may be secondary to a cause of stroke (e.g., endocarditis) or a complication of stroke (e.g., pneumonia).

Seizure Assessment

New-onset seizures at the time of the stroke should be treated with a short-acting agent such as lorazepam 4 mg IV if the seizure is not self-limited.

If the patient is properly oxygenated and is hemodynamically stable, then you must consider the next questions:

Is the event a stroke? Is the patient truly having a stroke, or are the patient's symptoms caused by a stroke mimicker?

The latter question is particularly important because a fibrinolytic agent administered to a patient with a *stroke mimicker* would be inappropriate and potentially harmful.

A stroke is caused by obstruction or damage to an artery or vein, or to bleeding in the brain, which results in a cerebral infarction. Stroke is usually manifested by a neurologic deficit of *abrupt* onset.

Warning signs of a stroke include the following:

- *Weakness:* sudden weakness, numbness, or tingling in the face, an arm, or a leg
- *Trouble speaking:* sudden temporary loss of speech or trouble understanding speech
- *Vision problems:* sudden loss of vision, particularly in one eye, or double vision
- *Headaches:* sudden severe and unusual headache
- *Dizziness:* sudden loss of balance, especially with any of the signs just listed

In *acute stroke*, you particularly need to know whether the patient has undergone an abrupt interruption of vascular supply to a specific brain region *as a result of a thrombus*. You need the answer to this question because rt-PA can reduce morbidity and mortality if given early in this situation.

There are other causes of stroke, with other pathophysiologic mechanisms, for which a fibrinolytic agent is not indicated. There are also conditions that *mimic* stroke, for which a fibrinolytic agent would also be inappropriate. Box 26.1 lists the common causes of strokes and stroke mimickers.

In determining whether the patient has had a stroke for which rt-PA should be considered, it is best to look at two main patterns of stroke involvement:

1. A *carotid artery stroke* usually results in one or more of the following: a hemiparesis, a hemianopsia, numbness or tingling in the face or one hand, and dysphasia or agnosia.
2. A *vertebrobasilar stroke* usually produces weakness or clumsiness, causes numbness on half of the body, and is often accompanied by cranial nerve and brain stem signs (e.g., double vision, vertigo, slurring of speech).

In this situation, it is not necessary to perform a meticulous hour-long neurologic examination involving pinprick and vibration sensing. At this point, look for obvious signs of stroke: trouble speaking or understanding, obvious *asymmetry* of the facial muscles (smile/grimace) or grip, *asymmetry* of arm and leg strength, and lack of coordination. If the patient does not have any of these abnormalities, the diagnosis of stroke is doubtful.

Once you have made the presumptive diagnosis of stroke, it is important to **call** your senior house staff or neurologist for help. This is necessary so that urgent arrangements can be set in motion (depending on the hospital, these may include calling in personnel involved with computed tomographic [CT] scanning, notifying an acute stroke team, arranging transfer to a stroke unit, and so forth), should the patient qualify for fibrinolytic therapy or thrombectomy. In the meantime, you can help by performing a more detailed physical examination to assess the severity of the stroke. This examination and its questions are specifically formulated to help you fill out the National Institutes of Health Stroke Scale (NIHSS). The stroke scale items should be administered in the order listed. Table 26.1 is an abbreviated version of the NIHSS.

This is also a good time to listen to the carotid arteries (for bruits), the heart (for aortic regurgitation murmur, which might raise the suspicion of an aortic dissection), and the lungs (for congestive heart failure).

If the event is a stroke, is it an acute ischemic stroke?

This question is best answered through brain imaging, particularly to determine whether the stroke is ischemic or hemorrhagic.

| BOX 26.1 | Causes of Strokes and Stroke Mimickers |

Ischemic Strokes
Lacunar Stroke
In situ cerebral thrombosis in small vessels (usual causes: hypertension, diabetes)

Occlusive Stroke
Embolism
- Carotid arterial thromboembolism
- Cardiogenic embolism
- Thromboembolism (e.g., left atrial thrombus in atrial fibrillation, left ventricular thrombus in cardiomyopathy, tumor embolism from left atrial myxoma, paradoxic embolism through a patent foramen ovale)
  Endocarditis
  Vasculitis
  Dissection

Hemorrhagic Strokes
Intracerebral Hemorrhage
Hypertensive hemorrhage
  Ruptured arteriovenous malformation
  Ruptured cavernous angioma
  Intratumor hemorrhage
  Embolism
  Vasculitis

Subarachnoid Hemorrhage
Ruptured saccular aneurysm
Trauma

Subdural and Epidural Hemorrhage
Trauma
Anticoagulant therapy

Stroke Mimickers
Hypoglycemia (look for a history of diabetes, low blood glucose levels, decreased level of consciousness) or severe *hyperglycemia*
  Complicated migraine (look for a history of similar events, headaches with aura)
  Postictal paralysis (look for a history of seizures or a witnessed seizure)
  Hypertensive encephalopathy (look for headache, delirium, significant hypertension, evidence of cerebral edema)
  Conversion disorder (look for a psychiatric history, neurologic findings that do not correspond to a vascular distribution, lack of cranial nerve findings)
  Meningitis/encephalitis
  Lower motor neuron facial nerve palsy (e.g., Bell palsy, trauma, tumor, infection)
  Spinal cord compression or inflammation (e.g., tumor, disk prolapse, infection, multiple sclerosis, vasculitis)

TABLE 26.1	National Institutes of Health Stroke Scale (Abbreviated Version)	

Tested Item	Title	Responses and Scores
1A	Level of consciousness	0—Alert 1—Drowsy 2—Obtunded 3—Coma/unresponsive
1B	Orientation questions (2)	0—Answers both correctly 1—Answers one correctly 2—Answers neither correctly
1C	Response to commands (2)	0—Performs both tasks correctly 1—Performs one task correctly 2—Performs neither
2	Gaze	0—Normal horizontal movements 1—Partial gaze palsy 2—Complete gaze palsy
3	Visual fields	0—No visual field defect 1—Partial hemianopia 2—Complete hemianopia 3—Bilateral hemianopia
4	Facial movement	0—Normal 1—Minor facial weakness 2—Partial facial weakness 3—Complete unilateral palsy
5	Motor function (arm) Left Right	0—No drift 1—Drift before 5 s 2—Falls before 10 s 3—No effort against gravity 4—No movement
6	Motor function (leg) Left Right	0—No drift 1—Drift before 5 s 2—Falls before 5 s 3—No effort against gravity 4—No movement
7	Limb ataxia	0—No ataxia 1—Ataxia in 1 limb 2—Ataxia in 2 limbs
8	Sensory	0—No sensory loss 1—Mild sensory loss 2—Severe sensory loss
9	Language	0—Normal 1—Mild aphasia 2—Severe aphasia 3—Mute or global aphasia

Continued

TABLE 26.1	National Institutes of Health Stroke Scale (Abbreviated Version)—cont'd	
Tested Item	**Title**	**Responses and Scores**
10	Articulation	0—Normal 1—Mild dysarthria 2—Severe dysarthria
11	Extinction or inattention	0—Absent 1—Mild (loss 1 sensory modality) 2—Severe (loss 2 modalities)

The type of brain imaging used will depend on local expertise and availability of emergency imaging techniques. Your hospital should already have imaging protocols in place for patients with acute ischemic stroke. Commonly this includes a non-contrast CT scan and a CT angiogram. The non-contrast CT scan is performed to rule out a hemorrhagic stroke. A normal non-contrast CT scan, particularly if performed soon after symptom onset, is common, and does not exclude an ischemic stroke. A CT angiogram can determine whether there is a large vessel occlusion, in which case thrombectomy may be indicated. This is important, as thrombectomy may be helpful for patients with large vessel occlusion up to 24 hours after symptom onset. More advanced imaging, such as a CT perfusion scan or MRI with diffusion and flare sequencing, helps determine how much brain tissue is infarcted and how much is salvageable. This is particularly useful in patients with symptom onset beyond 4.5 hours to determine whether they are candidates for late thrombolysis (up to 9 hours post-stroke in selected patients) or thrombectomy (up to 24 hours post-stroke in selected patients). If the non-contrast CT scan supports an acute *ischemic infarct,* the patient should be considered for fibrinolytic therapy immediately. If the scan is normal, the patient may nonetheless be having an acute ischemic stroke (particularly when the CT scan is obtained soon after the patient's symptoms begin and if the infarct is small).

Blood work should include electrolytes, glucose, CBC, INR, PTT, and creatinine. Depending on the history and physical exam, other blood work may include a toxicology screen, measurements of blood alcohol level, arterial blood gases, and a pregnancy test.

If the event is an acute ischemic stroke, is the patient eligible for fibrinolytic therapy?

Assess inclusion and exclusion criteria. The eligibility requirements for thrombolytic therapy in patients with acute ischemic stroke have become more individual specific and take into account the patient's age, time of symptom onset, stroke severity, stroke territory, history of diabetes or previous stroke, use of anticoagulants, and other factors. Since time is of the essence, it's critical to immediately involve your hospital's stroke team in this assessment.

Box 26.2 lists inclusion and exclusion criteria from the American Heart Association/American Stroke Association.

Management

If the patient is eligible for fibrinolytic therapy, how is this most safely accomplished?

If, after completion of this checklist, the patient is considered a candidate for thrombolytic therapy, and if your hospital has a stroke protocol or policy involving administration of a thrombolytic agent, then you should notify the appropriate personnel immediately. Strict adherence to the Stroke Council of the American Stroke Association/American Heart Association Guidelines (2019) is recommended. If a fibrinolytic agent is indicated, do not wait for the results of the bloodwork to administer it.

The recommended dosage of **rt-PA for patients weighing less than 100 kg is a total dose of 0.9 mg/kg, with 10% (0.09 mg/kg) given as an intravenous bolus over 1 minute and the remaining 90% (0.81 mg/kg) given as an intravenous infusion over 60 minutes.** For patients weighing more than 100 kg, load with 9 mg (10% of 90 mg) as an intravenous (IV) bolus over 1 minute, followed by 81 mg (90% of 90 mg) as a continuous infusion over 60 minutes. An alternative to r-tPA is **tenecteplase (TNKase) 0.25 mg/kg IV over 5 seconds (maximum total dose 25 mg)**; its advantage, unlike r-tPA, is that it can be given as a single bolus without a continuous infusion and it is less expensive.

Endovascular therapy is a potential alternative for patients who are ineligible for intravenous thrombolysis or have failed in recanalizing the occluded artery. Such neurointerventional approaches may offer higher recanalization rates than intravenous thrombolysis.

If your hospital does not have the resources or institutional commitment to safely administer alteplase or tenecteplase to victims of acute ischemic stroke or undertake more invasive interventions, but if it is possible to quickly and safely transfer the patient to an acute stroke facility with the necessary experience, then you should immediately organize such transfer.

If your hospital is not equipped to safely administer alteplase or tenecteplase, and there is no chance of urgently transferring the patient to an acute stroke facility, then the management of the acute stroke is largely supportive. In this case, your focus is on nonfibrinolytic measures to limit irreversible cerebral damage.

BOX 26.2	Eligibility Recommendations for IV Alteplase in Patients With AIS

Indications (COR I)

Within 3 h*	IV alteplase (0.9 mg/kg, maximum dose 90 mg over 60 min with initial 10% of dose given as bolus over 1 min) is recommended for selected patients who may be treated within 3 h of ischemic stroke symptom onset or patient last known well or at baseline state. Physicians should review the criteria outlined in this table to determine patient eligibility.[†] (COR I; LOE A)
Within 3 h-Age	For otherwise medically eligible patients ≥18 y of age, IV alteplase administration within 3 h is equally recommended for patients ≤80 and >80 y of age.[†] (COR I; LOE A)
Within 3 h-Severe stroke	For severe stroke, IV alteplase is indicated within 3 h from symptom onset of ischemic stroke. Despite increased risk of hemorrhagic transformation, there is still proven clinical benefit for patients with severe stroke symptoms.[†] (COR I; LOE A)
Within 3 h-Mild disabling stroke	For otherwise eligible patients with mild but disabling stroke symptoms, IV alteplase is recommended for patients who can be treated within 3 h of ischemic stroke symptom onset or patient last known well or at baseline state (COR;LOE B-R)[‡]
3-4.5 h*	IV alteplase (0.9 mg/kg, maximum dose 90 mg over 60 min with initial 10% of dose given as bolus over 1 min) is also recommended for selected patients who can be treated within 3 and 4.5 h of ischemic stroke symptom onset or patient last known well. Physicians should review the criteria outlined in this table to determine patient eligibility.[†] (COR I; LOE B-R)[§]
3-4.5 h-Age	IV alteplase treatment in the 3- to 4.5-h time window is recommended for those patients ≤80 y of age, without a history of both diabetes mellitus and prior stroke, NIHSS score ≤25, not taking any OACs, and without imaging evidence of ischemic injury involving more than one-third of the MCA territory.[†] (COR I; LOE B-R)[§]
Urgency	Treatment should be initiated as quickly as possible within the above-listed time frames because time to treatment is strongly associated with outcomes.[†] (COR I; LOEA)

BOX 26.2	Eligibility Recommendations for IV Alteplase in Patients With AI—cont'd

BP	IV alteplase is recommended in patients with BP <185/110 mmHg and in those patients whose BP can be lowered safely to this level with antihypertensive agents, with the physician assessing the stability of the BP before starting IV alteplase.[†] (COR I; LOE B-NR)[§]
Blood glucose	IV alteplase is recommended in otherwise eligible patients with initial glucose levels >50 mg/dL.[†] (COR I; LOE A)
CT	IV alteplase administration is recommended in the setting of early ischemic changes on NCCT of mild to moderate extent (other than frank hypodensity).[†] (COR I; LOE A)
Prior antiplatelet therapy	IV alteplase is recommended for patients taking antiplatelet drug monotherapy before stroke on the basis of evidence that the benefit of alteplase outweighs a possible small increased risk of sICH.[†] (COR I; LOE A)
	IV alteplase is recommended for patients taking antiplatelet drug combination therapy (e.g., aspirin and clopidogrel) before stroke on the basis of evidence that the benefit of alteplase outweighs a probable increased risk of sICH.[†] (COR I; LOE B-NR)[§]
End-stage renal disease	In patients with end-stage renal disease on hemodialysis and normal aPTT, IV alteplase is recommended.[†] (COR I; LOE C-LD)[§] However, those with elevated aPTT may have elevated risk for hemorrhagic complications.
Additional Recommendations for Treatment With IV Alteplase for Patients With AIS (COR IIa)	**And (COR IIb)**
3-4.5 h-Age	For patients >80 y of age presenting in the 3- to 4.5-h window, IV alteplase is safe and can be as effective as in younger patients.[†] (COR IIa; LOE B-NR)[§]
3-4.5 h-Diabetes mellitus and prior stroke	In AIS patients with prior stroke and diabetes mellitus presenting in the 3- to 4.5-h window, IV alteplase may be as effective as treatment in the 0- to 3-h window and may be a reasonable option.[†] (COR IIb; LOE B-NR)[§]

Continued

BOX 26.2	Eligibility Recommendations§ for IV Alteplase in Patients With AI—cont'd

3-4.5 h-Severe stroke	The benefit of IV alteplase between 3 and 4.5 h from symptom onset for patients with very severe stroke symptoms (NIHSS score >25) is uncertain.[†] *(COR IIb; LOE C-LD)*§
3-4.5 h-Mild disabling stroke	For otherwise eligible patients with mild disabling stroke, IV alteplase may be reasonable for patients who can be treated within 3 and 4.5 h of ischemic stroke symptom onset or patient last known well or at baseline state. *(COR IIb; LOE B-NR)*[‡]
Wake-up and unknown time of onset	IV alteplase (0.9 mg/kg, maximum dose 90 mg over 60 min with initial 10% of dose given as bolus over 1 min) administered within 4.5 h of stroke symptom recognition can be beneficial in patients with AIS who awake with stroke symptoms or have unclear time of onset >4.5 h from last known well or at baseline state and who have a DW-MRI lesion smaller than one-third of the MCA territory and no visible signal change on FLAIR. *(COR IIa; LOE B-R)*[‡]
Preexisting disability	Preexisting disability does not seem to independently increase the risk of sICH after IV alteplase, but it may be associated with less neurological improvement and higher mortality. Therapy with IV alteplase for acute stroke patients with preexisting disability (mRS score ≥2) may be reasonable, but decisions should take into account relevant factors, including quality of life, social support, place of residence, need for a caregiver, patients' and families' preferences, and goals of care.[†] *(COR IIb; LOE B-NR)*§
	Patients with preexisting dementia may benefit from IV alteplase. Individual considerations such as life expectancy and premorbid level of function are important to determine whether alteplase may offer a clinically meaningful benefit.[†] *(COR IIb; LOE B-NR)*§
Early improvement	IV alteplase treatment is reasonable for patients who present with moderate to severe ischemic stroke and demonstrate early improvement but remain moderately impaired and potentially disabled in the judgment of the examiner.[†] *(COR IIa; LOE A)*
Seizure at onset	IV alteplase is reasonable in patients with a seizure at the time of onset of acute stroke if evidence suggests that residual impairments are secondary to stroke and not a postictal phenomenon.[†] *(COR IIa; LOE C-LD)*§

BOX 26.2	Eligibility Recommendations for IV Alteplase in Patients With AI—cont'd

Blood glucose	Treatment with IV alteplase in patients with AIS who present with initial glucose levels <50 or >400 mg/dL that are subsequently normalized and who are otherwise eligible may be reasonable. (Recommendation modified from 2015 IV Alteplase to conform to text of 2015 IV Alteplase. [*COR IIb; LOE C-LD*])§
Coagulopathy	IV alteplase may be reasonable in patients who have a history of warfarin use and an INR ≤1.7 or a PT <15 s.† (*COR IIb; LOE B-NR*)§
	The safety and efficacy of IV alteplase for acute stroke patients with a clinical history of potential bleeding diathesis or coagulopathy are unknown. IV alteplase may be considered on a case-by-case basis.† (*COR IIb; LOE C-EO*)§
Dural puncture	IV alteplase may be considered for patients who present with AIS, even in instances when they may have undergone a lumbar dural puncture in the preceding 7 d.† (*COR IIb; LOE C-EO*)§
Arterial puncture	The safety and efficacy of administering IV alteplase to acute stroke patients who have had an arterial puncture of a noncompressible blood vessel in the 7 d preceding stroke symptoms are uncertain.† (*COR IIb; LOE C-LD*)§
Recent major trauma	In AIS patients with recent major trauma (within 14 d) not involving the head, IV alteplase may be carefully considered, with the risks of bleeding from injuries related to the trauma weighed against the severity and potential disability from ischemic stroke. (Recommendation modified from 2015 IV Alteplase to specify that it does not apply to head trauma. [*COR IIb; LOE C-LD*])§
Recent major surgery	Use of IV alteplase in carefully selected patients presenting with AIS who have undergone a major surgery in the preceding 14 d may be considered, but the potential increased risk of surgical site hemorrhage should be weighed against the anticipated benefits of reduced stroke related neurological deficits.† (*COR IIb; LOE C-LD*)§
GI and genitourinary bleeding	Reported literature details a low bleeding risk with IV alteplase administration in the setting of past GI/genitourinary bleeding. Administration of IV alteplase in this patient population may be reasonable.† (*COR IIb; LOE C-LD*)§ (Note: Alteplase administration within 21 d of a GI bleeding event is not recommended; see Contraindications.)

Continued

BOX 26.2	Eligibility Recommendations for IV Alteplase in Patients With AI—cont'd

Menstruation	IV alteplase is probably indicated in women who are menstruating who present with AIS and do not have a history of menorrhagia. However women should be warned that alteplase treatment could increase the degree of menstrual flow.[†] *(COR IIa; LOE C-EO)*[§]
	When there is a history of recent or active vaginal bleeding causing clinically significant anemia, then emergency consultation with a gynecologist is probably indicated before a decision about IV alteplase is made.[†] *(COR IIa; LOE C-EO)*[§]
	Because the potential benefits of IV alteplase probably outweigh the risks of serious bleeding in patients with recent or active history of menorrhagia without clinically significant anemia or hypotension, IV alteplase administration may be considered.[†] *(COR IIb; LOE C-LD)*[§]
Extracranial cervical dissections	IV alteplase in AIS known or suspected to be associated with extracranial cervical arterial dissection is reasonably safe within 4.5 h and probably recommended.[†] *(COR IIa; LOE C-LD)*[§]
Intracranial arterial dissection	IV alteplase usefulness and hemorrhagic risk in AIS known or suspected to be associated with intracranial arterial dissection remain unknown, uncertain, and not well established.[†] *(COR IIb; LOE C-LD)*[§]
Unruptured intracranial aneurysm	For patients presenting with AIS who are known to harbor a small or moderate-sized (<10 mm) unruptured and unsecured intracranial aneurysm, administration of IV alteplase is reasonable and probably recommended.[†] *(COR IIa; LOE C-LD)*[§]
	Usefulness and risk of IV alteplase in patients with AIS who harbor a giant unruptured and unsecured intracranial aneurysm are not well established.[†] *(COR IIb; LOE C-LD)*[§]
Intracranial vascular malformations	For patients presenting with AIS who are known to harbor an unruptured and untreated intracranial vascular malformation the usefulness and risks of administration of IV alteplase are not well established.[†] *(COR IIb; LOE C-LD)*[§]
	Because of the increased risk of ICH in this population of patients, IV alteplase may be considered in patients with stroke with severe neurological deficits and a high likelihood of morbidity and mortality to outweigh the anticipated risk of ICH.[†] *(COR IIb; LOE C-LD)*[§]

BOX 26.2	Eligibility Recommendations for IV Alteplase in Patients With AI—cont'd

CMBs
> In otherwise eligible patients who have previously had a small number (1–10) of CMBs demonstrated on MRI, administration of IV alteplase is reasonable. *(COR IIa; Level B-NR)*[‡]
>
> In otherwise eligible patients who have previously had a high burden of CMBs (>10) demonstrated on MRI, treatment with IV alteplase may be associated with an increased risk of sICH, and the benefits of treatment are uncertain. Treatment may be reasonable if there is the potential for substantial benefit. *(COR IIb; Level B-NR)*[‡]

Concomitant tirofiban, eptifibatide
> The efficacy of the IV glycoprotein IIb/II a inhibitors tirofiban and eptifibatide coadministered with IV alteplase is not well established. *(COR IIb; Level B-NR)*[‡]

Extra-axial intracranial neoplasms
> IV alteplase treatment is probably recommended for patients with AIS who harbor an extra-axial intracranial neoplasm. *(COR IIa; LOE C-EO)*[§]

Acute MI
> For patients presenting with concurrent AIS and acute MI, treatment with IV alteplase at the dose appropriate for cerebral ischemia, followed by percutaneous coronary angioplasty and stenting if indicated, is reasonable.[†] *(COR IIa; LOE C-EO)*[§]

Recent MI
> For patients presenting with AIS and a history of recent MI in the past 3 mo, treating the ischemic stroke with IV alteplase is reasonable if the recent MI was non-STEMI.[†] *(COR IIa; LOE C-LD)*[§]
>
> For patients presenting with AIS and a history of recent MI in the past 3 mo, treating the ischemic stroke with IV alteplase reasonable f the recent MI was a STEMI involving the right or inferior myocardium.[†] *(COR IIa; LOE C-LD)*[§]
>
> For patients presenting with AIS and a history of recent MI in the past 3 mo, treating the ischemic stroke with IV alteplase may be reasonable if the recent MI was a STEMI involving the left anterior myocardium.[†] *(COR IIb; LOE C-LD)*[§]

Acute pericarditis
> For patients with major AIS likely to produce severe disability and acute pericarditis, treatment with IV alteplase may be reasonable[†] *(COR IIb; LOE C-EO)*[§]; urgent consultation with a cardiologist is recommended in this situation.

Continued

BOX 26.2	Eligibility Recommendations for IV Alteplase in Patients With AI—cont'd

	For patients presenting with moderate AIS likely to produce mild disability and acute pericarditis, treatment with IV alteplase is of uncertain net benefit.[†] (COR IIb; LOE C-EO)[§]
Left atrial or ventricular thrombus	For patients with major AIS likely to produce severe disability and known left atrial or ventricular thrombus, treatment with IV alteplase may be reasonable.[†] (COR IIb; LOE C-LD)[§]
	For patients presenting with moderate AIS likely to produce mild disability and known left atrial or ventricular thrombus, treatment with IV alteplase is of uncertain net benefit.[†] (COR IIb; LOE C-LD)[§]
Other cardiac diseases	For patients with major AIS likely to produce severe disability and cardiac myxoma, treatment with IV alteplase may be reasonable.[†] (COR IIb; LOE C-LD)[§]
	For patients presenting with major AIS likely to produce severe disability and papillary fibro-elastoma, treatment with IV alteplase may be reasonable.[†] (COR IIb; LOE C-LD)[§]
Procedural stroke	IV alteplase is reasonable for the treatment of AIS complications of cardiac or cerebral angiographic procedures, depending on the usual eligibility criteria.[†] (COR IIa; LOE A)[§]
Systemic malignancy	The safety and efficacy of IV alteplase in patients with current malignancy are not well established.[†] (COR IIb; LOE C-LD)[§] Patients with systemic malignancy and reasonable (>6 mo) life expectancy may benefit from IV alteplase if other contraindications such as coagulation abnormalities, recent surgery, or systemic bleeding do not coexist.
Pregnancy	IV alteplase administration may be considered in pregnancy when the anticipated benefits of treating moderate or severe stroke outweigh the anticipated increased risks of uterine bleeding.[†] (COR IIb; LOE C-LD)[§]
	The safety and efficacy of IV alteplase in the early postpartum period (<14 d after delivery) have not been well established.[†] (COR IIb; LOE C-LD)[§]
Ophthalmological conditions	Use of IV alteplase in patients presenting with AIS who have a history of diabetic hemorrhagic retinopathy or other hemorrhagic ophthalmic conditions is reasonable to recommend, but the potential increased risk of visual loss should be weighed against the anticipated benefits of reduced stroke-related neurological deficits.[†] (COR IIa; LOE B-NR)[§]

BOX 26.2	Eligibility Recommendations for IV Alteplase in Patients With AI—cont'd

Sickle cell disease	IV alteplase for adults presenting with an AIS with known sickle cell disease can be beneficial.[†] (COR IIa; LOE B-NR)[‡]
Hyperdense MCA sign	In patients with a hyperdense MCA sign, IV alteplase can be beneficial.[†] (COR IIa, LOE B-NR)[‡]
Illicit drug use	Treating clinicians should be aware that illicit drug use may be a contributing factor to incident stroke. IV alteplase is reasonable in instances of illicit drug use–associated AIS in patients with no other exclusions.[†] (COR IIa; LOE C-LD)[§]
Stroke mimics	The risk of symptomatic intracranial hemorrhage in the stroke mimic population is quite low; thus, starting IV alteplase is probably recommended in preference over delaying treatment to pursue additional diagnostic studies.[†] (COR IIa: LOE B-NR)[§]
Contraindications (COR III: No Benefit)	**And (COR III: Harm)**
0- to 3-h window-Mild nondisabling stroke	For otherwise eligible patients with mild nondisabling stroke (NIHSS score 0-5), IV alteplase is not recommended for patients who could be treated within 3 h of ischemic stroke symptom onset or patient last known well or at baseline state. (COR III: No Benefit, LOE B-R)[‡]
3- to 4.5-h window-Mild nondisabling stroke	For otherwise eligible patients with mild nondisabling stroke (NIHSS score 0-5), IV alteplase is not recommended for patients who could be treated within 3 and 4.5 h of ischemic stroke symptom onset or patient last known well or at baseline state. (COR III: No Benefit, LOE C-LD)[‡]
CT	There remains insufficient evidence to identify a threshold of hypoattenuation severity or extent that affects treatment response to alteplase. However, administering IV alteplase to patients whose CT brain imaging exhibits extensive regions of clear hypoattenuation is not recommended. These patients have a poor prognosis despite IV alteplase, and severe hypoattenuation defined as obvious hypodensity represents irreversible injury.[†] (COR III: No Benefit; LOE A)[‖]
ICH	IV alteplase should not be administered to a patient whose CT reveals an acute intracranial hemorrhage.[†] (COR III: Harm; LOE C-EO)[§]
Ischemic stroke within 3 mo	Use of IV alteplase in patients presenting with AIS who have had a prior ischemic stroke within 3 mo may be harmful.[†] (COR III: Harm; LOE B-NR)[§,‖]

Continued

BOX 26.2	Eligibility Recommendations for IV Alteplase in Patients With AI—cont'd

Severe head trauma within 3 mo	In AIS patients with recent severe head trauma (within 3 mo), IV alteplase is contraindicated.† *(COR III: Harm; LOE C-EO)*§,‖
Acute head trauma	Given the possibility of bleeding complications from the underlying severe head trauma, IV alteplase should not be administered in posttraumatic infarction that occurs during the acute in-hospital phase.† *(COR III: Harm; LOE C-EO)*§,‖(Recommendation wording modified to match COR III stratifications.)
Intracranial/intraspinal surgery within 3 mo	For patients with AIS and a history of intracranial/spinal surgery within the prior 3 mo, IV alteplase is potentially harmful.† *(COR III: Harm; LOE C-EO)*§,‖
History of intracranial hemorrhage	IV alteplase administration in patients who have a history of intracranial hemorrhage is potentially harmful.† *(COR III: Harm;*LOE C-EO)§,‖
Subarachnoid hemorrhage	IV alteplase is contraindicated in patients presenting with symptoms and signs most consistent with an SAH.† *(COR III:Harm; LOE C-EO)*§,‖
GI malignancy or GI bleed within 21 d	Patients with a structural GI malignancy or recent bleeding event within 21 d of their stroke event should be considered high risk, and IV alteplase administration is potentially harmful.† *(COR III: Harm; LOE C-EO)*§,‖
Coagulopathy	The safety and efficacy of IV alteplase for acute stroke patients with platelets <100,000/mm³, INR >1.7, aPTT >40 S, or PT >15 S are unknown, and IV alteplase should not be administered.† *(COR III: Harm; LOE C-EO)*§,‖ (In patients without history of thrombocytopenia, treatment with IV alteplase can be initiated before availability of platelet count but should be discontinued if platelet count is <100,000/mm³. In patients without recent use of OACs or heparin treatment with IV, alteplase can be initiated before availability of coagulation test results but should be discontinued if INR is >1.7 or PT is abnormally elevated by local laboratory standards.) (Recommendation wording modified to match COR III stratifications.)
LMWH	IV alteplase should not be administered to patients who have received a full treatment dose of LMWH within the previous 24 h.† *(COR III: Harm; LOE B-NR)*§,‡ (Recommendation wording modified to match COR III stratifications.)

BOX 26.2	Eligibility Recommendations for IV Alteplase in Patients With AI—cont'd

Thrombin inhibitors or factor Xa inhibitors	The use of IV alteplase in patients taking direct thrombin inhibitors or direct factor Xa inhibitors has not been firmly established but may be harmful.[†] (COR III Harm; LOE C-EO)[§,ǁ] IV alteplase should not be administered to patients taking direct thrombin inhibitors or direct factor Xa inhibitors unless laboratory tests such as aPTT, INR, platelet count, ecarin clotting time, thrombin time, or appropriate direct factor Xa activity assays are normal or the patient has not received a dose of these agents for >48 h (assuming normal renal metabolizing function). (Alteplase could be considered when appropriate laboratory tests such as aPTT, INR, ecarin clotting time, thrombin time, or direct factor Xa activity assays are normal or when the patient has not taken a dose of these ACs for >48 h and renal function is normal.) (Recommendation wording modified to match COR III stratifications.)
Concomitant abciximab	Abciximab should not be administered concurrently with IV alteplase. (COR III: Harm; LOE B-R)[‡]
Concomitant IV aspirin	IV aspirin should not be administered within 90 min after the start of IV alteplase. (COR III: Harm; LOE B-R)[‡]
Infective endocarditis	For patients with AIS and symptoms consistent with infective endocarditis, treatment with IV alteplase should not be administered because of the increased risk of intracranial hemorrhage.[†] (COR III Harm; LOE C-LD)[§,ǁ] (Recommendation wording modified to match COR III stratifications.)
Aortic arch dissection	IV alteplase in AIS known or suspected to be associated with aortic arch dissection is potentially harmful and should not be administered.[†] (COR III: Harm; LOE C-EO)[§,ǁ] (Recommendation wording modified to match COR III stratifications.)
Intra-axial intracranial neoplasm	IV alteplase treatment for patients with AIS who harbor an intra-axial intracranial neoplasm is potentially harmful.[†] (COR III: Harm; LOE C-EO)[§,ǁ]

Unless otherwise specified, these eligibility recommendations apply to patients who can be treated within 0-4.5 hours of ischemic stroke symptom onset or patient last known well or at baseline state.

Clinicians should also be informed of the indications and contraindications from local regulatory agencies (for current information from the US Food and Drug Administration refer to http://www.accessdata.fda.gov/drugsatfda_docs/tabel/2015/103172s5203lbl.pal).

For a detailed discussion of this topic and evidence supporting these recommendations, refer to the American Heart Association (AHA) scientific statement on the rationale for inclusion and exclusion criteria for IV alteplase in AIS.

AC indicates anticoagulants; AIS, acute ischemic stroke; aPTT, activated partial thromboplastin time; BP, blood pressure; CMB, cerebral microbleed; COR, class of recommendation; CT, computed tomography; DW-MRI, diffusion-weighted magnetic resonance imaging; FLAIR, fluid-attenuated inversion recovery; GI, gastrointestinal; ICH, intracerebral hemorrhage; INR, international normalized ratio; IV, intravenous; LMWH, low-molecular-weight heparin; LOE, level of evidence; MCA, middle cerebral artery; MI, myocardial infarction; MRI, magnetic resonance imaging; mRS, modified Rankin Scale; NCCT, noncontrast computed tomography; NIHSS, National Institutes of Health Stroke Scale; OAC, oral anticoagulant; PT, prothromboplastin time; sICH, symptomatic intracerebral hemorrhage; and STEMI, ST-segment-elevation myocardial infarction.

*When uncertain, the time of onset time should be considered the time when the patient was last known to be normal or at baseline neurological condition.

†Recommendation unchanged or reworded for clarity from 2015 IV Alteplase. See Table XCV in online Data Supplement 1 for original wording.

‡See also the text of these guidelines for additional information on these recommendations.

§LOE amended to conform with American College of Cardiology/AHA 2015 Recommendation Classification System.

‖COR amended to conform with American College of Cardiology/AHA 2015 Recommendation Classification System.

Reprinted with permission. Stroke.2019;50:e344-e418 © American Heart Association, Inc.

What can be done to minimize further neurologic deficit in the acute situation in a patient with acute ischemic stroke?

Blood Pressure Control

Rapid lowering of BP in hypertensive patients with acute ischemic stroke is not known to be beneficial, and it may actually be harmful. Hypertension in the patient with acute stroke should not be treated unless the systolic BP is higher than 220 mm Hg and the diastolic BP exceeds 120 mm Hg. Box 26.3 is a guide for the approach to arterial hypertension in the patient with acute ischemic stroke who is being considered for fibrinolytic therapy.

Exercise considerable caution in deciding whether to lower BP in patients with acute ischemic stroke who are *not* being considered for fibrinolytic therapy. In this case, a more conservative approach is recommended: Agents and routes of administration should be chosen to minimize abrupt falls in BP. A reasonable target is to lower BP by 15% to 25% within the first day.

Arrhythmia Detection and Control

Patients with acute stroke should have cardiac monitoring for the first 24 hours.

BOX 26.3	Potential Approaches to Arterial Hypertension in Acute Ischemic Stroke Patients Who Are Candidates for Acute Reperfusion Therapy

Options to Treat Arterial Hypertension in Patients With AIS Who Are Candidates for Emergency Reperfusion Therapy*

COR IIb

Patient otherwise eligible for emergency reperfusion therapy except that BP is >185/110 mm Hg:

Labetalol 10–20 mg IV over 1–2 min, may repeat 1 time; or

Nicardipine 5 mg/h IV, titrate up by 2.5 mg/h every 5–15 min, maximum 15 mg/h; when desired BP reached, adjust to maintain proper BP limits; or

Clevidipine 1–2 mg/h IV, titrate by doubling the dose every 2–5 min until desired BP reached; maximum 21 mg/h

Other agents (e.g., hydralazine, enalaprilat) may also be considered

If BP is not maintained ≤185/110 mmHg, do not administer alteplase

Management of BP during and after alteplase or other emergency reperfusion therapy to maintain BP ≤180/105 mmHg:

Monitor BP every 15 min for 2 h from the start of alteplase therapy, then every 30 min for 6 h, and then every hour for 16 h

If systolic BP >180–230 mmHg or diastolic BP >105–120 mm Hg:

Labetalol 10 mg IV followed by continuous IV infusion 2–8 mg/min; or

Nicardipine 5 mg/h IV, titrate up to desired effect by 2.5 mg/h every 5–15 min, maximum 15 mg/h; or

Clevidipine 1–2 mg/h IV, titrate by doubling the dose every 2–5 min until desired BP reached; maximum 21 mg/h

If BP not controlled or diastolic BP >140 mmHg, consider IV sodium nitroprusside

AIS indicates acute ischemic stroke; BP, blood pressure; COR, class of recommendation; IV, intravenous; and LOE, level of evidence.

*Different treatment options may be appropriate in patients who have comorbid conditions that may benefit from rapid reductions in BP such as acute coronary event, acute heart failure, aortic dissection, or preeclampsia/eclampsia.

Data derived from Jauch et al.

Reprinted with permission. Stroke.2019;50:e344-e418 © American Heart Association, Inc.

Temperature Control

The source of any fever should be thoroughly investigated (see Chapter 12). Treating a fever with antipyretics or cooling devices may improve the prognosis of patients with stroke.

What other issues need to be considered as a result of the stroke deficit?

- Swallowing assessment
- Mobility assessment: risk for falls/injury

If the patient has an acute ischemic stroke and is not a candidate for thrombolytic therapy, administer **acetylsalicylic acid (ASA)**,

160 mg PO as a one-time loading dose. In dysphagic patients, the ASA may be administered by enteral tube or as a **rectal suppository in a dose of 300 mg PR.** In patients with acute ischemic stroke who are treated with rtPA, do not give ASA until after the 24-hour postthrombolysis scan has ruled out intracranial hemorrhage.

Hemorrhagic Strokes

If the noncontrast CT scan shows a *hemorrhagic infarction,* the patient is not a candidate for fibrinolytic therapy. In this case, seek expert advice, and evaluate the patient for causes of acute cerebral hemorrhage. Initial treatment includes identifying and reversing any clotting disorders, monitoring and managing increased intracranial pressure, and controlling BP. Consult a neurologist or neurosurgeon as appropriate. Cerebellar hemorrhage, intraventricular hemorrhage with hydrocephalus, and subarachnoid hemorrhage each necessitate urgent neurosurgical consultation.

Syncope

Syncope is a brief loss of consciousness as a result of sudden reduction in cerebral blood flow. Another term, *presyncope,* refers to the situation in which reduction in cerebral blood flow is sufficient to result in a sensation of impending loss of consciousness, although the patient does not actually pass out. Presyncope and syncope represent degrees of the same disorder and should be addressed as manifestations of the same underlying problem. Your task is to discover the cause of the syncopal attack. Although a diagnosis of syncope implies a cardiovascular etiology, other conditions such as hypoglycemia and seizure disorders can present as sudden loss of consciousness, and are important to consider in your evaluation of the patient.

PHONE CALL

Questions

1. Did the patient actually lose consciousness?
2. Is the patient still unconscious?
3. What are the patient's vital signs?
4. Is the patient diabetic?

    Although most syncope is due to a sudden drop in blood pressure, a sudden fall in cerebral nutrients, that is, hypoglycemia, can also cause loss of consciousness.

5. Was any seizure-like activity witnessed?

    A seizure causes sudden loss of consciousness because of abnormal activity in the fronto-parietal association cortex.

6. Was the patient recumbent, sitting, or standing when the episode occurred?

    Syncope while the patient is in the recumbent position almost always has a cardiac origin.

7. Why was the patient admitted?

    An admitting diagnosis of seizure disorder, transient ischemic attack (TIA), or cardiac disease may help direct you to the cause of the syncopal attack.

8. Has the patient sustained any evidence of injury?
9. What drugs is the patient on?

Orders

If the patient is still unconscious, order the following:

1. **Intravenous (IV) Hep-Lock immediately**, if an IV line is not already in place
2. Turn the patient onto the left side.

   📖 This maneuver prevents the patient's tongue from falling back into their throat and obstructing the upper airway, and it minimizes the risk of aspiration if vomiting occurs.
3. Stat 12-lead electrocardiographic (ECG) monitoring and rhythm strip

   📖 Although almost all patients with syncope regain consciousness within a few minutes, you are more likely to be able to document a cardiac dysrhythmia early, while the patient still has symptoms. The ECG may also show other baseline abnormalities such as epsilon waves in V1-V2 (arrhythmogenic right ventricular cardiomyopathy), right bundle branch block with ST elevation in V1-V3 (Brugada syndrome), and long (usually > 460 ms) or short (usually < 360 ms) QT syndrome, any of which may result in ventricular arrhythmias.
4. If the patient is diabetic, take a stat finger-prick blood glucose reading, and then administer 📖 **50% dextrose in water (D50W), 50 mL intravenously**.

If the patient has regained consciousness, if there is no evidence of head or neck injury, and if the vital signs are stable, do the following:

1. To return the patient to bed, ask the registered nurse (RN) to slowly raise the patient to a sitting position and then to a standing position.
2. The patient should be placed back in bed, with instructions to remain there until you are able to assess the problem.
3. Order an ECG and a rhythm strip. If the ward has telemetry capabilities, begin telemetry for the patient. If not, arrange to have the patient transferred to a ward with telemetry or continuous ECG monitoring capabilities.
4. Have the vital signs measured every 15 minutes until you arrive at the patient's bedside. Ask the RN to call you back immediately if the vital signs become unstable before you are able to assess the patient.

Informing the Registered Nurse

Tell the RN, "I will arrive at the bedside in . . . minutes."

If a patient has syncope, you must see the patient immediately if the patient is still unconscious or if the patient has abnormalities in the heart rate or blood pressure. If the patient is alert and conscious with normal vital signs (and if other more urgent problems require your attention), the RN should observe the patient and call you if a problem arises before you are able to get there.

ELEVATOR THOUGHTS

What causes syncope?

1. Cardiovascular causes
   a. Dysrhythmias
      i. Tachycardia
         (1) Supraventricular tachycardia (including atrial fibrillation and flutter)
         (2) Ventricular tachycardia
         (3) Ventricular fibrillation
      ii. Bradycardia
         (1) Sinus node disease
         (2) Atrioventricular (AV) node disease—usually with second- or third-degree AV block
   b. Pacemaker malfunction (e.g., failure to pace or capture)
   c. Syncope with exertion
      i. Aortic stenosis
      ii. Pulmonic stenosis
      iii. Hypertrophic obstructive cardiomyopathy
      iv. Subclavian steal syndrome
   d. Pulmonary embolism
   e. Neurally mediated (reflex) syncope
      i. Common faint (vasodepressor reaction)
      ii. Situational syncope (e.g., occurring after cough, micturition, defecation, sneezing, eating)
      iii. Carotid sinus syncope
   f. Orthostatic hypotension
      i. Drug induced
      ii. Volume depletion
      iii. Autonomic failure
      iv. Postural orthostatic tachycardia syndrome
2. Neurologic causes
   a. Brainstem TIA or stroke (drop attacks)
   b. Seizure
   c. Subarachnoid hemorrhage (SAH)
   d. Cervical spondylosis
3. Miscellaneous
   a. Hypoglycemia
   b. Hyperventilation
   c. Psychogenic pseudosyncope and psychogenic nonepileptic seizures

MAJOR THREAT TO LIFE

- Airway obstruction, aspiration pneumonia, or both

📖 Because most patients recover from syncopal attacks within a few minutes, the actual loss of consciousness is not the major problem. Of greater importance is that while the patient is unconscious, the tongue may block the oropharynx or the patient may aspirate oral or gastric contents into the lungs, which may result in the development of aspiration pneumonia or acute respiratory distress syndrome (ARDS). Therefore, in an unconscious patient your primary goal is to protect the airway until the patient regains consciousness and the cough reflexes are again effective.

- Recurrence of an unrecognized, potentially fatal cardiac dysrhythmia

📖 Once the patient has regained consciousness, the major threat to life is the recurrence of an unrecognized, potentially fatal cardiac dysrhythmia. This can best be identified and managed by transferring the patient to an intensive care unit/cardiac care unit (ICU/CCU) or other setting with ECG monitors if a dysrhythmia is suspected of causing the syncopal episode.

BEDSIDE

Quick-Look Test

Does the patient look well (comfortable), sick (uncomfortable or distressed), or critical (about to die)?

This simple observation helps determine the necessity for immediate intervention. Most patients who have had episodes of syncope and have regained consciousness look perfectly well.

Airway and Vital Signs

If the patient is still unconscious, ensure that the RN has placed them on the left side and that the patient's tongue has not fallen into the back of the throat. Most episodes of syncope are short-lived, and by the time you arrive at the bedside, the patient will probably have regained consciousness. Look for abnormalities in the vital signs, which may help you diagnose the specific cause of syncope.

What is the patient's heart rate?

Supraventricular or ventricular tachycardias should be documented on ECG tracings; if they occur, the patient should be treated immediately. (Refer to Chapter 15, page 156, for the treatment of supraventricular tachycardia, and page 159 for the treatment of ventricular tachycardia.)

Any patient with a transient or persistent supraventricular or ventricular tachycardia or a history of these arrhythmias should be transferred to the ICU/CCU or other setting with ECG monitoring for appropriate management if no other cause of syncope can be found.

What is the patient's blood pressure?

A patient with resting or orthostatic hypotension should be managed as outlined in Chapter 18.

📖 Remember that a massive internal hemorrhage (such as gastrointestinal bleeding or ruptured aortic aneurysm) occasionally manifests with a syncopal attack.

Hypertension, if found in association with headache and neck stiffness, may indicate SAH. A brief loss of consciousness is common at the onset of SAH and is often associated with dizziness, vertigo, or vomiting.

What is the patient's temperature?

Patients with syncope are rarely febrile. If fever is present, it is usually caused by a concomitant illness unrelated to the syncopal attack. However, be careful, especially if the syncopal attack was unwitnessed, to search for the possibility of a seizure secondary to meningitis, which may manifest as both *fever* and *syncope.*

Selective History and Chart Review

Has the patient experienced an episode of syncope before?

If the answer is yes, ask the patient whether a diagnosis was made after the previous attack.

What does the patient or witness recall about the time immediately before the syncope?

- Syncope that occurs while the patient is in the upright position after an emotional or painful stimulus and is preceded by nausea, diaphoresis, pallor, and a *gradual* loss of consciousness is typical of the common faint (vasodepressor syncope).
- Syncope that occurs while the patient changes from the supine or sitting position to the standing position is suggestive of orthostatic hypotension.
- An *aura,* although rare, is indicative of a seizure as the cause of syncope in an unwitnessed attack.
- *Palpitations* that precede an attack may be suggestive of a cardiac dysrhythmia as the cause of syncope.
- Syncope that occurs while or immediately after the patient performs a *Valsalva maneuver*—as happens with a bout of coughing, micturition, straining at stool, or sneezing—may result from transient reduction of venous return to the right atrium and neurally mediated reflex bradycardia.
- Syncope that occurs *after the patient turns the head to one side* (especially if the patient is wearing a tight collar) or during shaving may represent carotid sinus syncope. This condition is observed most often in elderly men.

- Syncope that occurs during *arm exercise* suggests subclavian steal syndrome.
- *Numbness and tingling* in the hands and feet are commonly experienced just before presyncope or syncope as a result of hyperventilation or anxiety.

Does the patient have a history of cardiac disease?

A patient with preexisting cardiac disease may have an increased risk of developing dysrhythmias.

Has the patient ever had a seizure?

An unwitnessed seizure may be perceived as a syncopal attack. Ask whether, during the attack, the patient bit his or her tongue or was incontinent of stool or urine; either event is suggestive of seizure activity. Hypoglycemia should be suspected as a possible cause of seizure or syncope in a diabetic patient who is taking oral hypoglycemic agents or insulin.

Has the patient ever had a stroke?

A patient with known cerebrovascular disease is vulnerable to a brainstem TIA or stroke. However, because atherosclerosis is a diffuse process, a patient with a history of stroke may also have coronary atherosclerosis, which may result in cardiac dysrhythmias.

What does the patient remember on waking from the syncopal attack?

Headache, drowsiness, and mental confusion are common sequelae of seizures but not of cardiac or orthostatic causes of syncope.

What medications is the patient taking?

Check the chart to see what medications the patient is being given.

- Digoxin, β-blockers, and calcium channel blockers may result in bradycardia. Digoxin, if present in toxic amounts, may also precipitate ventricular tachycardia.
- Anti-arrhythmia drugs (e.g., sotalol, dofetilide, amiodarone, quinidine, procainamide, disopyramide), tricyclic antidepressants, phenothiazines, and some of the *nonsedating* antihistamines may prolong the QTc interval, which leads to ventricular tachycardia (torsades de pointes; Fig. 27.1A) or the prolonged QT interval syndrome (see Fig. 27.1B).
- Agents that reduce afterload or preload (angiotensin-converting enzyme inhibitors, angiotensin-receptor blockers, calcium channel blockers, hydralazine, prazosin, nitroglycerin, nitrates, diuretics) may cause syncope, especially in elderly or volume-depleted patients.
- Phenothiazines, tricyclic antidepressants, alcohol, and cocaine lower the seizure threshold and may cause a seizure.
- Oral hypoglycemic agents and insulin may cause hypoglycemic seizures or syncope. Many factors can contribute to erratic glucose levels in hospitalized diabetic patients, including coexisting illnesses, changing activity levels, poor appetite, and medication interactions.

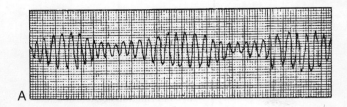

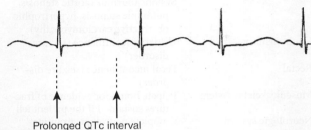

Prolonged QTc interval
(usually >0.46s)

B

FIG. 27.1 ECG representation of torsades de pointes (A) and prolonged QTc interval (B).

Selective Physical Examination

The physical examination is directed toward finding a cause for the syncope. If the patient fell during the syncopal attack, however, it is equally important to search for evidence of injuries sustained.

Vitals	Repeat measurements now; at this time, measure the patient's blood pressure in both arms.
	📖 A difference of more than 20 mm Hg may be indicative of subclavian steal syndrome.
Head, ears, eyes, nose, throat (HEENT)	Fundoscopy: look for subhyaloid hemorrhages; blood diffuses between the retinal fiber layer and the internal limiting membrane, forming a pocket of blood with sharp borders and often a fluid level.
	Tongue or cheek laceration (seizure disorder)
	Neck stiffness (meningitis leading to a seizure, SAH)
	Supraclavicular or subclavicular bruit (subclavian steal syndrome)
Respiratory system	Crackles, wheezes (aspiration during the syncopal episode)

Cardiovascular system	Pacemaker/automatic implantable cardioverter-defibrillator (ICD) (pacemaker failure to capture; tachyarrhythmias)
	Flat jugular venous pressure (volume depletion)
	Atrial fibrillation (vertebrobasilar embolism)
	Systolic murmur (aortic stenosis, pulmonic stenosis, hypertrophic obstructive cardiomyopathy)
Genitourinary	Urinary incontinence (seizure disorder)
Rectal	Fecal incontinence (seizure disorder)
Musculoskeletal system	Palpate bones for evidence of fractures sustained if the patient fell
Neurologic system	Complete neurologic examination: seek evidence of residual localizing signs that may indicate a TIA, completed stroke, SAH, space-occupying intracranial lesion, or Todd paralysis; vertebrobasilar TIAs or strokes are frequently accompanied by other evidence of brainstem dysfunction (i.e., cranial nerve abnormalities) such as diplopia, nystagmus, facial paralysis, vertigo, dysphagia, and dysarthria

Management

An immediate cause for syncope often cannot be found. Because treatment of the various causes of syncope is so different, the cause of a syncopal episode must be proved and documented before definitive treatment can proceed. Investigations may take several days to complete. Once you have assessed a patient with syncope, you must study the history, physical findings, and laboratory data to decide the most likely cause of syncope and to arrange for further investigation, if necessary.

Cardiovascular Causes

If a cardiovascular cause of syncope is suspected, whether related to a dysrhythmia, a valvular problem, or a pacemaker, the patient should be transferred to the CCU or to an intermediate-care unit where continuous ECG monitoring is available. If no ECG-monitored beds are available, and if ischemia-induced dysrhythmia is not suspected, 24-hour Holter monitoring should be arranged for the patient first thing in the morning.

Always consider a silent myocardial infarction with subsequent transient atrioventricular block, ventricular tachycardia, or ventricular fibrillation as the cause for syncope of cardiac origin.

Treatment of specific dysrhythmias, if still present when you are assessing the patient, is discussed in Chapter 15:

1. Tachycardias
   a. Ventricular tachycardia (page 159)
   b. Supraventricular tachycardia (page 156)
2. Bradycardias
   a. Sinus bradycardia (page 167)
   b. Atrioventricular blocks (page 168)
   c. Atrial fibrillation with slow ventricular response (page 168)

A pacemaker or automatic implantable cardioverter-defibrillator (AICD), if present, should be interrogated by the appropriate programmer. Interrogation yields helpful information as to whether the pacemaker or AICD is functioning properly. Many currently used pacemakers also have rhythm storage functions that may indicate whether a tachyarrhythmia was responsible for the patients syncopal episode. AICDs have even more sophisticated rhythm storage capabilities and provide more information regarding possible tachyarrhythmias as a cause for the patient's syncope.

If *aortic stenosis, pulmonic stenosis,* or *hypertrophic obstructive cardiomyopathy* is thought to be responsible for exertional syncope, arrange for an echocardiogram in the morning to document the suspected cardiac lesion, and ask for a cardiology consultation.

If a pulmonary embolism is thought responsible for the patient's syncope, refer to Chapter 24, page 296 for further evaluation and management.

Neurally Mediated (Reflex) Syncope

Most vasodepressor attacks can be managed without transfer to the ICU/CCU, as outlined in Chapter 18, page 197.

The definitive diagnosis of *carotid sinus syncope* requires potentially dangerous carotid sinus pressure, which should only be performed while the electrocardiogram is being monitored for cardiac dysrhythmias. Although the patient does not require ICU/CCU admission overnight, arrangements should be made in the morning to evaluate the cardiac rhythm during carotid sinus massage.

Orthostatic Hypotension

Syncope caused by *volume depletion* can be managed with IV fluid replacement, as outlined in Chapter 18, page 197.

Drug-induced orthostatic hypotension and *autonomic failure* are complex treatment problems. As long as the patient's volume status is normal, they can be addressed in the morning through consultation with a neurologist or clinical pharmacologist.

Until the underlying problem responsible for orthostatic hypotension is corrected, instruct patients that if they must get out of bed during the night, they should ask the RN for assistance and should move slowly from the supine to sitting position and then move slowly again from the sitting to standing position.

Neurologic Causes

Suspected *brainstem TIA* or *stroke* should be considered an emergency, and the patient should be evaluated for fibrinolytic therapy. Call your resident immediately for help. Your institution may have an acute stroke team with protocols in place to evaluate suspected acute stroke patients. Refer to Chapter 26 for the evaluation and management of suspected acute ischemic stroke.

If a *seizure* is suspected, you must first document the cause of the seizure, as outlined in Chapter 23, page 270.

If *SAH* is suspected, arrange for an urgent non-contrast CT scan of the head to look for blood in the subarachnoid space. A normal CT scan does not, however, rule out SAH, and a lumbar puncture may be necessary to look for xanthochromic cerebrospinal fluid. If such a lesion is identified, a neurosurgeon should be consulted for further investigation and management. A CTA, magnetic resonance angiography (MRA), or digital subtraction angiography will help determine if a cerebral aneurysm is responsible for the subarachnoid hemorrhage.

Miscellaneous

Syncope caused by *hypoglycemia* is usually due to oral or subcutaneous hypoglycemic agents, and should be managed with IV dextrose as per page 401. Once the blood glucose is corrected, review the patient's medications and make adjustments to prevent future recurrences.

Syncope caused by *hyperventilation* or *anxiety states* can be alleviated if the patient breathes into a paper bag when he or she begins to feel anxious or presyncopal. This step corrects hypocapnia and thereby prevents a syncopal attack.

REMEMBER

1. In an elderly patient, the main hazard of a syncopal attack is not necessarily the underlying disease but rather a fracture or other injury sustained during a fall.
2. Except for the Stokes-Adams attack (third-degree atrioventricular block), true syncope rarely occurs when a patient is in the recumbent position.

Transfusion Reactions

Blood transfusions are given around the clock in hospitals. Reactions to blood products may vary from severe to mild. An organized approach helps you sort out the nature of the reaction and what to do about it.

PHONE CALL

Questions

1. What symptoms does the patient have?
   Fever, chills, chest pain, back pain, diaphoresis, and shortness of breath can all be manifestations of a transfusion reaction.
2. What are the vital signs including temperature?
3. Which blood product is being transfused, and how long ago was it started?
4. Why was the patient admitted?

Orders

1. Stop the transfusion immediately if the patient has any of the following symptoms:
   • Sudden onset of hypotension
   • Chest or back pain with tachypnea
   • Shortness of breath
   • Any symptom (even fever, chills, or urticaria) occurring within minutes of the start of the transfusion
   • Fever in a patient who has never before received a blood transfusion or who has never been pregnant; this symptom may represent an acute hemolytic reaction

   An acute hemolytic transfusion reaction can appear with any of the aforementioned symptoms. Such reactions, although rare, are associated with an extremely high mortality rate, which is proportionate to the volume of blood infused. In previously pregnant patients or patients who have previously received transfusions, fever may be a nonhemolytic febrile reaction.
2. If the blood transfusion has been stopped, keep the intravenous line open with normal saline.

Informing the Registered Nurse

Tell the registered nurse (RN), "I will arrive at the bedside in … minutes."

Any patient with suspected hemolytic or anaphylactic transfusion reaction must be evaluated immediately.

ELEVATOR THOUGHTS

What causes transfusion reactions?

1. Immune reactions
   a. Nonhemolytic febrile reaction, which is the most common transfusion reaction and is believed to be caused by antibodies directed against contaminating white blood cells. It is usually manifested by fever, chills, and sometimes mild dyspnea 1 to 6 hours after transfusion of red blood cells (RBCs) or platelets. It can be treated by stopping the transfusion (primarily to determine that a more serious hemolytic reaction is not taking place) and administering antipyretics.
   b. Acute hemolytic reaction, in which errors in identification of the patient or labeling of the blood result in transfusion of mismatched RBCs. Acute hemolytic reaction is caused by rapid hemolysis of donor RBCs by preformed recipient antibodies, usually as a result of ABO incompatibility. Such errors are exceedingly rare but may occur in emergency situations (e.g., in the postanesthetic stage, operating room, or emergency room), if usual procedures for patient identification and blood labeling are breached.
   c. Delayed hemolytic reaction, which develops as a consequence of prior exposure to foreign red cell antigens (i.e., pregnancy or previous transfusion) and is usually caused by Kidd or Rh antibodies. Re-exposure to these antigens results in an anamnestic rise in alloantibodies that were not detectable at the time of the original crossmatch. Hemolysis occurs 2 to 10 days after transfusion and may be accompanied by fever and hemolysis, which is usually milder than in the acute hemolytic reactions.
   d. Anaphylaxis (immunoglobulin G response to immunoglobulin A [IgA] antibodies), which may result from transmission of IgA antibodies from the donor's blood into a presensitized IgA-deficient patient.
      Congenital IgA deficiency is a common (1 per 1000), asymptomatic disorder. The first transfusion that an IgA-deficient patient receives will contain IgA antibodies, which are recognized by the patient's immune system as foreign antigens. Thus the IgA-deficient patient becomes

sensitized and develops anti-IgA antibodies, which, in subsequent transfusions, may cause anaphylaxis or urticaria.

There are two known IgA allotypes (genetic variations in the structure of the immunoglobulin). Anaphylactic reactions are more common in patients who lack both allotypes of IgA, but they have been reported in patients who lack only one allotype. Individuals with IgA molecules of one allotype may develop antibodies against the other allotype, and subsequent transfusion reactions manifest as urticaria or, on occasion, anaphylaxis.

   e. Simple allergic reactions, including urticaria, can be caused by transmission of antigens (e.g., food allergens such as shrimp) from the donor's blood. This may also occur when IgA antibodies are infused into an IgA-deficient patient (i.e., deficiency in one of the two allotypes).

   f. Posttransfusion purpura, which is an unusual immune thrombocytopenia that occurs 5 to 10 days after transfusion of a platelet-containing product (and can occur not only with platelet transfusions but also with RBC transfusions and granulocyte concentrates). The thrombocytopenia occurs in patients previously sensitized to a foreign antigen by pregnancy or prior transfusion, and it results in destruction of both donor and recipient platelets. A second (also rare) mechanism for posttransfusion purpura is thrombocytopenia caused by passive transfer of antiplatelet antibodies from a previously immunized donor.

2. Nonimmune hemolysis, which may occur if the blood has been overheated or has undergone trauma. Trauma to blood products occurs (1) by excessive hand squeezing or pumping of the infusion bag during the rapid administration of blood in an emergency or (2) by delivery through a needle that is too small.

3. Pulmonary edema
   a. Transfusion-associated circulatory overload (TACO)—Volume overload may be induced in a patient with a history of congestive heart failure (CHF) because blood transfusions expand the intravascular volume.
   b. Transfusion-related acute lung injury (TRALI). Noncardiogenic pulmonary edema can result from immune reactions related to antibodies directed against human leukocyte antigens.

4. Septic (bacterial contamination) reactions
   Platelet concentrates are particularly susceptible because of the storage conditions at 20°C to 24°C.

MAJOR THREAT TO LIFE

- Anaphylaxis
- Acute hemolytic reaction
- Hypoxia from pulmonary edema (from either TACO or TRALI)

Anaphylaxis and acute hemolytic reactions are rare, but when they do occur, they can be fatal. *Anaphylaxis* may cause death through severe laryngospasm or bronchospasm or through profound peripheral vasodilatation and cardiovascular collapse. An *acute hemolytic reaction* is a medical emergency because of the possible development of acute renal failure, disseminated intravascular coagulation (DIC), or both. TACO and TRALI may both cause *pulmonary edema* resulting in hypoxia.

BEDSIDE

Quick-Look Test

Does the patient look well (comfortable), sick (uncomfortable or distressed), or critical (about to die)?

A patient with impending anaphylaxis may look sick (agitated, restless, or short of breath). A patient with pulmonary edema secondary to a transfusion reaction may look critically ill, with severe shortness of breath.

Airway and Vital Signs

What is the patient's respiratory rate?

Tachypnea may be a manifestation of CHF or, particularly if associated with audible wheezing, may be a sign of impending anaphylaxis.

What is the patient's blood pressure?

Hypotension is an ominous sign. Ensure that the transfusion has been stopped. Hypotension is seen in acute hemolytic reactions and in anaphylactic reactions. However, if the transfusion is undertaken for volume depletion, as in acute blood loss, hypotension may represent continued loss of intravascular volume from uncontrolled bleeding.

Have the blood tag and patient's wristband been checked?

Compare the identification tag on the blood with that on the patient's wristband.

Selective Physical Examination

Head, ears, eyes, nose, throat (HEENT)	Flushed face (hemolytic reaction or anaphylaxis)
	Facial or pharyngeal edema (anaphylaxis)
Respiratory system	Wheezing (anaphylaxis)

Neurologic system	Decreased level of consciousness (anaphylaxis or hemolytic reaction)
Skin	Heat along the vein being used for the transfusion (hemolytic reaction)
	Oozing from intravenous sites may be the only sign of hemolysis in an unconscious or anesthetized patient; DIC is a late manifestation of an acute hemolytic transfusion reaction.
Urine	Check the urine color: free hemoglobin turns urine red or brown and is indicative of a hemolytic reaction

If the patient shows evidence of anaphylaxis or hemolysis, stop the transfusion and immediately begin emergency treatment (see the Management section in this chapter).

Selective History

Has the patient developed any symptoms since the initial telephone call?

- Fever or chills (acute hemolytic reaction, nonhemolytic febrile reaction, or septic reaction)
- Headache, chest pain, back pain, or diaphoresis (hemolytic reaction)
- Shortness of breath (volume overload or pulmonary leukoagglutinin reaction): a leukoagglutinin reaction in an elderly patient is often misdiagnosed as cardiogenic pulmonary edema. *Has the patient had previous transfusion reactions?*

Chills and fever are most common in a patient who has received multiple transfusions or who has had several pregnancies.

Management

Anaphylaxis

1. Ensure that the transfusion has been stopped.
2. Epinephrine is the most important drug for any anaphylactic reaction.

   Through its α-adrenergic action, epinephrine reverses peripheral vasodilatation, and through its β-adrenergic action, it reduces bronchoconstriction and increases the force of cardiac contraction. In addition it suppresses release of histamine and leukotrienes.

   Two strengths of epinephrine are available for injection. Make sure that you are using the correct strength.

   For profound anaphylactic shock that is immediately life-threatening, use the intravenous route. Administer epinephrine 1 mg (10 mL of the 0.1 mg/mL solution) every 3 to 5 minutes. Follow each dose with a 20 mL flush, and elevate the arm for 10 to 20 seconds after each dose. Higher doses may be required. See page 426 for alternative doses and routes of administration.

For less severe situations, epinephrine can be given intramuscularly (IM). Note the different concentration. Administer **epinephrine, 0.5 mg (0.5 mL of the 1 mg/mL solution) IM;** repeat after 5 minutes in the absence of improvement or if deterioration occurs. Several doses may be necessary.

3. **Hydrocortisone, 500 mg by slow intravenous infusion or by intramuscular injection,** followed by 100 mg intravenously (IV) or intramuscularly (IM) every 6 hours to help avert late sequelae.

   📖 This is particularly important in asthmatic patients who have been treated previously with corticosteroids.

4. **Salbutamol, 2.5 mg per 3 mL of normal saline by nebulizer.**

   📖 This is an adjunctive measure if bronchospasm is a major feature.

5. Intubation if necessary.

Acute Hemolytic Reaction

1. Ensure that the transfusion has been stopped.
2. Replace all intravenous tubing.
3. **Normal saline, 500 mL IV,** as fast as possible, followed by an infusion of normal saline, 100 to 200 mL/hour. Aim for a urine output of 100 to 200 mL/hour to prevent acute renal failure.
4. Draw 20 mL of the patient's blood (from a limb other than the one in which the transfusion was given), and send the sample for the following laboratory work:
   a. Repeat type and crossmatch
   b. Coombs test, plasma free hemoglobin
   c. Complete blood cell count, RBC structure
   d. Measurements of platelets, prothrombin time, activated partial thromboplastin time, and fibrin degradation products
   e. Measurements of urea and creatinine levels
   f. Unclotted blood for a stat spin (hemolysis is demonstrated when the plasma remains pink despite spinning for 5 minutes: i.e., hemoglobinemia)
5. Obtain a urine sample for free hemoglobin. Urine can also be tested with dipsticks. If hemoglobinuria is present, the dipstick results will be positive for hemoglobin and negative for RBCs.
6. Send the blood product bag back to the blood bank for the following:
   a. Repeat crossmatch
   b. Coombs test
   c. Culture

7. If oliguria develops despite adequate intravenous fluids and appropriate diuretics, acute renal failure should be suspected. (For management of acute renal failure, see Chapter 9, page 85.)

Pulmonary Edema

1. If transfusion-associated cardiac overload (TACO) is the cause for pulmonary edema, stop the transfusion or slow the rate of transfusion, unless the patient urgently needs blood.
2. **Furosemide, 40 mg IV.** If the patient is already receiving a diuretic or if there is renal insufficiency, a higher dose of furosemide may be required.
3. For the management of CHF, refer to Chapter 24, pages 291–293. Volume overload, with subsequent pulmonary edema, should be anticipated in a patient with a history of CHF. This problem may be prevented by administering a diuretic (e.g. **furosemide, 40 mg IV**) during the transfusion.
4. Treatment of TRALI is supportive and may involve intubation and mechanical ventilation.

Urticaria

1. Do not stop the transfusion.
   Hives alone are rarely serious, but hives with hypotension is considered an anaphylactic reaction until proved otherwise.
2. **Diphenhydramine, 50 mg orally or IV (not IM).**

Fever

1. Stop the transfusion until a hemolytic reaction can be ruled out. Fever developing within minutes of the start of a blood transfusion is probably a symptom of a hemolytic reaction.
2. For a suspected septic reaction send the blood product bag for culture and initiate antibiotics
   Vancomycin 15 to 20 mg/kg IV q 8 to 12 h with Ceftaroline 600 mg IV q8 to 12 h
3. For a nonhemolytic, nonseptic febrile reaction, usually no treatment is required. If the fever is high and the patient is distressed, however, an antipyretic drug, such as **acetaminophen, 650 mg orally**, is usually effective.

Laboratory-Related Problems: The Common Calls

Acid–Base Disorders

Most cases of acidemia or alkalemia are first discovered from measurement of arterial hydrogen ion concentration (pH).

ACIDEMIA (pH ≤7.35)

First decide whether the acidemia is a respiratory acidemia (i.e., caused by hypoventilation) or a metabolic acidemia (i.e., caused by acid gain or bicarbonate [HCO_3] loss).

Respiratory Acidemia

- pH ≤ 7.35
- Partial pressure of carbon dioxide (Pco_2) ↑
- HCO_3 normal or ↑

Metabolic Acidemia

- pH ≤ 7.35
- Pco_2 normal or ↓
- HCO_3 ↓

The normal response to respiratory acidemia is an increase in HCO_3. An immediate increase in HCO_3 occurs because the increase in Pco_2 results in the generation of HCO_3, according to the law of mass action:

$$CO_2 + H_2O \leftrightarrow H + HCO_3$$

Later, renal tubular preservation of HCO_3 occurs to buffer the change in pH. The expected increase in HCO_3 in *acute respiratory acidemia* is 0.1 mEq/L (ΔPco_2). The expected increase in HCO_3 in *chronic respiratory acidemia* is 0.4 mEq/L (ΔPco_2). When the HCO_3 level is lower than expected, a mixed respiratory and metabolic acidemia should be suspected. An HCO_3 level higher than expected is suggestive of a combination of respiratory acidemia and metabolic alkalemia.

The normal respiratory response to metabolic acidemia is hyperventilation, with a decrease in Pco_2. The expected decrease in Pco_2 in uncomplicated metabolic acidemia is 1 to 1.5 mEq/L

(ΔHCO_3). When the Pco_2 is higher than expected, a mixed metabolic and respiratory acidemia should be suspected. When the Pco_2 is lower than expected, a combination of metabolic acidemia and respiratory alkalemia should be suspected.

RESPIRATORY ACIDEMIA

- pH ≤ 7.35
- Pco_2 ↑
- HCO_3 normal or ↑

Causes

1. Depression of the central nervous system respiratory center
   a. Drugs (e.g., morphine)
   b. Lesions of the respiratory center
2. Compromised respiratory muscle function
   a. Drugs (e.g., succinylcholine)
   b. Muscular disease (amyotrophic lateral sclerosis, Guillain-Barre syndrome, muscular dystrophy)
   c. Hypokalemia, hypophosphatemia
   d. Neuropathies
3. Respiratory disorders
   a. Acute airway obstruction (chronic obstructive pulmonary disease, asthma)
   b. Severe interstitial lung disease
   c. Pleural effusion
   d. Pneumothorax
4. Thoracic cage limitation (obesity hypoventilation syndrome-Pickwickian syndrome)

Manifestations

Respiratory acidemia occurs when a failure (either acute or chronic) in ventilation occurs. The manifestations of respiratory acidemia are often overshadowed by those of the accompanying hypoxia. Symptoms and signs directly attributable to CO_2 retention—which are uncommon when Pco_2 is lower than 70 mm Hg—include the following:

- Bradypnea
- Drowsiness
- Confusion
- Papilledema
- Asterixis

Management

Mild

The pH ranges from 7.30 to 7.35. A patient with mild respiratory acidemia can be observed while reversible causes are sought and corrected. Repeat arterial blood gas measurements should be obtained, depending on the patient's clinical condition and course. In a patient with an acute asthmatic attack, however, a normal or, certainly, an elevated P_{CO_2} is a warning sign of impending respiratory failure.

Moderate

The pH ranges from 7.20 to 7.29. A patient with moderate respiratory acidemia must be monitored carefully. Any further decrease in pH would render the patient susceptible to life-threatening ventricular dysrhythmias. If a readily reversible cause can be found, the patient can be monitored carefully while treatment measures are instituted. Such a patient should not be left alone until it is determined that his or her condition is improving. Sequential determinations of pH should be guided by the patient's clinical condition and course.

Severe

The pH is 7.19 or lower. A patient with severe respiratory acidemia is at high risk for cessation of respiration, life-threatening ventricular dysrhythmias, or both. Call your resident for help immediately. The patient probably requires transfer to the intensive care unit (ICU) for monitoring, intubation, and mechanical ventilation while reversible causes are sought.

METABOLIC ACIDEMIA

- pH ≤7.35
- P_{CO_2} normal or ↓
- HCO_3 ↓

Causes

The metabolic acidemias occur in two varieties: *normal anion gap* and *high anion gap*. The normal anion gap is (Na + K serum concentrations) − (Cl + HCO_3 serum concentrations) = 10–12 mmol/L. Most of the normal anion gap is accounted for by negatively charged plasma proteins. Remember that for every decline in serum albumin of 10 g/L you must add 4 to the calculated anion gap. If hypoalbuminemia is not corrected, serious acidemias of the high anion gap type may be overlooked.

Normal Anion Gap Acidemia

1. Loss of HCO_3
   a. Diarrhea, ileus, fistula
   b. High-output ileostomy
   c. Renal tubular acidosis
   d. Carbonic anhydrase inhibitors

2. Addition of H^+
   a. Ammonium chloride (NH_4Cl), found in household cleaning products
   b. Hydrochloride (HCl), found in bleaching agents

High Anion Gap Acidemia

1. Lactic acidemia
2. Ketoacidosis (type 1 diabetes, alcohol, starvation, sodium glucose co-transporter-2 (SGLT2) inhibitors)
3. Renal failure
4. Drugs (aspirin, ethylene glycol, methyl alcohol, toluene, paraldehyde)
5. High-flux dialysis acetate buffer
6. Severe dehydration

The change in anion gap should equal the change in HCO_3. Any deviation from this signifies a mixed acid-base disorder. Always remember to *calculate the osmolar gap* (see Chapter 35, page 418) in high anion gap acidemias to determine whether ingestions have contributed to the abnormalities.

On occasion, the pH may be normal, but the presence of a wide anion gap may be a clue to underlying metabolic acidemia.

Manifestations

The signs and symptoms of metabolic acidemia are nonspecific and include the following:

- Hyperventilation (in an effort to blow off CO_2)
- Fatigue
- Confusion progressing to stupor and then to coma
- Decreased cardiac contractility
- Peripheral vasodilation progressing to hypotension

Management

Mild

The pH ranges from 7.30 to 7.35.

Moderate

The pH ranges from 7.20 to 7.29.

Severe

The pH is 7.19 or lower.

For all causes of metabolic acidemia, management involves reversal of the underlying cause. In most cases of mild or moderate metabolic acidemia, the acid-base disorder can be treated effectively by reversing the underlying condition. However, in some conditions (e.g., chronic renal failure), the condition is not easily reversed. In this situation, mild or moderate metabolic acidemia does not necessitate treatment. Severe metabolic acidemia result-ing from chronic renal failure can be treated with **oral or intrave-nous sodium bicarbonate ($NaHCO_3$)**, but you must be careful not to precipitate volume overload.

For other causes of metabolic acidemia, it is occasionally neces-sary to raise the blood pH by administering $NaHCO_3$, but this ac-tion is usually reserved only for severe metabolic acidemias. Some important precautions should be considered:

1. The amount of $NaHCO_3$ given depends on the pH and how effective and rapid the therapy for reversing the underlying cause is going to be. For instance, metabolic acidemia with a pH of 6.9 is a medical emergency, and an initial dose of 150 mmol of intravenous (IV) $NaHCO_3$ may be required while other resuscitation measures are instituted. In meta-bolic acidemia with a pH of 7.10 in a patient with diabetic ketoacidosis, only 50 mmol of IV $NaHCO_3$ may be required while insulin and fluids are administered. You can estimate the amount of bicarbonate required by calculating the extra-cellular buffer deficit, as follows:

$$\text{Buffer deficit} = (\text{normal serum } HCO_3 - \text{measured serum } HCO_3)(\text{body weight in kg}) \ (0.4),$$

where 0.4 is a correction factor representing the proportion of body weight that is composed of extracellular fluid (0.2) and the buffering provided by intracellular components. The initial dose of HCO_3 should be approximately half of the calculated buffer deficit. Full correction should not be attempted within the first 24 hours because of the risk of delayed compensation and al-kalemia with tetany, seizures, and ventricular dysrhythmias. The HCO_3 should be diluted (50 to 150 mmol/L is achieved by adding one to three 50-mmol vials to 1 L of 5% dextrose in water [D5W]) and given slowly, because undiluted $NaHCO_3$ infused directly can cause fatal ventricular dysrhythmias.

2. In the presence of cardiac arrest, metabolic acidemia can be treated with HCO_3, but only after alveolar ventilation is en-sured, because further depression of respiration can result from a shift in intracellular pH in the respiratory control center in the CNS. When ventilation is ensured, an initial dose of HCO_3, 1 mmol/kg body weight can be administered by rapid IV in-jection, with repeated doses of 0.5 mmol/kg body weight every 10 minutes during continued cardiac arrest.

📖 Remember that IV $NaHCO_3$ is a significant sodium load and may lead to congestive heart failure (CHF). Do not substitute one problem for another.

ALKALEMIA (pH ≥ 7.45)

First decide whether the patient has a respiratory or a metabolic alkalemia.

Respiratory Alkalemia

- pH ≥ 7.45
- P_{CO_2} ↓
- HCO_3 ↓

Metabolic Alkalemia

- pH = 7.45
- P_{CO_2} normal or ↑
- HCO_3 ↑

The normal response to respiratory alkalemia is a decrease in HCO_3. The HCO_3 decreases immediately as a result of the decrease in P_{CO_2}, according to the law of mass action:

$$CO_2 + H_2O \leftrightarrow H + HCO_3$$

Later, renal tubular loss of HCO_3 occurs to buffer the change in pH. The expected decrease in HCO_3 in acute respiratory alkalemia is 0.2 mEq/L (ΔP_{CO_2}). The expected decrease in HCO_3 in chronic respiratory alkalemia is 0.4 mEq/L (ΔP_{CO_2}). When the HCO_3 level is higher than expected, a combined respiratory and metabolic alkalemia should be suspected. When the HCO_3 level is lower than expected, a combined respiratory alkalemia and metabolic acidemia should be suspected.

The normal response to metabolic alkalemia is hypoventilation, with an increase in the P_{CO_2}. The expected increase in uncomplicated metabolic alkalemia is 0.6 mEq/L (ΔHCO_3). When the P_{CO_2} is higher than expected, a combined metabolic alkalemia and respiratory acidemia should be suspected. When the P_{CO_2} is lower than expected, a combined metabolic and respiratory alkalemia should be suspected.

RESPIRATORY ALKALEMIA

- pH ≥ 7.45
- P_{CO_2} ↓
- HCO_3 ↓

Causes

1. Physiologic conditions (pregnancy, high altitude)
2. CNS disorders (anxiety, pain, fever, tumor)
3. Drugs (aspirin, nicotine, progesterone)

4. Pulmonary disorders (CHF, pulmonary embolism, asthma, pneumonia)
5. Miscellaneous conditions (hepatic failure, hyperthyroidism)

Manifestations

- Confusion
- Numbness, tingling, paresthesias (perioral, hands, feet)
- Lightheadedness
- Tetany in severe cases

Management

Mild

The pH ranges from 7.45 to 7.55.

Moderate

The pH ranges from 7.56 to 7.69.

Severe

The pH is 7.70 or higher.

Mild respiratory alkalemia commonly occurs in certain physiologic conditions (pregnancy, high altitude) and, in these cases, necessitates no treatment. Any of the other causes listed may result in mild respiratory alkalemia, and many patients can be treated symptomatically (e.g., a febrile patient can be treated with antipyretics, a patient in pain can be treated with analgesics, and an anxious patient can be treated with reassurance or sedatives). In addition to these measures, more pronounced degrees of respiratory alkalemia caused by anxiety can be treated by rebreathing into a paper bag. The only effective treatment for the other causes listed is eliminating the underlying condition.

METABOLIC ALKALEMIA

- pH ≥ 7.45
- Pco_2 normal or ↑
- HCO_3 ↑

Causes

1. With extracellular volume depletion and low urinary chloride (usually <10 mEq/L)
   a. Gastrointestinal losses
      i. Vomiting
      ii. Gastrointestinal drainage (nasogastric suction)
      iii. Chloride-wasting diarrhea
      iv. Villous adenoma

b. Renal losses
   i. Diuretic therapy
   ii. Posthypercapnia status
   iii. Nonreabsorbable anions
   iv. Penicillin, carbenicillin, ticarcillin
2. With extracellular volume expansion and the presence of urinary chloride (usually >20 mEq/L)
   a. Mineralocorticoid excess
      i. Endogenous
         (1) Hyperaldosteronism
         (2) Cushing syndrome
         (3) Genetic causes: Bartter, Gitelman, Liddle and mineralocorticoid excess syndromes
      ii. Exogenous
         (1) Glucocorticoids
         (2) Mineralocorticoids
         (3) Carbenoxolone
         (4) Licorice excess
   b. Alkali ingestion
   c. Poststarvation feeding

Manifestations

Metabolic alkalemia has no specific signs or symptoms. Severe alkalemia may result in the following:

- Apathy
- Confusion or stupor

Management

Mild

The pH ranges from 7.45 to 7.55.

Moderate

The pH ranges from 7.56 to 7.69.

Severe

The pH is 7.70 or higher.

Beyond correction of the underlying cause, specific treatment is rarely required for mild or moderate metabolic alkalemia. *Metabolic alkalemia associated with extracellular fluid volume depletion* usually responds to an infusion of normal saline, which enhances renal HCO_3 excretion.

Associated electrolyte abnormalities (particularly hypokalemia) may be more threatening to the patient's well-being than the metabolic alkalemia is. Attention to concomitant electrolyte disorders is very important.

For *diuretic-induced alkalemia,* administration of potassium chloride (KCl) may improve the patient's condition.

If the patient has both *volume overload* and a metabolic alkalemia, **acetazolamide, 250 to 500 mg orally or intravenously every 8 hours,** enhances the renal HCO_3 excretion and may be helpful.

In *Bartter syndrome,* the alkalemia may respond to prostaglandin synthetase inhibitors, such as indomethacin.

It is very unusual to require an acidifying agent, such as NH_4Cl or dilute HCl, even for severe metabolic alkalemia. Such agents should be administered only under the direct guidance of your resident and the patient's attending physician.

Anemia

The serum hemoglobin (Hb) value is one of the most common laboratory measurements in hospitalized patients.

	Normal Hg level	Hg level in anemia
Men	13.6–17.2 g/100 ml	<13.2 g/100 ml
Women	12–15 g/100 ml	<11.6 g/100 ml

Remember that Hb is a *concentration*, and its value can be modified by both a change in its *content* and a change in its *diluent* (plasma). For instance, a patient's Hb may be elevated (i.e., in the *normal* range) despite a sudden loss of intravascular volume, as occurs in an acute hemorrhage. Because of the possibility of transfusion-related illnesses, you must avoid automatically initiating red blood cell (RBC) transfusions to correct a low Hb level. *Remember to treat the patient, not the laboratory value.*

CAUSES OF ANEMIA

1. Blood loss
   a. Acute
      i. Gastrointestinal (GI) hemorrhage
      ii. Trauma
      iii. Concealed hemorrhage
         (1) Ruptured aortic aneurysm
         (2) Ruptured fallopian tube (ectopic pregnancy)
         (3) Retroperitoneal hematoma
         (4) Postsurgical bleeding
   b. Chronic
      i. GI bleeding
      ii. Uterine bleeding
2. Inadequate production of RBCs
   a. Anemia of chronic disease (chronic inflammation, uremia, endocrine failure, liver disease)
   b. Iron deficiency
   c. Megaloblastic anemias (vitamin B_{12} and folate deficiency, drug effects, inherited disorders)

    d. Sideroblastic anemias (drug effects, alcohol effects, malignancy, rheumatoid arthritis, inherited disorders)

    e. Acquired disorders of marrow stem cells (aplastic anemia, myelodysplastic syndromes, chemotherapy, drug effects)

3. Hemolysis

    a. Extrinsic factors (immune hemolysis, splenomegaly, mechanical trauma, infection, microangiopathic hemolytic anemia)

    b. Membrane defects (e.g., hereditary spherocytosis, paroxysmal nocturnal hemoglobinuria)

    c. Internal RBC defects (e.g., thalassemia, sickle cell disease)

    d. Acute or delayed RBC transfusion reactions

Manifestations

The manifestations of anemia depend on the underlying medical conditions, the severity of the anemia, and the rapidity with which it develops. The body's reaction to an acute reduction in RBC mass is usually manifested by compensatory alterations in the cardiovascular and respiratory systems.

Acute anemias caused by hemorrhage result in symptoms and signs of intravascular volume depletion, including the following:

- Pallor, diaphoresis, tachypnea
- Cold, clammy extremities
- Hypotension, tachycardia
- Shock

Anemias that develop slowly over weeks or months are not usually accompanied by signs of intravascular volume depletion. In these cases, symptoms and signs are often not so obvious and may vary, depending on the presence of disease in other organ systems.

Common Symptoms

- Fatigue, lethargy, weakness
- Dyspnea
- Palpitations
- Worsening of symptoms in patients with angina pectoris or claudication, or onset of symptoms with a transient ischemic attack (TIA)
- Gastrointestinal disturbances (caused by shunting of blood from the splanchnic bed): anorexia, nausea, bowel irregularity
- Vertigo, headaches, tinnitus lack of libido

Signs

- Pallor
- Tachypnea
- Tachycardia, wide pulse pressure, hyperdynamic precordium
- Jaundice or splenomegaly (in hemolytic anemias)

Management

Assess the Severity

The severity of the situation should be determined according to the Hb level, the patient's volume status, the rapidity with which the anemia developed, and the likelihood that the underlying process will continue unabated.

Treatment of a Patient Who Is in Shock or Has Volume Depletion

Acute anemia caused by blood loss (and thus intravascular volume depletion) results in compensatory tachycardia and tachypnea. If full hemodynamic compensation is inadequate, hypotension or shock results. In your assessment of the patient's volume status, check for postural changes (see Chapter 3, page 10), which may be the earliest manifestation of acute blood loss.

1. Notify your resident.
2. Ensure that at least one large-bore (size 16 if possible) intravenous (IV) line is in place. Two such lines are preferable.
3. If active bleeding is evident, ensure that your hospital has blood on hold. If it does not, order stat crossmatch for 2, 4, or 6 units of packed RBCs, depending on your estimate of blood loss.
4. Replenish intravascular volume by administering IV fluids. The best immediate choice is a crystalloid (normal saline or Ringer's lactate), which stays in the intravascular space at least temporarily. Albumin or banked plasma can be given, but they are expensive, carry a risk of virus transmission, and are not always available. When a new, severe anemia is associated with intravascular volume depletion, the assumption is that blood has been lost from the intravascular space; therefore ideally, blood should be replaced. If your hospital has no blood on hold for the patient, a stat crossmatch usually takes 50 minutes. If blood is on hold, it should be available at the patient's bedside in 30 minutes. In an emergency, O-negative blood may be administered, although this practice is usually reserved for acute trauma victims. If the patient refuses blood or blood products, refer to Chapter 13, page 122. Transfusion-related infections can be minimized by transfusing only when necessary.
5. Order the appropriate IV rate, which depends on the patient's volume status. Shock necessitates IV fluid wide open through at least two large-bore IV sites. Elevating the IV bag, squeezing the IV bag, or using IV pressure cuffs may help speed the rate of delivery of the solution. Mild or moderate volume depletion can be treated with 500 to 1000 mL of normal saline, given as rapidly as possible, with serial determinations of volume status and assessment of cardiac status. If blood is not at the patient's bedside within 30 minutes, delegate someone to find the reason for the delay.

Note: Aggressive volume replacement in a patient with a history of congestive heart failure may result in pulmonary edema. Do not overshoot the goal of volume repletion.

6. Determine the site of hemorrhage.
   a. Look for obvious signs of external bleeding: from IV entry sites, skin lesions, hematemesis, menstrual bleeding.
   b. Examine for signs of occult blood loss.
      i. Perform a rectal examination to look for melena.
      ii. Occult blood loss should be suspected if swelling is found at biopsy or surgical sites (e.g., flank swelling after renal biopsy, ascites after liver biopsy) or if flank or periumbilical ecchymoses are visible (possible hemoperitoneum).
      iii. If the patient is a woman in her childbearing years, a ruptured fallopian tube (ectopic pregnancy) must be considered. A pelvic examination, if indicated, should be performed by an experienced physician.
      iv. If a ruptured thoracic or abdominal aortic aneurysm is likely, immediate surgical referral is necessary.
7. Review the chart for exacerbating factors that may contribute to ongoing hemorrhage (e.g., administration of antiplatelet agents, anticoagulants, or fibrinolytic agents or the presence of coagulopathies) and for recent pertinent laboratory values (activated partial thromboplastin time, prothrombin time, platelet count).
8. Request surgical consultation when appropriate.

Treatment of a Patient Who Is Normovolemic

Patients can tolerate even severe anemia (Hb level, <7 g/100 ml) if it develops slowly. Mild chronic anemias (Hb level, 10 to 12 g/100 ml) in the context of normal intravascular volume often do not alter the vital signs. If the patient is normovolemic, transfusion therapy is seldom warranted on an urgent basis. If you have excluded the presence of active hemorrhage, the anemia must be caused by (1) chronic blood loss, (2) inadequate production of RBCs, or (3) hemolysis.

1. An unexpected Hb <10 g/100 ml merits a repeat measurement to exclude laboratory error while other assessments are being performed. An asymptomatic patient with mild anemia (Hb level, 10 to 12 g/100 ml) and normal vital signs usually can wait if you must attend to other problems of higher priority. Always keep in mind, however, that if active bleeding is responsible for the anemia, a stable patient may become unstable very quickly.
2. What is the patient's usual Hb level? Look in the current or old chart to determine whether the anemia is a new finding. If the current Hb level is more than 1 or 2 g/100 ml lower than previous values, assume that the underlying cause of anemia has worsened or a second factor has developed (e.g., a patient with a chronic disease, such as systemic lupus erythematosus, may normally have an

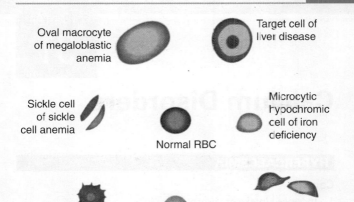

FIG. 30.1 **Findings on a blood smear that are diagnostic features associated with specific anemias.**

Hb of 9.0 g/100 ml; a new value of 7.5 g/100 ml may represent further marrow suppression, hemolysis, or new onset of bleeding).

3. If the patient is comfortable, the cardiovascular examination yields normal findings, and your examination reveals no suspicion of active bleeding, further investigation can take place in the morning. Several baseline studies are helpful in pointing you in the right direction to diagnose the cause of the anemia:

   a. Measurement of RBC volume. The mean corpuscular volume is useful in classifying the anemias caused by decreased RBC production (microcytic, normocytic, macrocytic).

   b. Examination of the blood smear. This study is more accurate than other measurements.

   c. Technologies in recognizing altered RBC structure often providing valuable clues for diagnosing specific anemias (Fig. 30.1).

   d. Reticulocyte count. Marrow erythropoiesis is assessed by this test. An elevated reticulocyte count is suggestive of hemolysis, recent hemorrhage, or a recently treated chronic anemia (e.g., vitamin B_{12} deficiency). An inappropriately low reticulocyte count is suggestive of a failure to produce RBCs (e.g., untreated iron deficiency, vitamin B_{12} deficiency, folate deficiency, or anemia of chronic disease).

   e. Serum bilirubin and lactic dehydrogenase that are elevated in hemolysis and normal in blood loss

   f. Vitamin B_{12} and folate, iron and iron binding capacity

Calcium Disorders

HYPERCALCEMIA

Causes

1. Increased intake or absorption
   a. Vitamin D or A intoxication
   b. Excessive calcium supplementation
   c. Milk-alkali syndrome (excessive antacid ingestion)
   d. Sarcoidosis and other granulomatous diseases
2. Increased production or mobilization from bone
   a. Primary hyperparathyroidism
   b. Neoplasm*: There are four mechanisms for hypercalcemia of malignancy:
      i. Bony metastasis (prostate, thyroid, kidney, breast, lung)
      ii. Parathyroid hormone-like substance elaborated by tumor cells (lung, kidney, ovary, colon)
      iii. Prostaglandin E2, which increases bony resorption (multiple myeloma)
      iv. Osteoclast-activating factor (multiple myeloma, lymphoproliferative disorders)
   c. Severe secondary hyperparathyroidism associated with renal failure
   d. Paget's disease
   e. Immobilization
   f. Hyperthyroidism
   g. Adrenal insufficiency
   h. Acromegaly
   i. Sarcoidosis: in addition to increased absorption from the gastrointestinal (GI) tract, conversion of 25(OH) vitamin D to the active form, $1,25(OH)_2$ vitamin D, is increased.
   j. Chronic lithium use
3. Decreased excretion
   a. Thiazide diuretics
   b. Familial hypocalciuric hypercalcemia

---

* Primary hyperparathyroidism and tumors account for 90% of cases of hypercalcemia.

Manifestations

The manifestations of hypercalcemia are numerous and nonspecific, often referred to as "bones, stones, and groans."

Head, ears, eyes, nose, throat (HEENT)	Corneal calcification (band keratopathy)
Cardiovascular system (CVS)	Short QT interval, prolonged PR interval (Fig. 31.1), dysrhythmias, digoxin sensitivity, hypertension
GI	Anorexia, nausea, vomiting, constipation, abdominal pain, pancreatitis ("groans")
Genitourinary system (GU)	Polyuria, polydipsia, nephrolithiasis ("stones")
Neurologic system	Restlessness, delirium, dementia, psychosis, lethargy, coma
Musculoskeletal system (MSS)	Muscle weakness, hyporeflexia, bone pain, fractures ("bones")
Miscellaneous	Hyperchlorhydric metabolic acidosis

Management

How severe is the situation?

The severity of the situation should be determined according to the serum calcium concentration, the rate of progression, and the presence or absence of symptoms. Most laboratories measure total serum calcium (ionized plus albumin bound), but the primary determinant of the physiologic effect is the ionized component.

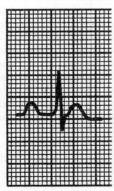

FIG. 31.1 Hypercalcemia (short QT interval, prolonged PR interval).

If the patient is hypoalbuminemic, a correction factor can be used to estimate the total calcium concentration. For every 10 g/L of hypoalbuminemia, add 0.2 mmol/L to the serum calcium value; for example if the measured serum calcium value is 2.6 mmol/L (the upper limit of normal) but the serum albumin value is low at 30 g/L (whereas a normal concentration of 40 g/L would be anticipated), the correct serum calcium value is 0.2 + 2.6 = 2.8 mmol/L (mild elevation).

Treatment should be aimed both at lowering the serum calcium and where possible treating the underlying cause.

How high is the serum calcium level?
- Normal range: 2.2 to 2.6 mmol/L
- Mild elevation: 2.6 to 2.9 mmol/L
- Moderate elevation: 2.9 to 3.2 mmol/L
- Severe elevation: higher than 3.2 mmol/L

Does the patient have a progressive cause that is likely to result in further increases?

If the situation is progressive, the patient requires immediate treatment.

Does the patient have symptoms?

Any patient with symptoms of hypercalcemia or potentially lethal manifestations such as arrhythmia or metabolic acidosis requires immediate treatment.

Treatment of Severe Hypercalcemia

Severe hypercalcemia (serum calcium level >3.2 mmol/L) requires immediate treatment because a fatal cardiac dysrhythmia may develop.

1. *Correct volume depletion and expand extracellular volume.* Administer normal saline, at a rate of 200 to 500 ml per hour adjusting the rate to maintain a urinary output of 100 to 250 ml per hour. This should restore intravascular volume with a consequent increase in calcium excretion. If the patient has a history of congestive heart failure, this volume expansion should be undertaken in the intensive care unit/cardiac care unit (ICU/CCU) to allow close monitoring of the volume status. Calcitonin 4 to 8 international units/kg IM or SC should be given and can be repeated in 12 hr for up to 48 hours. Thereafter tachyphylaxis reduces its effect. A bisphosphonate should be added: zoledronic acid 4 mg IV over 15 minutes. The maximum effect is in 2 to 4 days. Both calcitonin and bisphosphonates inhibit bone resorption by interfering with osteoclast function.

2. *If necessary, institute dialysis.* On occasion, when the serum calcium level is extremely high (e.g., >4.5 mmol/L) and saline diuresis cannot be achieved, hemodialysis or peritoneal dialysis is required.

TABLE 31.1	**Interventions**		
Intervention	**Trade Name**	**Dose**	**Comment**
Saline		200–500 ml IV per h	Hypercalcemia is accompanied by volume depletion
Calcitonin	Miacalcin	4–8 IU/kg IM or SC q 12h for up to 48 h	With hydration should lower serum calcium in 24–48 h
Bisphosphonates			
Zoledronic acid	Zoneta	4 mg IV over 15 minutes	Bisphosphonate of first choice
Pamidronate	Pamisol	60 mg IV or SC over 24 h	SC route may be useful in hospice patients
Ibandronate	Boniva	2 mg IV over 2 h	Useful in hypercalcemia of malignancy
Clodronate	Casteon	1600–2400 mg PO once daily	Useful in hypercalcemia of malignancy
Alendronate	Fosamax	5-10 mg PO once daily	Potent
Risedronate	Actonel	5 mg PO once daily	Potent
Others			
Cinacalcet	Sensipar	30–90 mg PO bid to qid	For hyperparathyroidism
Denosumab	Prolia	60–120 mg SC	Useful in face of resistance to bisphosphonates
Prednisone		20–40 mg PC od	Useful in hypercalcemia due to excess vitamin D
Dialysis			For patients in renal or heart failure

3. *If hypercalcemia is secondary to neoplasm,* in addition to the administration of normal saline (as previously discussed), one of the following medications may be of value (Table 31.1):

   a. Corticosteroids: **prednisone, 20 to 40 mg orally (PO) daily.**
      📖 Steroids antagonize the peripheral action of vitamin D (decreased absorption, decreased mobilization from bone, and decreased renal tubular reabsorption of calcium).

   b. **Plicamycin, 25 mcg/kg in 1 L of 5% dextrose in water (D5W), or in 1 L normal saline IV over 4 to 6 hours.**
      Plicamycin inhibits bone resorption. The onset of action is 48 hours.

   c. Bisphosphonates: These inhibit bone resorption and are effective agents in the control of cancer-associated hypercalcemia. **Zoledronic acid 4 mg IV over 15 minutes.** Alternatively, administer **pamidronate, 60 to 90 mg in 1 L of normal saline or D5W IV over 2 to 24 hours.**

Treatment of Moderate Hypercalcemia or Symptomatic Mild Hypercalcemia

Moderate hypercalcemia (serum calcium level, 2.9 to 3.2 mmol/L) or symptomatic mild hypercalcemia (2.6 to 2.9 mmol/L) should be managed as follows:

1. *Correct volume depletion and expand extracellular fluid volume* with **normal saline, 500 mL IV, administered over 1 to 2 hours.** More normal saline can be given at a rate to maintain slight volume expansion.
2. **Oral phosphate, 0.5 to 3 g/day**, depending on GI tolerance (without excessive flatulence or diarrhea), may be given to patients with low or normal serum phosphate levels.

Treatment of Asymptomatic Mild Hypercalcemia

Asymptomatic mild hypercalcemia (serum calcium level, 2.6 to 2.9 mmol/L) does not necessitate immediate treatment. The appropriate investigations can be ordered in the morning.

HYPOCALCEMIA

Causes

1. Decreased intake or absorption
   a. Malabsorption
   b. Intestinal bypass surgery
   c. Short bowel syndrome
   d. Vitamin D deficiency
2. Decreased production or mobilization from bone
   a. Hypoparathyroidism (after subtotal thyroidectomy or parathyroidectomy)
   b. Pseudohypoparathyroidism (parathyroid hormone resistance)
   c. Vitamin D deficiency: decreased production of 25(OH) vitamin D or $1,25(OH)_2$ vitamin D
   d. Acute hyperphosphatemia (tumor lysis, acute renal failure, rhabdomyolysis)
   e. Acute pancreatitis
   f. Hypomagnesemia
   g. Alkalosis (hyperventilation, vomiting, fistula)
   h. Neoplasm

      i. Paradoxic hypocalcemia associated with osteoblastic metastasis (lung, breast, prostate)

     ii. Medullary carcinoma of the thyroid (calcitonin-producing tumor)

   iii. Rapid tumor lysis with phosphate release

3. Increased excretion

  a. Chronic renal failure

  b. Drugs (aminoglycosides, loop diuretics)

Manifestations

The earliest symptoms are paresthesia of the lips, fingers, and toes.

HEENT	Papilledema, diplopia
CVS	Prolonged QT interval without U waves (Fig. 31.2)
GI	Abdominal cramps
Neurologic system	Confusion, irritability, depression
	Hyperactive tendon reflexes
	Carpopedal spasm, laryngospasm (stridor), tetany
	Generalized tonic-clonic seizures
	Paresthesia of lips, fingers, toes
Special tests	*Chvostek sign* (Fig. 31.3): facial muscle spasm elicited by tapping the facial nerve immediately anterior to the earlobe and below the zygomatic arch (this is a normal finding in 10% of the population)

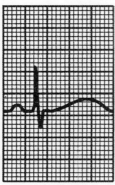

FIG. 31.2 Hypocalcemia (long QT interval).

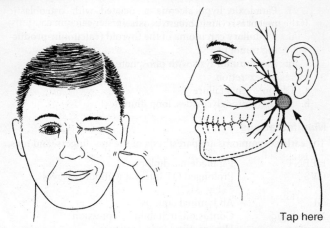

Tap here

FIG. 31.3 Chvostek sign: facial muscle spasm elicited by tapping the facial nerve immediately anterior to the earlobe and below the zygomatic arch.

Management

How severe is the situation?

The severity of the situation should be determined on the basis of the serum calcium and phosphate concentrations and the presence or absence of symptoms. If the serum albumin concentration is not within the normal range, a correction factor can be used to estimate the total serum calcium (ionized plus albumin bound). See page 362 for a discussion of this correction factor.

How low is the serum calcium level?

- Normal range, 2.2 to 2.6 mmol/L
- Mild depletion, 1.9 to 2.2 mmol/L
- Moderate depletion, 1.5 to 1.9 mmol/L
- Severe depletion, lower than 1.5 mmol/L

What is the serum phosphate concentration?

If the serum phosphate concentration is markedly elevated (>6 mmol/L) in severe hypocalcemia, hyperphosphatemia must be corrected with intravenous glucose and insulin before calcium is given, to avoid metastatic calcification.

Is the patient symptomatic?

Hypocalcemic patients who are asymptomatic do not require urgent correction with intravenous calcium.

Is the patient receiving digoxin?

If the patient is receiving digoxin, administer calcium cautiously because calcium potentiates the action of digoxin. Ideally, if intravenous calcium administration is required, the patient should have continuous electrocardiographic monitoring.

Treatment of Severe Symptomatic Hypocalcemia

A patient with severe symptomatic hypocalcemia (serum calcium levels <1.5 mmol/L) requires immediate treatment because of the danger of respiratory failure from laryngospasm.

1. If the patient's phosphate (PO_4) level is normal or low, administer 10 to 20 mL (93 mg elemental calcium/10 mL) of 10% solution of calcium gluconate IV in 100 mL of D5W over 30 minutes. If the patient has evidence of tetany or laryngeal stridor, the same dose should be given over 2 minutes as a direct injection: that is, calcium gluconate 10% solution, 10 to 20 mL IV, over 2 minutes. Oral calcium can be started immediately: 1 to 2 g of elemental calcium PO three times a day. If the corrected serum calcium value is lower than 1.9 mmol/L 6 hours after this treatment is initiated, a calcium infusion is required. Add 10 mL (93 mg elemental calcium) of a 10% calcium gluconate solution to 500 mL of D5W, and infuse over 6 hours. If the serum calcium value is not within the normal range after 6 hours of this infusion, 5 mL (46.5 mg elemental calcium) of calcium gluconate can be added to the initial infusion dose every 6 hours until a satisfactory serum calcium level is achieved. A patient who has undergone parathyroidectomy may require 100 to 150 mg of elemental calcium per hour. Once a satisfactory response has been achieved with intravenous calcium gluconate, oral replacement with elemental calcium may begin in doses of 0.5 to 2 g three times a day.

2. If the patient is hyperphosphatemic (PO_4 >6 mmol/L), correction with glucose and insulin is required before intravenous calcium is administered. Consult the nephrology services immediately.

Treatment of Mild and Moderate Asymptomatic Hypocalcemia

Patients with mild or moderate asymptomatic hypocalcemia do not require urgent intravenous calcium replacement. Oral calcium replacement with elemental calcium, 1000 to 1500 mg/day, can be started to achieve a corrected serum calcium level in the range of 2.2 to 2.6 mmol/L. Long-term treatment with oral calcium or vitamin D depends on the cause, which can be evaluated in the morning.

Coagulation Disorders

While on call, you will be confronted with abnormal results of tests of hemostasis. These must always be interpreted in the clinical context in which the measurements were made. Bleeding is the most common clinical manifestation of a coagulation disorder, and the type of bleeding can alert you to the probable type of disorder present.

Patients with *vessel* or *platelet abnormalities* may have petechiae or purpura, or they may bruise easily. The bleeding is characteristically superficial (e.g., oozing from mucous membranes or intravenous sites). The bleeding of scurvy is observed only rarely in North America and is usually manifested by perifollicular hemorrhages, although gingival bleeding and intramuscular hematomas also may occur.

Bleeding caused by *coagulation factor deficiencies* may occur spontaneously and in deeper organ sites (e.g., visceral hemorrhages) and hemarthroses, and it tends to be slowly progressive and prolonged. Bleeding associated with fibrinolytic agents is usually manifested by continuous oozing from intravenous sites.

Tests to Assess Hemostasis

Three tests are commonly used to assess hemostasis: prothrombin time (PT), activated partial thromboplastin time (aPTT), and platelet count. A fourth test, bleeding time, is used infrequently because it is rarely helpful for making a specific diagnosis, and it carries the risk of accidental exposure to hepatitis and human immunodeficiency virus (HIV). Laboratory features of the common coagulation disorders are listed in Table 32.1.

Prothrombin Time

The one-stage PT is a measurement that reflects the *extrinsic coagulation system* (Fig. 32.1). It is affected by deficiencies in factors I, II, V, VII, and X. However, antagonists of the extrinsic system—including unfractionated heparin, activated antithrombin III, and fibrin degradation products—can prolong the PT.

TABLE 32.1   Laboratory Features of Common Coagulation Disorders

Disorder	Diagnostic Laboratory Test				
	Activated Partial Thromboplastin Time	Prothrombin Time	Platelets	Bleeding Time	Other
Vessel Abnormalities					
Vasculitis	Normal	Normal	Normal	Normal or ↑	C3, C4 C1Q binding
Increased vascular fragility	Normal	Normal	Normal	↑	—
Hereditary connective tissue disorders	Normal	Normal	Normal	↑	—
Paraproteinemias	Normal	Normal	Normal	↑	—
Platelet Disorders					
Thrombocytopenia	Normal	Normal	↓	Normal or ↑[a]	—
Impaired platelet function	Normal	Normal	Normal	↑	—
Coagulation Factor Abnormalities					
Unfractionated heparin	↑	↑ or normal	Normal or ↓	Normal or ↑	—
LMWH	Normal	Normal	Normal	Normal or ↑	—
Warfarin	Normal or ↑	↑	Normal	Normal	—
Dabigatran	↑	↑	Normal	Normal	—
Rivaroxaban	↑	↑	Normal	Normal	—
Apixaban	↑	↑	Normal	Normal	—
Edoxaban	↑	↑	Normal	Normal	—
Vitamin K deficiency	↑	↑	Normal	Normal	—

Continued

TABLE 32.1 Laboratory Features of Common Coagulation Disorders —cont'd

DIC	↑	↑	→	Normal or ↑[a]	↑ Fibrin degradation products ↓ Fibrinogen
Factor VIII deficiency	↑	Normal	Normal	Normal	↓ Value on factor VIII assay
Factor IX deficiency	↑	Normal	Normal	Normal	Normal factor IX assay
von Willebrand disease	Normal or ↑	Normal	Normal	Normal or ↑	Normal or ↓ value on factor VIII assay ↓ Factor VIII antigen ↓ Ristocetin cofactor
Liver disease	↑	↑	Normal or ↓	Normal or ↑	—

DIC, Disseminated intravascular coagulation; *LMWH,* low-molecular-weight heparin.

[a] Depends on degree of thrombocytopenia.

DISORDERS ASSOCIATED WITH PROTHROMBIN TIME PROLONGATION

- Coagulation factor abnormalities
- Oral anticoagulants
- Vitamin K deficiency
- Liver disease
- Disseminated intravascular coagulation (DIC)
- Unfractionated heparin

Activated Partial Thromboplastin Time

The aPTT is a measurement that reflects the *intrinsic coagulation system* (see Fig. 32.1). It is most sensitive to deficiencies and abnormalities in the sequence of procoagulant activities that occur before factor X activation.

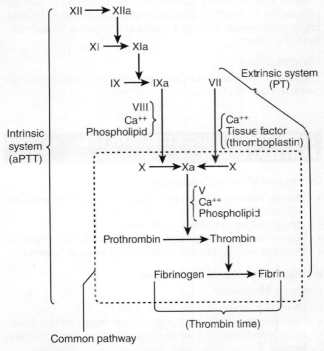

FIG. 32.1 **The coagulation cascade.** *aPTT*, Activated partial thromboplastin time; *PT*, prothrombin time.

DISORDERS ASSOCIATED WITH ACTIVATED PARTIAL THROMBOPLASTIN TIME PROLONGATION

- Circulating anticoagulant
- Unfractionated heparin
- Factor VIII, factor IX deficiency
- von Willebrand disease
- DIC
- Vitamin K deficiency
- Oral anticoagulants

One cause of aPTT prolongation is the presence of an acquired anticoagulant, such as the lupus erythematosus anticoagulant. This situation is differentiated from a factor deficiency in that the aPTT fails to normalize when a sample of the plasma of a patient with an acquired anticoagulant is mixed with normal plasma in a ratio of 50:50.

Note that low-molecular-weight heparin (LMWH) does not prolong the PT or aPTT. It exerts its anticoagulant effect by binding to antithrombin III, which results in anti–factor Xa and anti–factor IIa activity.

Platelet Count

The platelet count is a reflection of the production and destruction (sequestration) of platelets.

DISORDERS ASSOCIATED WITH LOW PLATELET COUNT

Decreased Marrow Production

- Marrow replacement by tumor, granuloma (e.g., tuberculosis, sarcoid), fibrous tissue
- Storage disease (e.g., Gaucher disease)
- Marrow injury by drugs (e.g., sulfonamides, chloramphenicol)
- Defective maturation (e.g., vitamin B_{12} or folate deficiency)

Increased Peripheral Destruction
Immune Mediated

- Drugs (e.g., quinine, quinidine, heparin)
- Connective tissue disorders (e.g., systemic lupus erythematosus)
- Lymphoproliferative disorders (e.g., chronic lymphocytic leukemia)
- HIV infection

- Idiopathic
- Posttransfusion purpura

Nonimmune Mediated

- Consumption (e.g., DIC, thrombotic thrombocytopenic purpura [TTP], prosthetic valves)

  📖 TTP characteristically occurs with a combination of hemolytic anemia, thrombocytopenia, fever, neurologic disorders, and renal dysfunction. The *hemolytic uremic syndrome* has a manifestation similar to that of TTP but without the neurologic manifestations. These two syndromes are distinct from DIC, which is characterized by prolonged aPTT and PT, reduced fibrinogen level, and elevated levels of fibrin degradation products. DIC most often occurs in the context of infection (e.g., gram-negative sepsis), obstetric catastrophe, malignancy (e.g., prostate cancer), and tissue damage or shock.
- Dilutional (e.g., massive transfusion)

Sequestration

- For instance, any cause of splenomegaly

Factitious Thrombocytopenia

Some patients have platelets that are susceptible to clumping when exposed to edetate disodium (EDTA), a preservative used in the lavender-topped blood collection tubes. This platelet clumping causes the platelet count to be falsely low when the blood specimen is read by an autoanalyzer. To diagnose factitious thrombocytopenia, verify platelet clumping by direct examination of the blood smear. An accurate platelet count can be obtained from these patients by collecting a blood sample in a sodium citrate (blue-topped) tube.

Vessel or Platelet Function Abnormalities

If the patient has a normal PT, aPTT, and platelet count and is not receiving LMWH, bleeding can still occur. This may be a result of *vessel abnormalities* or *abnormal platelet function*.

Vessel Abnormalities (Vascular Factor)

HEREDITARY DISORDERS

- Hereditary hemorrhagic telangiectasia
- Ehlers-Danlos syndrome
- Marfan syndrome
- Pseudoxanthoma elasticum
- Osteogenesis imperfecta

ACQUIRED DISORDERS

Vasculitis

- Schönlein-Henoch purpura
- Systemic lupus erythematosus
- Polyarteritis nodosa
- Rheumatoid arthritis
- Cryoglobulinemia

Increased Vascular Fragility

- Senile purpura
- Cushing syndrome
- Scurvy

Impaired Platelet Function

HEREDITARY DISORDERS

- von Willebrand disease
- Bernard-Soulier disease
- Glanzmann thrombasthenia

ACQUIRED DISORDERS

- Drugs (e.g., aspirin; clopidogrel; ticlopidine; prasugrel; ticagrelor; glycoprotein IIb/ IIIa inhibitors; nonsteroidal anti-inflammatory drugs [NSAIDs]; antibiotics such as high-dose penicillin, cephalosporins, nitrofurantoin)
- Uremia
- Paraproteins (e.g., amyloidosis, multiple myeloma, Waldenström macroglobulinemia)
- Myeloproliferative and lymphoproliferative disease (e.g., chronic granulocytic leukemia, essential thrombocytosis)
- Post–cardiopulmonary bypass status

Bleeding in Coagulation Disorders

MANIFESTATIONS

Bleeding in a patient with a coagulation disorder is of concern for two reasons:

1. Progressive loss of intravascular volume, if uncorrected, may lead to hypovolemic shock, with inadequate perfusion of vital organs.
2. Hemorrhage into specific organ sites may produce local tissue or organ injury (e.g., intracerebral hemorrhage, epidural hemorrhage with spinal cord compression, hemarthrosis).

MANAGEMENT

Vessel Abnormalities

Treatment of bleeding that results from vessel abnormalities usually consists of treatment of the underlying disorder.

1. Serious bleeding caused by *hereditary disorders of connective tissue* and by hereditary hemorrhagic telangiectasia most often necessitates local mechanical or surgical measures at the site of hemorrhage to control blood loss. In some patients with hereditary hemorrhagic telangiectasia, bleeding may be controlled with aminocaproic acid.
2. In the vasculitides, control of bleeding is best achieved by the use of corticosteroids, other immunosuppressive agents, or both.
3. There is no good treatment for the increased vascular fragility that results in senile purpura. Purpura caused by *Cushing syndrome* is preventable with normalization of plasma cortisol levels. However, in a patient receiving therapeutic corticosteroids, the underlying indication for therapy often prevents a significant reduction in steroid levels. Hemorrhages associated with scurvy do not recur after adequate dietary supplementation of ascorbic acid.

Coagulation Factor Abnormalities

Treatment of coagulation factor abnormalities is dependent on the specific factor deficiency or deficiencies.

1. *Specific factor deficiencies* should always be treated in consultation with a hematologist. Factor VIII deficiency (hemophilia A) can be treated with fresh-frozen plasma or cryoprecipitate, but factor VIII concentrate is the treatment of choice. Nonblood products may also be of benefit, such as desmopressin acetate (DDAVP) injection or aminocaproic acid. Factor IX deficiency (hemophilia B) may be treated with fresh-frozen plasma or prothrombin complex concentrate, but factor IX concentrate is the treatment of choice.
2. Active bleeding in patients with *liver disease* and an elevated PT, aPTT, or international normalized ratio (INR) should be managed with fresh-frozen plasma. Because many patients with liver disease also have vitamin K deficiency, it is worthwhile to administer vitamin K, 10 mg subcutaneously (SC), intramuscularly (IM), or orally (PO) daily for 3 days. Intravenous vitamin K occasionally causes an anaphylactic reaction. Factor IX concentrates carry a risk of thrombosis and are contraindicated in liver disease.
3. *Vitamin K deficiency* can be treated in a manner identical to that outlined later for the correction of warfarin coagulopathy.

Ideally, however, you should identify and treat the underlying cause of vitamin K deficiency.

4. The treatment of DIC is both complicated and controversial. All medical authorities agree, however, that definitive management involves treating the underlying cause. In addition, a patient with DIC often requires coagulation factor and platelet support in the form of fresh-frozen plasma, cryoprecipitate, and platelet transfusions.

5. Bleeding that results from *anticoagulant therapy* can be reversed slowly or rapidly, depending on the clinical status of the patient and the site of bleeding.

   a. *Unfractionated heparin* has a half-life of only 1½ hours; therefore, simply discontinuing a heparin infusion should normalize the aPTT and correct a heparin-induced coagulopathy involving minor episodes of bleeding. LMWH, however, has a longer half-life, and it may be necessary to reverse the heparin effect with protamine sulfate. This may also be necessary in cases of serious bleeding associated with unfractionated heparin. The usual dose of **protamine sulfate is approximately 1 mg per 100 U of unfractionated heparin by slow intravenous infusion**. Determine the dosage by estimating the amount of circulating heparin; for example, for a patient receiving a maintenance infusion of 1000 U of unfractionated heparin per hour intravenously, the heparin infusion should be stopped and sufficient protamine should be given to neutralize approximately half of the preceding hour's dose—a total protamine dose of 5 mg. No more than 50 mg per single dose in a 10-minute period should be given. Side effects of protamine include hypotension, bradycardia, flushing, and bleeding.

   b. Protamine does not completely neutralize anti–factor Xa activity, and excessive protamine doses may worsen bleeding; therefore in patients receiving LMWH, it should only be used to neutralize LMWH effect if there is significant bleeding.

   c. The *warfarin* effect can be reversed rapidly, as may be required in life-threatening hemorrhages, by administration of prothrombin complex concentrates, with the dose dependent on the patient's INR. If unavailable, *plasma* (e.g., 2 units at a time) may be used, with subsequent redetermination of INR. Although both fresh-frozen plasma and banked plasma contain the vitamin K–dependent clotting factors, banked plasma is considerably less expensive and is thus preferred. For severe bleeding (e.g., intracranial hemorrhage), urgent hematologic consultation is needed. When prolonged reversal of anticoagulant effect is desired, **vitamin K, 10 mg PO, SC, or IM, may be given daily for 3 days.**

In patients taking warfarin, minor bleeding complications may necessitate temporary discontinuation of this drug. Intravenous vitamin K occasionally causes an anaphylactic reaction and should be administered with caution.

d. The anticoagulant effect of the *direct oral anticoagulants* (DOACS) can be reversed rapidly by prothrombin complex concentrate as described above for warfarin. Plasma (e.g., 2 units at a time) may be used if prothrombin complex concentrate is unavailable. Additionally, if the DOAC was ingested within 2 hours of your evaluating the patient, one dose of activated charcoal can be given orally. The monoclonal antibody, idarucizumab, is available for reversal of *dabigatran* effect, and dabigatran is also dialyzable. The anticoagulant effect of Factor Xa inhibitors (apixaban, rivaroxaban, edoxaban) can be reversed with andexanetalfa, which is a recombinant human Factor Xa variant which binds to oral Factor Xa inhibitors. Ciraparantag, an antidote for rivaroxaban, apixaban, and edoxaban, is under development. Factor Xa inhibitors are not dialyzable.

6. For *bleeding caused by fibrinolytic agents*, localized oozing at sites of invasive procedures can often be controlled by local pressure dressings; such oozing can be prevented by avoiding invasive procedures. For more serious hemorrhage, the agent must be discontinued. Fibrinolytic agents that are not fibrin specific cause systemic fibrinogenolysis; therefore fresh-frozen plasma may be needed to replace fibrinogen. Cryoprecipitate can also be used to replace fibrinogen and replenish factor VIII levels. **Aminocaproic acid**, which is an inhibitor of plasminogen activator, has also been used (**20 to 30 g/day**) but should not be initiated before hematologic consultation.

Platelet Abnormalities

Treatment of bleeding in a thrombocytopenic patient varies, depending on the presence of either an abnormality in platelet production or an increase in platelet destruction.

1. *Decreased marrow production* of platelets is treated in the long term by identification and, if possible, correction of the underlying cause (e.g., chemotherapy for tumor, removal of marrow toxins, vitamin B_{12} or folate supplementation when indicated). In the short term, however, a serious bleeding complication should be treated by platelet transfusion (e.g., 6 to 8 units at a time). One unit of platelets can be expected to increase the platelet count by $1000/\mu L$ in a patient with inadequate marrow production of platelets. Check the response to transfusion by ordering a 1-hour posttransfusion platelet count.

2. *Increased peripheral destruction* of platelets is best managed by identification and correction of the underlying problem. Often, this involves the use of systemic corticosteroids or other immunosuppressive agents. Such patients tend to have less serious bleeding manifestations than do those with inadequate marrow production of platelets, but platelet transfusion may be required for life-threatening bleeding episodes. Significant bleeding in patients with *idiopathic thrombocytopenic purpura* may respond to intravenous immune globulin, followed by platelet transfusions. Platelet transfusion therapy should not be used to treat thrombocytopenia in a patient with TTP, because it may actually worsen the condition. The platelet abnormality in TTP is best treated with plasma infusion or, preferably, plasma exchange.

3. *Dilutional thrombocytopenia* caused by massive transfusion of red blood cells and intravenous fluid therapy is treated with platelet transfusion as required. Dilutional thrombocytopenia can usually be prevented by a transfusion of 8 units of platelets for every 10 to 12 units of RBCs transfused. (Because massive transfusion may also result in consumption and dilution of coagulation factors in the recipient, plasma should be administered if the patient shows evidence of bleeding and if PT, aPTT, or INR is significantly elevated.)

4. *von Willebrand disease* may be treated with factor VIII concentrates or cryoprecipitate. DDAVP injection is useful in type 1 von Willebrand disease but may exacerbate thrombocytopenia in type 2 disease.

5. Bleeding disorders resulting from *acquired platelet dysfunction* are best managed by identification and correction of the underlying problem. Temporary treatment of bleeding disorders caused by these conditions may involve platelet transfusion or other more specialized measures (e.g., cryoprecipitate, DDAVP injection, plasmapheresis, conjugated estrogens, intensive dialysis in uremia).

CHAPTER

33

Glucose Disorders

The management of glucose disorders has become increasingly complex because of the proliferation of insulin types, the popular use of new insulin-delivery and glucose-monitoring devices, the two types of units to measure blood glucose—mmol/L and mg/dl and the variety of agents used in the chronic management of type 2 diabetes (Table 33.1).

It is important to be familiar with the insulin brands commonly used in your institution and to have an understanding of the various insulin delivery devices. Comparative durations of action of insulin preparations are listed in the Formulary, page 509.

Abnormalities in glucose metabolism characterize the disorder diabetes mellitus (diabetes = siphon or pass through; mellitus = sweet). Type 1 diabetes is an autoimmune disease resulting in the production of too little insulin. Type 2 diabetes is a result of obesity, diet, and inactivity resulting in resistance to insulin and relatively too little insulin production.

Insulin is the treatment of choice for type 1 diabetes. Type 2 diabetes is treated by lifestyle changes including diet, weight loss, and exercise as well as antihyperglycemic agents.

Insulin may be administered intravenously (usually reserved for emergencies) or subcutaneously. The subcutaneous (SC) route may involve direct injection, a pen device, or a continuous infusion system (the *insulin pump*). Insulin pens are available through a variety of manufacturers and often contain particular types of insulin or premixtures. Usually, the patient is familiar with the use and limitations of their pen. If simple adjustments cannot be made and you must change a patient's insulin dosage, it is best to use direct injection with a needle and syringe or consult your resident or a diabetes education nurse. The insulin pump is a more complex method of continuous insulin delivery. Principles of insulin use with the insulin pump are described in Box 33.1. Unless you are familiar with this device, it is best to contact your resident or attending physician before you make changes in the patient's insulin regimen.

391

TABLE 33.1	Conversion Table
mmol/L	**mg/100 ml**
0.6	10
2.8	50
6.1	**110**
7.0	126
11.1	**195**
13.75	250
22.5	**405**

Insulin conversion: 1 mg per 100 ml = 0.0555 mmol/L
1 mmol/L = 18.018 mg per 100 ml

BOX 33.1	The Insulin Pump

An insulin pump is a small mechanical device that delivers insulin subcutaneously by means of an infusion set. The pump is worn outside the body in a pouch or on a belt. The infusion set is a long, thin plastic tube connected to a flexible plastic cannula that is inserted into the skin at the infusion site, usually in the SC abdominal tissue. The infusion set remains in place for 2 to 4 days and is then replaced; a new location is used each time.

When a patient with an insulin pump is admitted to the hospital, the pump should remain on the patient at all times, unless other arrangements are made for insulin replacement. These patients have been trained in insulin pump therapy and, in most situations, can aid in maintaining glycemic control with the pump, together with the diabetes education nurse and the attending physician. If the patient is unconscious, in most cases the pump can be removed (*do not cut the tubing:* just detach the pump and infusion set from the patient), and insulin can be administered by alternative methods.

The insulin pump is not an artificial pancreas. It is a computer-controlled unit that delivers insulin in precise amounts at preprogrammed times. Only Humalog or NovoLog (NovoRapid) insulin is used. The pump is not automatic; the patient has to decide, on the basis of blood glucose results and the amount of food that will be consumed, how much insulin should be administered.

The device contains a small reservoir of insulin (up to 3 mL), a small battery-powered pump, and a computer to control its operation. The pump is set to deliver insulin in two ways:
1. Basal rate: a small, continuous flow of insulin delivered automatically every 15 min. The basal rate is programmed by the operator and may vary at different times of the day.
2. Bolus dose: designed to supplement the food eaten during a meal or to correct elevated blood glucose levels. Bolus doses can be programmed at any time, which gives the patient greater flexibility with regard to when and what he or she eats.

Blood glucose can be continuously monitored using a continuous glucose monitor (CGM) The monitor displays sugar levels at 1-, 5-, 10-, or 15-minute intervals. If glucose drops to a dangerously low level or a high preset level, the monitor will sound an alarm. Fortunately, most blood glucose meters are prefixed to measure in mmol/L or mg/dl. This avoids accidental switching—which could be fatal.

A variety of oral antihyperglycemic agents are used in the treatment of Type 2 diabetes (see Formulary).

Hyperglycemia

CAUSES

Patients With Documented Diabetes Mellitus

- Poorly controlled type 1 or type 2 diabetes mellitus
- Stress (surgery, infection, severe illness)
- Drugs (corticosteroids, thiazides, β-blockers, phenytoin, nicotinic acid, opiates, protease inhibitors)
- Total parenteral nutrition (TPN) administration
- Pancreatic injury (pancreatitis, trauma, surgery)
- Insulin delivery problems with insulin pumps (e.g., programming errors, pump or alarm malfunctions, reservoir problems, problems with infusion set or injection site)

Patients Without Previously Documented Diabetes Mellitus

- New onset of diabetes mellitus
- Stress (surgery, infection, severe illness)
- Drugs (corticosteroids, thiazides, β-blockers, phenytoin, nicotinic acid, opiates, protease inhibitors)
- TPN administration
- Pancreatic injury (pancreatitis, trauma, surgery)

ACUTE MANIFESTATIONS

Mild Hyperglycemia

The fasting blood glucose level ranges from 6.1 to 11.0 mmol/L (110 to 195 mg/100 ml)

- May be asymptomatic
- Polyuria, polydipsia, thirst

Moderate Hyperglycemia

The fasting blood glucose level ranges from 11.1 to 22.5 mmol/L (195 to 405 mg/ 100 ml)

- Volume depletion (tachycardia, decreased jugular venous pressure [JVP], with or without hypotension)
- Polyuria, polydipsia, thirst
- May be asymptomatic

Severe Hyperglycemia

The fasting blood glucose level exceeds 22.5 mmol/L (over 405 mg/100 ml)

Type 1 Diabetes Mellitus

- Musty odor of breath (ketone breath)
- Kussmaul breathing (deep, pauseless respirations seen when the hydrogen ion concentration pH <7.2)
- Volume depletion (tachycardia, decreased JVP, with or without hypotension)
- Anorexia, nausea, vomiting, abdominal pain (may mimic a "surgical abdomen")
- Ileus, gastric dilation
- Hyporeflexia, hypotonia, delirium, coma

Type 2 Diabetes Mellitus

- Polyuria, polydipsia
- Volume depletion
- Confusion, coma

MANAGEMENT

Assess the Severity

The severity of the situation should be determined on the basis of the blood glucose level (Table 33.2) and the patient's symptoms.

Treatment of Mild, Asymptomatic Hyperglycemia

Regardless of whether a patient is taking oral hypoglycemics or an insulin preparation, urgent treatment is not required for mild, asymptomatic hyperglycemia. If the patient is not known to be diabetic, it may be useful to take the initial steps to determine

TABLE 33.2	Blood Glucose Levels	
	Blood Glucose Level	
Glycemic Level	**Fasting or Preprandial (mmol/L) and mg/dL**	**2-Hour Postprandial (mmol/L and mg/dL)**
Normal range	3.5-6.0 mmol/L, or 63-108 mg/dL	<11.0 mmol/L, or <198 mg/dL
Mild hyperglycemia	6.1-11.0 mmol/L, or 110-198 mg/dL	11.1-16.5 mmol/L, or 200-297 mg/dL
Moderate hyperglycemia	11.1-22.5 mmol/L, or 200-405 mg/dL	16.6-27.5 mmol/L, or 299-495 mg/dL
Severe hyperglycemia	>22.5 mmol/L, or >405 mg/dL	>27.5 mmol/L or >495 mg/dL

whether the patient does have diabetes, impaired fasting glucose, or impaired glucose tolerance. Order the following:

1. Fasting blood glucose measurement in the morning. A fasting blood glucose level higher than 7.0 mmol/L (126 mg/100 ml) on more than one occasion confirms the diagnosis of diabetes mellitus. Make sure that the patient is not receiving glucose-containing intravenous (IV) solutions, which would make these results invalid. In addition the diagnosis of diabetes mellitus cannot be made in the setting of stress (e.g., infection, surgery, severe illness). Any one of the following criteria is diagnostic for diabetes mellitus:
   a. Fasting blood glucose level >7.0 mmol/L (126 mg/100 ml) × 2 (venous plasma)
   b. A glucose tolerance test with a 2-hour postprandial blood glucose measurement of >11.1 mmol/L (200 mg/100 ml) (venous plasma)
   c. A hemoglobin A1C of ≥6.5%
   d. The hemoglobin A1C level is a measure of the average blood sugar over the last 3 months.
   e. Symptoms of diabetes (polyuria, polydipsia, blurred vision, weight loss) and a random blood glucose level >11.1 mmol/L (110 mg/100 ml) × 2 (venous plasma)
2. Finger-prick blood glucose (FPBG) readings before meals and at bedtime. If the readings are higher than 25 mmol/L (450 mg/100 ml) or lower than 2.8 mmol/L (50 mg/100 ml), a stat blood glucose sample should be drawn and a physician informed.

Treatment of Moderate Hyperglycemia

For a patient with moderate hyperglycemia who is already taking insulin, the insulin dosage may have to be adjusted. Whenever possible, a patient's insulin regimen should be adjusted according to the same insulin preparations and the same delivery device that the patient is already using. Examine the diabetic record for the past 3 days.

A sample adjustment in insulin dosage is presented in Table 33.3. The SC insulin dose given is indicated in parentheses (e.g., 20/10 indicates that 20 U of neutral protamine Hagedorn [NPH] and 10 U of rapid or short-acting insulin have been given).

You may be called at night because of, for example, an FPBG reading of 25 mmol/L (450 mg/dL). Order the following:

1. Stat random blood glucose measurement to confirm the FPBG reading.
2. Rapid or short-acting insulin, 5 to 10 U subcutaneously, immediately.

  📖 It is not your job to devise a schedule that will achieve perfect blood glucose control for the rest of the patient's hospital

TABLE 33.3   Sample Insulin Dosage Adjustment

	Before Breakfast		Before Lunch		Before Supper		At Bedtime	
Date	Finger-Prick Blood Glucose Reading	Neutral Protamine Hagedorn/ Rapid or Short-Acting Insulin (mmol/L)	Finger-Prick Blood Glucose Reading	Neutral Protamine Hagedorn/ Rapid or Short-Acting Insulin (mmol/L)	Finger-Prick Blood Glucose Reading	Neutral Protamine Hagedorn/Rapid or Short-Acting Insulin (mmol/L)	Finger-Prick Blood Glucose Reading	Neutral Protamine Hagedorn/ Rapid or Short-Acting Insulin (mmol/L)
August 1	16.7	20/10	13.9	0/0	16.7	10/10	18.1	0/0
August 2	13.9	20/10	16.7	0/4	8.3	10/10	19.4	0/0
August 3	16.7	20/10	15.2	0/0	13.1	10/10	25.0	0/0

stay. Short-term control of blood glucose levels has not been shown to decrease complications in diabetic patients. When the blood glucose level is elevated at night, your aim is to prevent the development of ketoacidosis in a patient with type 1 diabetes mellitus or the development of the hyperosmolar state in a patient with type 2 diabetes mellitus without causing symptomatic hypoglycemia with your treatment. In general, for most noncritical hospitalized patients with diabetes, a preprandial glucose <7.8 mmol/L (140 mg/dL) and all random glucose levels <10 mmol/L (180 mg/dL) are advised.

3. An 0300 FPBG reading. Determining the reason for poor control of blood glucose before breakfast may aid in the ongoing adjustment of the patient's insulin.

   📖 If hypoglycemia is documented at 3 a.m., then prebreakfast hyperglycemia may reflect hyperglycemic rebound (the Somogyi effect), which is correctly managed by reducing the before-supper NPH insulin dose. If hyperglycemia is documented at 3 a.m., then pre-breakfast hyperglycemia may reflect inadequate insulin coverage overnight. This is correctly managed by increasing the before-supper NPH insulin dose.

For a patient with moderate hyperglycemia who is not taking insulin, a corrective dose of rapid or short-acting insulin may be given (e.g., rapid or short-acting insulin, 5 to 10 U SC for a random glucose reading of 25 mmol/L [450 mg/dL]). If the patient is taking oral hypoglycemics or injectable GL1-P receptor agonists, particularly if they are not eating, consider holding these agents.

Sliding-scale insulin is not recommended except in the short term (1 to 2 days). The basal-bolus (prandial) insulin regimen is a better approach because it addresses basal insulin requirements, meal-related requirements, and supplemental (e.g., unexpected glucose elevations due to stress, infection, etc.). A useful formula to remember is that for an insulin-naïve patient, the recommended total daily insulin dose should start between 0.3 to 0.5 units/kg, with lower doses in the elderly and those with impaired renal function.

Treatment of Severe Hyperglycemia

Severe hyperglycemia necessitates urgent treatment. In most cases, this involves temporarily stopping the patient's previous diabetic medications and administering IV hydration and insulin.

Diabetic Ketoacidosis

This complication may occur in a patient with poorly controlled type 1 diabetes mellitus. It is caused by an absolute insulin deficit and results in impaired resynthesis of long-chain fatty acids from acetate, with subsequent conversion to the acidic ketone bodies (ketosis).

1. *Order bloodwork—serum glucose, electrolytes, ketones, Cr level, and arterial blood gas.*

     Repeat the measurements for ABGs and potassium level in 2 hours and thereafter as required.

     Hyperglycemic patients can have metabolic acidemia and hypokalemia. As normal saline and insulin are administered, the acidemia is corrected, and the potassium shifts into the cells from the extracellular fluid. This can result in a worsening of hypokalemia.

2. *Correct volume depletion.* Administer **500 to 1000 mL of normal saline intravenously** over the first hour; subsequent IV rates are guided by reassessment of volume status.

     📖 Patients with diabetic ketoacidosis often have a 3- to 5-L volume deficit. It is therefore not unusual for such patients to require normal saline at rates of 500 mL/hour for an additional 2 to 8 hours to restore euvolemia. If a patient has a history of congestive heart failure (CHF), weighs less than 50 kg, or is 80 years of age or older, normal saline should be given cautiously, to avoid iatrogenic CHF.

3. *Correct serum potassium levels*

     Once adequate renal function (patient producing approximately 50 ml urine/hour) has been established, correct serum potassium deficits. If serum K < 3.3 mEq/L, give **KCl 20 to 40 mEq IV/hour** until serum K is >3.3 mEq/L. If the serum potassium is 3.3 to 5.3 mEq/L, add **KCl 20 to 30 mEq per L of IV fluid** to maintain serum K in the 4 to 5 mEq/L range. If serum K >5.3 mEq/L, give no added potassium.

4. *Begin an insulin infusion.* Administer a single dose of **0.1 units/ kg of IV regular insulin** by direct slow injection, followed by an infusion rate that is based on close monitoring of blood glucose. Start the insulin infusion at **0.1 U/kg per hour in normal saline**.

     📖 Regular insulin can bind to the plastic IV tubing. To ensure accurate insulin delivery, 30 to 50 mL of the infusion solution should be run through the IV tubing and discarded before the tubing is connected to the patient. Discontinue the standing order for SC insulin or oral hypoglycemics before you begin the insulin infusion.

5. *Monitor blood glucose level hourly* by FPBG measurements. When the blood glucose level has fallen to 14 mmol/L (252 mg/100 ml), continue the insulin infusion but switch the delivery solution from normal saline to 5% dextrose in water (D5W). Continue the insulin infusion until the blood glucose level remains stable at 8 to 10 mmol/L (144 to 180 mg/100 ml). As the blood glucose level falls, the rate of insulin infusion should be slowed (e.g., from 0.025 to 0.05 U/kg per hour).

📖 The rate of fall of the blood glucose level should be approximately 2 mmol/L per hour; more aggressive treatment of hyperglycemia may result in severe hypokalemia and cerebral edema.

6. When the glucose level has stabilized at 8 to 10 mmol/L (144 to 189 mg/ 100 ml), *restart SC insulin,* remembering that the insulin infusion must be continued for 1 to 2 hours after the injection of SC insulin; otherwise, ketogenesis will be reactivated. Continue to monitor the bedside glucose level every 4 hours, adding supplemental rapid or short-acting insulin to keep blood glucose between 8 and 10 mmol/L.

7. Monitor blood glucose level, serum electrolyte levels, and arterial blood gas (ABG) measurements.

8. *Search for the precipitating cause.* Common precipitating factors include the following:
   a. Infection
   b. Inadequate insulin dosage
   c. Dietary indiscretion
   d. Pancreatitis

Hyperosmolar, Hyperglycemic, Nonketotic State

This condition may occur in a patient with poorly controlled type 2 diabetes mellitus. It is a syndrome of profound volume depletion that results from a sustained hyperglycemic diuresis without compensatory fluid intake. The condition in the vernacular is known as HONC or HONK (hyperosmolar nonketotic coma). Typical patients are 50 to 70 years old. Many have no history of diabetes mellitus. The precipitating event is often stroke, infection, pancreatitis, or drug use. The blood glucose level is often very high (>55 mmol/L [1000 mg/ 100 ml]), but significant ketosis is absent.

1. *Order baseline measurements of electrolytes, urea level, creatinine level, and glucose level.* Repeat the measurements of blood glucose level and electrolytes in 2 hours and thereafter as required.

2. *Correct volume depletion and water deficit.* The objectives of fluid therapy in the nonketotic hyperosmolar state are to correct the volume deficit and to resolve the hyperosmolarity. These objectives can be achieved by administering **normal saline, 500 to 1000 mL intravenously over 1 to 2 hours**; subsequent IV rates are guided by reassessment of volume status. Once the volume deficit is corrected with normal saline, remaining water deficits—as indicated by persistent hypernatremia or hyperglycemia—are best corrected with hypotonic IV solutions, such as 1/2 normal saline.

3. *Correct serum potassium levels*
   Once adequate renal function (patient producing approximately 50 ml urine/hour) has been established, correct serum

potassium deficits. If serum K < 3.3 mEq/L, give **KCl 20 to 30 mEq IV/hour** until serum K is >3.3 mEq/L. If the serum potassium is 3.3 to 5.3 mEq/L, add **KCl 20 to 30 mEq per L of IV fluid** to maintain serum K in the 4 to 5 mEq/L range. If serum K >5.3 mEq/L, give no added potassium.

4. *Begin an insulin infusion.* See the previous discussion of the treatment of diabetic ketoacidosis. Rehydration alone often produces a substantial fall in blood glucose level through renal excretion. As a result, patients with the hyperosmolar, hyperglycemic, nonketotic state generally require less insulin than a patient with type 1 diabetes and ketoacidosis.

5. Search for *the* precipitating cause:
   a. Infection
   b. Inadequate fluid intake
   c. Other acute illnesses (myocardial infarction, stroke)

Hypoglycemia

CAUSES

Patients With Documented Diabetes Mellitus

- Excess insulin, or oral hypoglycemics
- Decreased caloric intake
- Missing meals or missing snacks
- Increased exercise

Patients Without Documented Diabetes Mellitus

- Surreptitious intake of insulin or oral hypoglycemic agents
- Insulinoma
- Supervised 72-hour fasting for the investigation of hypoglycemia
- Drugs (ethanol, pentamidine, disopyramide, monoamine oxidase [MAO] inhibitors)
- Hepatic failure
- Adrenal insufficiency

MANIFESTATIONS

Adrenergic Response (Catecholamine Release Caused by Rapid Decrease in Glucose Level)

- Diaphoresis
- Palpitations
- Tremulousness
- Tachycardia
- Hunger
- Acral and perioral numbness

- Anxiety
- Combativeness
- Confusion
- Coma

Central Nervous System Response

Response may develop slowly over 1 to 3 hours.
- Headache
- Diplopia
- Bizarre behavior
- Focal neurologic deficits
- Confusion
- Seizures
- Coma

The adrenergic response does not always precede the central nervous system response, and some patients may progress directly from confusion or inability to speak, to seizure or coma.

MANAGEMENT

Assess the Severity

Any symptomatic patient with suspected hypoglycemia requires treatment. Symptoms may be precipitated by either a rapid fall in blood glucose level or an absolute low level of blood glucose.

1. *Draw 1 mL of blood* for blood glucose testing to confirm the diagnosis. If the cause of hypoglycemia is not clear, draw 10 mL and ask the laboratory to save an aliquot for later measurement of insulin and C peptide. *Do not wait* to receive the blood glucose results before beginning treatment.

    📖 Insulin produced endogenously includes the C peptide fragment; commercial preparations of insulin do not. Thus a high insulin level in association with a high C peptide level and hypoglycemia is suggestive of endogenous production of excess insulin (e.g., insulinoma), whereas a high insulin level in association with a low C peptide level and hypoglycemia is suggestive of surreptitious or therapeutic administration of exogenous insulin.

2. If the patient is awake and cooperative, oral glucose in the form of sweetened fruit juice can be given. If the patient is unable to take oral fluids or is unconscious, **D50W, 50 mL intravenously**, should be given by direct, slow injection. If the patient has no IV access and is unable to take oral fluids (e.g., is unconscious), **glucagon, 1 mg subcutaneously or intramuscularly**, should be administered. After glucagon administration, vomiting may develop; therefore a patient who is not fully conscious should be monitored carefully to prevent aspiration.

3. If ongoing hypoglycemia is anticipated, or if the patient's symptoms were severe (e.g., seizure), begin a maintenance IV infusion of D5W or D10W at a rate of 100 mL/hour. Ask the registered nurse to reassess the patient in 1 hour. In addition, remeasure the blood glucose level in 2 to 4 hours to ensure that a hypoglycemic relapse has not occurred. If the patient has hypoglycemia caused by oral hypoglycemic agents, repeated doses of D50W may be required because these drugs are metabolized and excreted slowly.

Potassium Disorders

Hyperkalemia

CAUSES

Excessive Intake

- K^+ supplements (oral or intravenous)
- Salt substitutes
- High-dose intravenous therapy with K^+ salts of penicillin
- Blood transfusions
- Diet high in potassium (dried figs, molasses, seaweed, avocados)

Decreased Excretion

- Renal failure (acute or chronic)
- Drugs
- K^+-sparing diuretics (spironolactone, eplerenone, triamterene, amiloride)
- Angiotensin-converting enzyme (ACE) inhibitors
- Angiotensin receptor blockers (ARBs)
- Angiotensin receptor neprolysin inhibitors
- Nonsteroidal anti-inflammatory drugs (NSAIDs)
- Trimethoprim-sulfamethoxazole
- Pentamidine
- Cyclosporine
- Addison disease, hypoaldosteronism
- Distal tubular dysfunction (i.e., type IV renal tubular acidosis [RTA])

Shift From Intracellular to Extracellular Fluid

- Acidemia (especially nonanion gap)
- Insulin deficiency (uncontrolled hyperglycemia)
- Tissue destruction (hemolysis, crush injuries, rhabdomyolysis, extensive burns, tumor lysis)
- Drugs (succinylcholine, digoxin, arginine, β-blockers)
- Hyperkalemic periodic paralysis

Factitious

- Prolonged tourniquet placement for venipuncture
- Blood sample hemolysis
- Leukocytosis
- Thrombocytosis

MANIFESTATIONS

Cardiac

- Fatal ventricular dysrhythmias

The progressive electrocardiographic (ECG) changes observed in hyperkalemia are peaked T waves → depressed ST segments → decreased amplitude of R waves → prolonged PR interval → small or absent P waves → wide QRS complexes → biphasic sine wave pattern (Fig. 34.1). Dysrhythmias associated with hyperkalemia include bradycardia, complete heart block, ventricular fibrillation, and asystole.

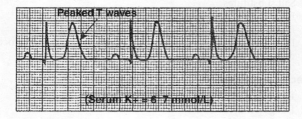

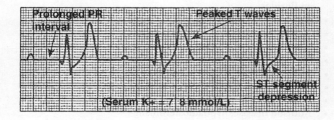

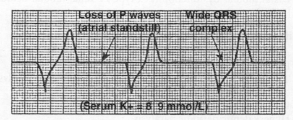

FIG. 34.1 Progressive ECG manifestations of hyperkalemia.

Neuromuscular

- Weakness, often beginning in the lower extremities
- Paresthesias
- Depressed tendon reflexes

MANAGEMENT

Electrocardiographic Monitoring

Fatal ventricular dysrhythmias can occur at any time during treatment; therefore continuous ECG monitoring is required if the K^+ level exceeds 6.0 mmol/L.

Assess the Severity

The severity of the patient's condition is not based solely on the serum K^+ concentration; it also takes into account the presence of neurological (weakness or paralysis) or cardiac (arrhythmias) symptoms and signs, the ECG findings, and whether the underlying cause is immediately remediable.

If Severe

- Neurological or cardiac findings attributable to hyperkalemia.
- Serum K^+ concentration exceeds 6.5 mmol/L.
- ECG findings due to hyperkalemia.
- Cause is not immediately remediable.
  In cases of severe hyperkalemia, take the following actions:
1. Notify your resident.
2. Initiate continuous ECG monitoring of the patient.
3. Correct contributing factors (acidemia, hypovolemia).
4. Administer one or more of the following:
   a. **Calcium gluconate, 5 to 10 mL of a 10% solution intravenously (IV) over 2 minutes.** This treatment temporarily antagonizes the cardiac and neuromuscular effects of hyperkalemia. The onset of action of calcium gluconate is immediate, and its effect lasts 1 hour. It does not, however, reduce the serum K^+ concentration. Caution: In a patient taking digoxin, calcium administration may precipitate ventricular dysrhythmias as a result of the combined effects of digoxin and calcium.
   b. **Fifty percent dextrose in water (D50W), 50 mL IV, followed by regular insulin, 5 to 10 units IV.** This treatment shifts K^+ from the extracellular fluid (ECF) to the intracellular fluid (ICF). The onset of action is immediate, and the effect lasts 1 to 2 hours. If the patient is already hyperglycemic (serum glucose > 11.1 mmol/L, 110 mg/100 ml), the D50W should be omitted. Subsequent serum glucose levels should be measured to determine whether additional doses of insulin are required and to ensure that hypoglycemia does not occur.

c. β-adrenergic agonists can reduce elevated serum potassium within 30 minutes by stimulating cyclic adenosine monophosphate (AMP) and shifting potassium from the ECF to the ICF. Administer **10 to 20 mg of nebulized salbutamol**, which may be repeated after 1 to 2 hours, or 0.5 to 2.5 mg IV.

d. **Sodium bicarbonate (NaHCO$_3$), 1 ampule (44.6 mmol) IV.** This treatment is helpful if the patient has a metabolic acidosis and works by shifting K$^+$ from the ECF to the ICF. The onset of action is immediate, and the effect lasts 1 to 2 hours.

e. Glucose-insulin-bicarbonate (HCO$_3$) "cocktail": D10W, 1000 mL, with 3 ampules of NaHCO$_3$ and 20 units of regular insulin at 75 mL/hour. This treatment should be continued until more definitive measures are taken.

f. A novel potassium binder such as sodium zirconium cyclosilicate (Lokelma) 10 g PO three times per day. An alternative is patiromer (Veltassa) 8.4 g PO one to three times per day, but its onset of action is slower. Sodium polystyrene sulfonate (Kayexalate) should be avoided because of the potential complication of intestinal necrosis, especially in patients with constipation, ileus, intestinal obstruction, or underlying bowel disease. However if the patient has life-threatening hyperkalemia, none of the intestinal conditions listed above, and a novel potassium binder is unavailable, kayexalate may be considered at a dose of 15 to 30 g (4 to 8 teaspoons) orally every 3 to 4 hours or 50 g in 200 mL D20W rectally by retention enema for 30 to 60 minutes every 4 hours. Potassium binders remove K$^+$ from the total body pool. If using sodium zirconium cyclosilicate or sodium polystyrene sulfonate, watch carefully for evidence of volume overload, because these agents work by exchanging Na$^+$ for K$^+$. Patiromer exchanges Ca^{++} for K$^+$.

5. Temporarily discontinue medications that contribute to hyperkalemia.

6. Hemodialysis. This treatment should be considered on an urgent basis if the aforementioned measures have failed or if the patient is in acute or chronic oliguric renal failure.

7. Monitor the serum K$^+$ concentration every 1 to 2 hours until it is lower than 6.0 mmol/L.

If Moderate

- Serum K$^+$ concentration is between 6.0 and 6.4 mmol/L.
- ECG findings due to hyperkalemia.
- Cause is not progressive.

In cases of moderate hyperkalemia, take the following actions:

1. Initiate continuous ECG monitoring of the patient.

2. Correct contributing factors (acidemia, hypovolemia).

3. Administer one or more of the following in the dosages previously outlined:

a. Calcium gluconate, 5 to 10 mL of a 10% solution intravenously (IV) over 2 minutes.
b. $NaHCO_3$ if the patient is acidotic
c. Glucose and insulin
d. A novel potassium binder such as sodium zirconium cyclosilicate.

4. Temporarily discontinue medications that contribute to hyperkalemia.
5. Monitor the serum K^+ concentration every 1 to 2 hours until it is lower than 6.0 mmol/L.

If Mild

- Serum K^+ concentration is lower than 6.0 mmol/L.
- No ECG findings of hyperkalemia.
- Cause is not progressive.
  In cases of mild hyperkalemia, take the following actions:
1. Correct contributing factors (acidemia, hypovolemia).
2. Temporarily discontinue medications that contribute to hyperkalemia.
3. Remeasure the serum K^+ concentration 4 to 6 hours later, depending on the cause.

Hypokalemia

CAUSES

Renal Losses (Urine K^+ Loss >20 mmol/Day)

- Diuretics, osmotic diuresis
- Antibiotics (carbenicillin, ticarcillin, nafcillin, amphotericin, aminoglycosides)
- RTA (classic type I)
- Hyperaldosteronism
- Mineralocorticoids (fludrocortisone, licorice, carbenoxolone)
- Glucocorticoid excess
- Magnesium deficiency
- Chronic metabolic alkalosis
- Bartter syndrome
- Fanconi syndrome
- Ureterosigmoidostomy
- Vomiting, nasogastric suction (hydrogen ions are lost with vomiting and nasogastric suction, which induces alkalosis that, in turn, results in renal K^+ wasting)

Extrarenal Losses (Urine K^+ Loss <20 mmol/Day]

- Chronic diarrhea
- Intestinal fistula

Inadequate Intake

- Over 1 to 2 weeks

Shift From Extracellular to Intracellular Space

- Acute alkalosis
- Drugs
- Insulin overdose
- Vitamin B$_{12}$ therapy
- β-agonists
- Lithium
- Hypokalemic periodic paralysis
- Hypothermia

MANIFESTATIONS

Cardiac

- Premature atrial contractions
- Premature ventricular contractions (PVCs)
- Digoxin toxicity
- ECG changes (Fig. 34.2)
  T wave flattening
  U waves
  ST segment depression

Neuromuscular

- Weakness
- Depressed deep tendon reflexes
- Paresthesias
- Ileus

Miscellaneous

- Nephrogenic diabetes insipidus
- Metabolic alkalosis
- Worsening of hepatic encephalopathy

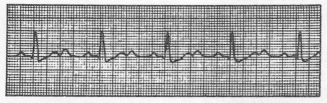

FIG. 34.2 ECG manifestations of hypokalemia.

MANAGEMENT

If possible, correct the underlying cause.

Assess the Severity

The severity of the patient's condition is based on the serum K^+ concentration, the ECG findings, and the clinical setting in which hypokalemia is occurring.

If Severe

- Serum K^+ concentration is lower than 3.0 mmol/L with PVCs in the setting of myocardial ischemia or digoxin toxicity.

  In cases of severe hypokalemia, take the following actions:

1. Notify your resident.
2. Initiate continuous ECG monitoring of the patient.
3. Intravenous replacement therapy may be required: **10 mmol KCl in 100 mL normal saline IV over 1 hour**. Repeat once or twice as necessary.

   KCl in small volumes should be administered through central intravenous lines, because these high concentrations of K^+ are sclerosing to peripheral veins.

   Further replacement can be achieved with maintenance therapy containing up to 40 to 60 mmol of KCl per liter of intravenous fluid at a maximum rate of 20 mmol/hour. K^+ can also be given by administering the liquid salt by nasogastric tube or by oral supplementation.
4. Check magnesium levels. If patient is hypomagnesemic, give 4 ml MgSO4 50% (8 mmol) diluted in 10 ml of NaCl 0.9% over 20 minutes, then start KCL infusion.
5. Recheck serum K^+ concentration after each 20 to 30 mmol of intravenous KCl has been administered.

If Moderate

- Serum K^+ is 3.0 mmol/L or lower with premature atrial contractions but no (or infrequent) PVCs and no digoxin toxicity.

  In cases of moderate hypokalemia, take the following actions:

1. Notify your resident.
2. Oral K^+ supplementation is usually adequate: **Slow-K** tablets each contain 8 mmol of KCl; **Kay Ciel Elixir** is composed of 20 mmol/15 mL; and **K-Lyte** contains 25 mmol per packet.
3. In this situation, intravenous replacement therapy should be reserved for patients with marked hypokalemia or for those who are unable to take oral supplements (see recommendations for severe hypokalemia).
4. Recheck serum K^+ concentration in the morning or sooner if clinically indicated.

If Mild

- Serum K^+ concentration is between 3.1 and 3.5 mmol/L, the patient has no (or infrequent) PVCs, and the patient is asymptomatic.

  In cases of mild hypokalemia, take the following actions:

1. Oral supplementation is usually adequate (see recommendations for moderate hypokalemia).
2. Recheck serum K^+ concentration in the morning or sooner if clinically indicated.

REMEMBER

1. Serious hyperkalemia can occur as a result of K^+ supplementation. Therefore serum K^+ levels should be closely monitored during treatment. Be particularly cautious in patients with renal impairment.
2. Hypokalemia and hypocalcemia may coexist. Correction of hypokalemia without accompanying correction of hypocalcemia may increase the risk of ventricular dysrhythmias.
3. Hypokalemia and hypomagnesemia may coexist. Correction of hypokalemia may be unsuccessful unless hypomagnesemia is corrected simultaneously.

Sodium Disorders

Hypernatremia

CAUSES

1. Inadequate intake of water
   a. Coma
   b. Hypothalamic dysfunction
2. Excessive water losses
   a. Renal losses
      i. Diabetes insipidus (nephrogenic or pituitary)
      ii. Osmotic diuresis (hyperglycemia, mannitol administration, urea)
   b. Extrarenal losses
      i. Gastrointestinal losses (vomiting, nasogastric suction, diarrhea)
      ii. Insensible losses (burns, febrile illness, tachypnea)
3. Excessive sodium gain
   a. Iatrogenic (excessive sodium administration)
   b. Primary hyperaldosteronism

MANIFESTATIONS

Hypernatremia most often results from depletion of extracellular fluid (ECF) volume as a result of hypotonic fluid loss (e.g., vomiting, diarrhea, sweating, osmotic diuresis). Symptoms are dependent on the absolute increase in serum osmolality and on the rate at which it develops. The manifestations of hypernatremia are caused by acute brain cell shrinkage from an outward shift of intracellular water, which results from the increased osmolality of ECF. These manifestations range from confusion and muscle irritability to seizures, respiratory paralysis, and death.

MANAGEMENT

Assess the Severity

The severity of the patient's condition is based on the patient's symptoms, the serum sodium concentration, the serum osmolality, and the ECF volume.

1. Osmolality can be measured in the laboratory. However, information may be sufficient for you to calculate it on the basis of the major osmotically active substances in the extracellular fluid, as follows:

   Serum osmolality (mmol/kg) =
   (2 × Na concentration [mmol/L]) = urea concentration
   (mmol/L) + glucose concentration(mmol/L)

   The normal range for osmolality is 281 to 297 mmol/kg.

2. Most patients with hypernatremia have an accompanying extracellular volume deficit that can compromise perfusion of vital organs. Assess the volume status of the patient (see Chapter 3).

3. Most patients with hypernatremia have relatively few symptoms and are not at immediate risk of dying.

Correct the Cause

The cause of hypernatremia is usually evident from the history and physical findings and should be corrected, if possible.

Correct Volume and Water Deficits

The choice of fluid is dependent on the severity of the extracellular volume deficit.

1. In patients who have volume depletion, hypernatremia can be corrected by administration of **intravenous normal saline** until the patient is hemodynamically stable and then changing to **½ normal saline or 5% dextrose in water (D5W)** to correct the remaining water deficit.

2. In patients who do not have volume depletion, **½ normal saline or D5W** can be used to correct the water deficit. You can estimate the volume of water required, remembering that the deficit is in total body water (TBW), which is approximately 60% of body weight:

$$\text{Water deficit} = \frac{(\text{Observed serum Na concentration} - \text{normal serum Na concentration}) \times (0.6 \times \text{body weight [kg]})}{\text{Normal serum sodium concentration}}$$

Example: A 65-year-old man is admitted to the hospital after being found in his apartment 2 days after falling and fracturing his hip. He has moderate volume depletion, and his serum sodium value is 156 mmol/L. His weight is 70 kg. The volume of water needed to correct the serum sodium is calculated as follows:

$$\text{Free water deficit} = \dfrac{156 \text{ mmol/L} - 140 \text{ mmol/L} \times (0.6 \times 70 \text{ L})}{140 \text{ mmol/L}} = 4.8 \text{ L}$$

📖 Remember to correct the osmolality abnormality at a rate similar to that at which it developed. Biological systems are more responsive to rates of change than to absolute amounts of change. It is safest to correct half the deficit and then reevaluate the patient's condition. Corrections in serum sodium in amounts larger than 1 to 2 mmol/L can lead to brain swelling, resulting in the development of confusion, seizures, or coma.

3. In an occasional patient with hypernatremia who has volume overload, you can correct the hypernatremia by initiating a diuresis with **furosemide, 20 to 40 mg intravenously**, and repeating it at intervals of 2 to 4 hours as necessary. Once the extracellular volume has returned to normal, if the serum sodium level is still elevated, diuresis should be continued, with urinary volume losses replaced with D5W until the serum sodium level is again in the normal range.

Hyponatremia

CAUSES

Hyponatremia With Decreased Extracellular Fluid Volume

1. Renal loss of sodium
   a. Diuretic excess
   b. Sodium-losing nephropathies
   c. Diuretic phase of acute tubular necrosis
   d. Bartter syndrome
   e. Hypoaldosteronism
2. Extrarenal losses of sodium
   a. Vomiting, nasogastric suction
   b. Diarrhea
   c. Sweating
   d. Burns
   e. Pancreatitis

Hyponatremia With Excess Extracellular Fluid Volume and Edema

1. Renal failure
2. Nephrotic syndrome
3. Congestive heart failure
4. Cirrhosis of the liver

Hyponatremia With Normal Extracellular Fluid Volume

1. Syndrome of inappropriate antidiuretic hormone (arginine vasopressin) (SIADH)
   a. Tumors
      i. Small cell carcinoma of the lung
      ii. Pancreatic carcinoma
      iii. Duodenal adenocarcinoma
      iv. Lymphosarcoma
   b. Central nervous system disorders
      i. Brain tumor
      ii. Brain trauma
      iii. Meningitis
      iv. Encephalitis
      v. Subarachnoid hemorrhage
      vi. Guillain-Barré syndrome
   c. Pulmonary disorders
      i. Tuberculosis
      ii. Pneumonia
   d. Drugs
      i. Hypoglycemic agents (chlorpropamide, tolbutamide)
      ii. Neuroleptic agents (e.g., haloperidol, trifluoperazine, fluphenazine)
      iii. Antidepressants (e.g., SSRIs, tricyclics, serotonin, and norepinephrine reuptake inhibitors)
      iv. Antineoplastic drugs (cyclophosphamide, vincristine)
      v. Narcotics
      vi. Clofibrate
      vii. Carbamazepine
      viii. Nicotine
   e. The postoperative state (particularly in premenopausal women)
2. Primary polydipsia (water intoxication)
3. Pseudohyponatremia
   a. Hyponatremia with normal serum osmolality
      i. Hyperlipidemia
      ii. Hyperproteinemia
   b. Hyponatremia with increased serum osmolality
      i. Excess urea
      ii. Hyperglycemia
      iii. Mannitol
      iv. Ethanol
      v. Methanol
      vi. Ethylene glycol
      vii. Isopropyl alcohol

4. Endocrine disorders
   a. Hypothyroidism
   b. Addison disease

MANIFESTATIONS

Manifestations of hyponatremia depend on the absolute decrease in serum osmolality, the rate of development of hyponatremia, and the volume status of the patient. When associated with a decreased serum osmolality, hyponatremia may cause the following:

- Confusion
- Lethargy
- Weakness
- Nausea and vomiting
- Seizures
- Coma
- Muscle cramps
- Headache

When hyponatremia develops gradually, a patient may tolerate a serum sodium concentration of less than 110 mmol/L with only moderate confusion or lethargy. However when the serum sodium concentration decreases rapidly from 140 to 115 mmol/L, the patient may experience a seizure.

MANAGEMENT

Assess the Severity

The severity of the patient's condition is based on the patient's symptoms, the serum sodium concentration, the serum osmolality, and the ECF.

Remember that when you attempt to correct disorders manifested by hyponatremia, brain cells try to maintain their volume in dilutional states by losing solutes (e.g., potassium). If the serum sodium level is corrected too rapidly (i.e., to levels >120 to 125 mmol/L), the serum may become hypertonic in relation to brain cells, which results in an outward shift of water and subsequent central nervous system damage caused by acute brain shrinkage (osmotic demyelination syndrome).

Correct the Cause (if possible)

Urinary electrolyte measurements may be helpful in identifying the primary cause of hyponatremia when more than one cause is possible. The renal response to salt and water loss depends on the cause of hyponatremia. When extrarenal losses of sodium and water occur through the skin (e.g., sweating, burns) or as a result of third-space losses (e.g., pancreatitis), the renal response is to conserve sodium (urine sodium level, <20 mmol/L) and to conserve water through secretion of antidiuretic hormone (high urine osmolality). However, if volume loss results from vomiting or nasogastric suction, primarily hydrochloride is lost from gastric secretions. The kidneys generate and excrete sodium bicarbonate ($NaHCO_3$) to maintain the acid-base balance, which causes urine to have a normal level (>20 mmol/L) of sodium but a low level (<20 mmol/L) of chloride. If volume loss is caused by diarrhea, primarily $NaHCO_3$ is lost in the stools. The kidneys generate and excrete ammonium chloride (NH_4Cl) to maintain the acid-base balance; as a result, urine has low levels of sodium but not of chloride.

Hyponatremia with ECF excess and edema may be accompanied by a low level (<20 mmol/L) of urinary sodium (e.g., nephrotic syndrome, congestive heart failure, cirrhosis of the liver) or a normal level of urinary sodium (renal failure).

Assess and Correct the Volume Status (see Chapter 3)

1. If the patient has volume depletion, correct the ECF volume with **normal saline**. Aim for a jugular venous pressure of 2 to 3 cm H_2O above the sternal angle. In this case, you can calculate the amount of sodium needed to improve the serum sodium concentration with the following formula:

$$(\text{Desired serum Na concentration} - \text{observed serum Na concentration}) \times \text{TBW}$$

where TBW = $0.6 \times$ weight (in kg).

📖 Remember that biological systems are more responsive to rates of change than to absolute amounts of change. Make corrections at a rate similar to that at which the abnormality developed. It is safest to correct half the deficit and then reassess the patient's condition.

Example: To raise the serum sodium level from 120 to 135 mmol/L in a man who weighs 70 kg, the amount of sodium required is calculated as follows:

$$(135 \text{ mmol/L} - 120 \text{ mmol/L}) \times (0.6 \times 70 \text{ L})$$
$$= (15 \text{ mmol/L}) \times (42 \text{ L})$$
$$= 630 \text{ mmol NA}$$

Because 1 L of normal saline contains 154 mmol of sodium, approximately 4 L of normal saline is needed to raise the patient's serum level to 135 mmol/L.

2. If the patient has *extracellular volume excess and edema,* treat the volume excess and hyponatremia with water restriction (e.g., 1 L per day) and diuretics. Because most of these states

are accompanied by secondary hyperaldosteronism, spirono-lactone is a reasonable choice of diuretic, as long as the patient is not hyperkalemic. Remember that the diuretic effect of this drug may be delayed for 3 to 4 days. The dose of spironolactone ranges from 25 to 200 mg daily in adults and can be given once daily or in divided doses. In this situation, strict intake-output charts can be useful. To raise the serum sodium level, the daily water intake should be less than the daily urine output.

3. If the patient has a normal ECF volume, SIADH, primary poly-dipsia, pseudohyponatremia, or an endocrine disorder should be considered.

Syndrome of Inappropriate Antidiuretic Hormone

The diagnosis of SIADH has stringent criteria:
1. Hyponatremia with serum hypo-osmolality
2. Urine that is less than maximally dilute in comparison with serum osmolality (i.e., a simultaneous urine osmolality that is higher than the serum osmolality)
3. Inappropriately large amounts of urine sodium (>20 mmol/L)
4. Normal renal function
5. Normal thyroid function
6. Normal adrenal function
7. Patient not taking diuretics

MANAGEMENT

SIADH should be treated as follows:
1. Correction of the underlying cause or contributory factors (e.g., drugs), if present.
2. Water restriction, usually to less than insensible losses (e.g., 500 to 1000 mL/day).
3. In addition to the first two measures, patients with severe symp-tomatic hyponatremia (serum sodium level <115 mmol/L) may benefit from furosemide-induced diuresis, with hourly replacement of urinary sodium and potassium losses using normal saline. In very rare cases, 3% saline is required. Too rapid a correction of hyponatremia can result in central pon-tine myelinolysis (osmotic demyelination syndrome) and other undesirable side effects. Correct the serum sodium level slow-ly. Once the serum sodium level exceeds 120 to 125 mmol/L, many of the symptoms of hyponatremia begin to lessen.
4. Demeclocycline, 300 to 600 mg orally twice a day, is occa-sionally useful in patients with chronic symptomatic SIADH in whom water restriction has been unsuccessful.
5. Urea, 15 to 30 g of a 99% solution in 50 ml of water PO. Re-peat every 6 to 8 hours to a maximum of 180 g per day. Urea

promotes sodium reabsorption in the ascending loop of Henle, thus inducing water elimination.

6. **Vaptans** (e.g., tolvaptan, satavaptan, lixivaptan, conivaptan) block vasopressin type 2 receptors in the collecting duct and have been used successfully to treat hyponatremia in patients with excessive vasopressin by effecting an aquaresis. However, they can lead to overcorrection and should only be instituted when other measures have failed and with the guidance of your resident or attending physician. They are not indicated for the treatment of hypovolemic hyponatremia.

Primary Polydipsia

Water intoxication should be suspected in a patient with a psychiatric disorder, particularly when excessive drinking and polyuria interfere with sleep or are noticed by the ward staff. The hyponatremia is often exacerbated by the effects of neuroleptic or antidepressant medications that the patient is taking.

MANAGEMENT

Immediate treatment involves fluid restriction, but this is only temporarily effective if not coupled with psychiatric assessment. **Demeclocycline, 300 to 600 mg orally twice a day**, may reduce the severity of hyponatremic episodes in patients with this disorder.

Pseudohyponatremia

You can establish the diagnosis of pseudohyponatremia by demonstrating the following:

1. Normal serum osmolality in the presence of hyperlipidemia or hyperproteinemia
2. A significant (>10 mmol/kg) osmolar gap

A significant osmolar gap is indicative of the presence of additional osmotically active solutes, which can falsely lower the serum sodium level. You can demonstrate this gap by first having the laboratory measure serum osmolality. You should then calculate serum osmolality by using the following formula:

$$\text{Serum osmolality (mmol/kg)} = (2 \times \text{Na concentration [mmol/L]}) + \text{glucose concentration)} \text{ (mmol/L)} + \text{urea concentration (mmol/L)}$$

If the *measured* serum osmolality is more than 10 mmol/kg higher than the calculated serum osmolality, the hyponatremia is at least partially caused by the presence of osmotically active solutes, such as excess lipids or plasma proteins.

MANAGEMENT

Treatment of pseudohyponatremia is restricted to correction of the underlying cause.

In cases of hyperglycemia, the true serum sodium concentration can be estimated by the following formula:

([Observed glucose concentration − normal glucose concentration] × [1.4]/normal glucose) + observed serum Na

The factor 1.4 is an arithmetic approximation to account for the shift of water that follows glucose into the extracellular compartment, thereby diluting sodium.

Example: A 35-year-old woman in diabetic ketoacidosis is admitted with the following laboratory results:
- Glucose concentration: 80 mmol/L
- Sodium concentration: 127 mmol/L
- Urea concentration: 25 mmol/L
- Creatinine concentration: 274 mmol/L

The true serum sodium concentration, for a normal glucose concentration that is assumed to be 5 mmol/L, is calculated as follows:

([180 mmol/L − 5 mmol/L] × 1.4/5 mmol/L)/127 mmol/L
= 21 mmol/L + 127 mmol/L
= 148 mmol/L

Endocrine Disorders

Hypothyroidism and *Addison disease* can be diagnosed from their typical clinical features in association with confirmatory laboratory studies.

MANAGEMENT

Hyponatremia in either of these conditions responds to treatment of the underlying endocrine disorder.

Blood Products

The maximum time over which blood products can be administered is 4 hours for 1 unit, because of the danger of bacterial infection and red blood cell hemolysis. For the same reasons, if the flow is interrupted for more than 30 minutes, the unit must be discarded. Blood products are generally well tolerated; however, acute reactions can occur. If so:

1. Stop the transfusion.
2. Maintain IV access using 0.9% saline through a new tubing.
3. Check vital signs.
4. Check ID band, blood label, and transfusion identification band (Table A1).

Packed Red Blood Cells, Leukocyte-Reduced Red Blood Cells, Red Cell Concentrate

- Volume: 300 ± 25 mL containing 55 g hemoglobin
- Maximum administration time: 4 hours
- Rate of infusion: Dependent on patient's clinical condition
- Administration: Standard blood set for each unit hung, plus a filter (filter not required if red blood cells are washed)
- Indications: Prevention or alleviation of inadequate oxygen delivery due to red blood cell deficiency or malfunction.

Frozen Red Blood Cells (Deglycerolized)

- Volume: Approximately 200 mL
- Maximum administration time: 4 hours
- Rate of infusion: Dependent on patient's clinical condition
- Administration: Standard blood set for each unit hung
- Indications: Storing of samples of rare blood groups and for autotransfusion
- *Note:* Use only in special situations.

Plasma (Fresh Frozen Plasma)

- Volume: Approximately 200 mL
- Maximum administration time: 4 hours
- Rate of infusion: Dependent on patient's clinical condition

TABLE A.1   Acute Transfusion Reactions

Reaction	Symptoms	Mechanism	Treatment
Simple allergic	Rash, itching, hives	Allergens or antibodies in donor blood react with recipient's antibodies	Antihistamines
Anaphylactic	Hives, flushed skin, wheezing, vomiting, diarrhea, cyanosis	Recipient IgA antibodies react with donor IgA antibodies	Epinephrine
Febrile nonhemolytic (FNHTR)	Fever >38°C Chills	Recipient WBC response to donor blood	Aspirin or acetaminophen
Acute hemolytic	Chills, hypotension, back pain, renal failure	Donor is of the wrong blood type	IV fluids
Septic	Fever, chills, hypotension	Bacterial contamination of donor blood	Antibiotics, IV fluids
Transfusion related acute lung injury (TRALI)	Severe dyspnea, fever	Recipient WBC response to donor blood	Respiratory support
Transfusion associated circulatory overload (TACO)	Severe dyspnea, tachycardia,	Heart failure due to volume overload	Diuretics, respiratory support

Delayed transfusion reactions include hemolytic, graft versus host reactions, and posttransfusion purpura.

- Administration: Standard blood set
- Indications: As a source of coagulation factors. Frozen plasma is frozen within 24 hours of collection and contains higher levels of labile coagulation factors (V and VIII). Nonlabile factors are well maintained in both frozen and stored (banked) plasma. Plasma may be used for the following:
  1. Significant hemorrhage that results from a deficiency of coagulation factors
  2. Immediate hemostasis in a patient taking warfarin
  3. Abnormal clotting tests and active bleeding in a patient with severe liver disease or massive transfusion (whole blood volume replaced within 24 hours)
  4. Thrombotic thrombocytopenic purpura (TTP), hemolytic uremic syndrome (HUS)
  5. Prophylaxis before an invasive procedure associated with a significant bleeding risk
- Outcome measurement: Prothrombin time (PT), activated partial thromboplastin time (aPTT), or both within 4 hours of transfusion

Platelets (Pooled Platelets, Apheresis Platelets)

- Volume: Approximately 300 mL
- Rate of infusion: As rapidly as tolerated by patient
- Administration: Blood component recipient set
- Indications: Prevention or treatment of bleeding due to platelet deficiency or dysfunction. Platelet use should be considered in the following situations:
  1. Patients with platelet counts of less than 20×10^9 on the basis of decreased platelet production
  2. Patients with consumptive thrombocytopenia (e.g., immune thrombocytopenia; disseminated intravascular coagulation [DIC]) only when bleeding is significant
  3. Patients with significant platelet dysfunction
- Outcome measurement: Platelet count 1 hour after transfusion
- *Note:* Mild allergic reactions are common but usually mild. In patients with a history of reactions, the use of acetaminophen, 650 mg orally, and diphenhydramine, 50 mg intravenously (IV), may prevent reactions. Narcotics (morphine, 5 to 10 mg IV) or steroids (hydrocortisone, 100 mg IV) also may be helpful. If these measures fail, leukocyte-reduced platelets are recommended. Transfusion associated circulatory overload (TACO) may occur.

In patients who are unresponsive to random donor platelets (defined by a <5-g/L increment in platelet count 1 hour after transfusion on two successive transfusions), platelets collected from a single donor by apheresis should be considered.

Cryoprecipitate, Leukocyte Reduced (Cryo)

- Volume: 5 to 10 mL
- Rate of infusion: As rapidly as possible
- Administration: Blood component recipient set
- Indications: Cryoprecipitate contains significant amounts of factor VIII (100 U per unit of cryoprecipitate), fibrinogen (250 mg per unit of cryoprecipitate), and von Willebrand factor. It is therefore useful in the treatment of mild hemophilia A and von Willebrand disease and in the repletion of fibrinogen (e.g., DIC, dilutional coagulopathy). The dose is dependent on body mass, the indication for use, and the severity of the preexisting deficiency.
- Outcome measurement: Factor VIII level and aPTT (hemophilia A); von Willebrand factor antigen level, bleeding time, or both (von Willebrand disease); fibrinogen level (DIC, dilutional coagulopathy)—all within 4 hours of transfusion.

Recombinant Factor VIIa Concentrate (NiaStase RT)

- Lyophilized, fractionated plasma product
- Supplied in 1, 2, and 5 mg single-use vials
- Must be reconstituted before use
- Indications: Uncontrollable bleeding in hemophilia patients (with factor VIII or IX deficiency) who have developed inhibitors against replacement factor VIII, Glanzmann thrombasthenia, congenital factor VII deficiency

Recombinant Factor VIII (Antihemophilic Factor)

- Lyophilized, fractionated plasma product
- Available in 500, 1000, 2000, 3000 IU vials
- Must be reconstituted before use
- Indications: Moderate to severe factor VIII deficiency and low titer of factor VIII inhibitors
- *Note:* Not for use in von Willebrand disease. Consult a hematologist before administration.

Recombinant Factor IX Complex (BeneFIX)

- Lyophilized, fractionated plasma product
- Available in 500, 1000, 2000, and 5000 IU. Factor IX content and storage conditions stated on labels
- Must be reconstituted before use
- Indications: Factor IX deficiency, hemophilia B. Consult a hematologist before administration

Albumin (Human)

- Concentrates of 25% in vials of 100 mL and 5% in vials of 250 and 500 mL
- Sodium content of approximately 145 mmol/L

- Indications: Hypoproteinemia with peripheral edema (give 25%); volume depletion when intravenous normal saline is contraindicated (give 5%). Not indicated in an asymptomatic hypoproteinemic patient

Granulocytes
- Half-life of 24 hrs
- Maintenance therapy in patients with severe neutropenia

Reading Electrocardiograms

Rate

Multiply the number of QRS complexes in a 6-second period (30 large squares) by 10 to obtain the number of beats per minute (Fig. B.1).

- Normal: rate = 60 to 100 beats/minute
- Tachycardia: rate greater than 100 beats/minute
- Bradycardia: rate less than 60 beats/minute

Rhythm

Is the rhythm regular?

Does a P wave precede every QRS complex? Does a QRS complex follow every P wave?

1. Yes: sinus rhythm
2. No P waves with irregular rhythm: atrial fibrillation
3. No P waves with regular rhythm: junctional rhythm; look for retrograde P waves in all leads

Axis

Fig. B.2.

P-Wave Configuration

NORMAL P WAVE

Look at all leads (Fig. B.3A).

LEFT ATRIAL ENLARGEMENT

The peak of the wave is often notched (see Fig. B.3B).

- Duration: 120 ms (three small squares in lead II); the notch is indicative of P mitrale.
- Amplitude: negative terminal P wave in lead V_1 greater than 1 mm in depth and greater than 40 ms (one small square)

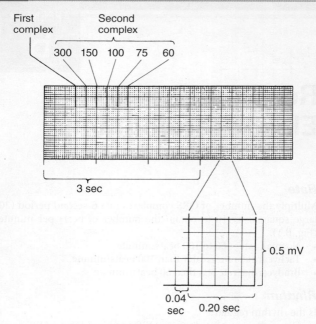

First complex

Second complex

300 150 100 75 60

3 sec

0.5 mV

0.04 sec   0.20 sec

FIG. B.1 **Rate.**

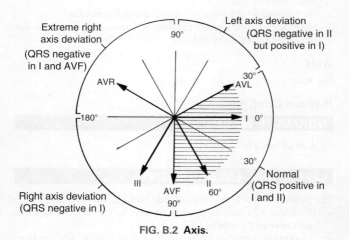

Extreme right axis deviation (QRS negative in I and AVF)

Left axis deviation (QRS negative in II but positive in I)

90°

30°

AVL

AVR

180°   I 0°

30°

III

AVF

II 60°

90°

Normal (QRS positive in I and II)

Right axis deviation (QRS negative in I)

FIG. B.2 **Axis.**

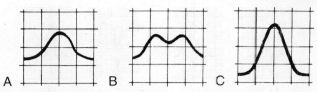

FIG. B.3 P-wave configuration in lead II. (*A*) Normal P wave. (*B*) Abnormal wave indicative of left atrial enlargement. (*C*) Abnormal wave indicative of right atrial enlargement.

RIGHT ATRIAL ENLARGEMENT

The peak of the wave is exaggerated (see Fig. B.3C).

- Amplitude: 2.5 mm in lead II, III, or aVF (i.e., tall peaked P wave of P pulmonale); 1.5 mm in the initial positive deflection of the P wave in lead V_1 or V_2.

QRS Configuration
LEFT VENTRICULAR HYPERTROPHY

1. Increased QRS voltage (S wave in lead V_1 or V_2 plus either R wave >35 mm in V_5 or R wave ≥11 mm in aVL)
2. ST-segment depression and negative T wave in left lateral leads are common.

RIGHT VENTRICULAR HYPERTROPHY

1. R wave greater than S wave in V_1
2. Right-axis deviation (>+90 degrees)
3. ST-segment depression and negative T wave in right precordial leads

Conduction Abnormalities
FIRST-DEGREE BLOCK

- PR interval is greater than or equal to 0.20 seconds (equal to one large square)

SECOND-DEGREE BLOCK

- Occasional absence of QRS complex and T wave after a P wave of sinus origin
- Type I (Wenckebach phenomenon): progressive prolongation of the PR interval before the missed QRS complex (see Fig. 15.18)

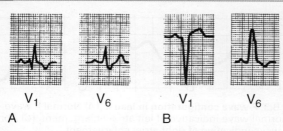

V_1 V_6 V_1 V_6

A   B

FIG. B.4 QRS configuration. (*A*) Complete right bundle branch block. (*B*) Complete left bundle branch block.

TABLE B.1	Patterns in Myocardial Infarction
Location of Infarct	**Patterns of Changes (Q Waves, ST Elevation or Depression, T Wave Inversion)[a]**
Inferior	Q wave in leads II, III, aVF
Inferoposterior	Q wave in leads II, III, aVF, and V_6 R wave > S wave and positive T wave in V_1
Anteroseptal	Q wave in leads V_1 to V_4
Anterolateral to posterolateral	Q wave in leads V_1 to V_5; Q wave in leads I, aVL, and V_6
Posterior	R wave > S wave in lead V_1, positive T wave, and Q wave in lead V_6

[a]A significant Q wave is greater than 40 ms wide or more than one-third of the QRS height. ST-segment or T-wave changes in the absence of significant Q waves may represent a non-Q wave infarction.

- Type II: absence of progressive prolongation of the PR interval before the missed QRS complex (see Fig. 15.19)

THIRD-DEGREE BLOCK

- Absence of any relationship between P waves of sinus origin and QRS complexes (see Fig. 15.20)

LEFT ANTERIOR HEMIBLOCK

- Left-axis deviation, Q wave in leads I and aVL, and a small R wave in lead III, in the absence of left ventricular hypertrophy

LEFT POSTERIOR HEMIBLOCK

- Right-axis deviation, a small R wave in lead I, and a small Q wave in lead III, in the absence of right ventricular hypertrophy

COMPLETE RIGHT BUNDLE BRANCH BLOCK

Examples of electrocardiographic readings for complete right bundle branch block are depicted in Fig. B.4A.

COMPLETE LEFT BUNDLE BRANCH BLOCK

Examples of electrocardiographic readings for complete left bundle branch block are depicted in Fig. B.4B.

VENTRICULAR PREEXCITATION

1. PR interval less than 0.11 seconds with widened QRS (>0.12 seconds) as a result of a delta wave is indicative of Wolff-Parkinson-White syndrome.
2. PR interval less than 0.11 seconds with a normal QRS complex is indicative of Lown-Ganong-Levine syndrome.

Miscellaneous

Calculation of Creatinine Clearance

Creatinine Clearance (CrCl) (mL/s) = 140 − age in years

1.5 (for men)/Serum creatine concentration (mmol/L)

Calculation of Alveolar–Arterial Oxygen Gradient [P(A − a)o₂]

The $P(A - a)O_2$ can be calculated easily from the arterial blood gas (ABG) values. It is useful in confirming the presence of a shunt:

$$P(A - a)O_2 = PAO_2 - PaO_2$$

where
- PAO_2 = alveolar oxygen tension, calculated as shown subsequently
- PaO_2 = arterial oxygen tension measured from ABG determinations

PAO_2 can be calculated by the following formula:

$$PAO_2 = (PB - PH_2O)(FiO_2) \, PaCO_2/R$$

where
- PB = barometric pressure (760 mm Hg at sea level).
- PH_2O = partial pressure of water vapor in the lung = 47 mm Hg.
- FiO_2 = fraction of O_2 in inspired gas.
- $PaCO_2$ = arterial CO_2 tension measured from ABG determinations.
- R = respiratory quotient (0.8).

Normal $P(A - a)O_2$ ranges from 12 mm Hg in a young adult to 20 mm Hg at age 70.

In pure ventilatory failure, the $P(A - a)O_2$ remains 12 to 20 mm Hg. In oxygenation failure, it increases.

Sputum Gram Stain

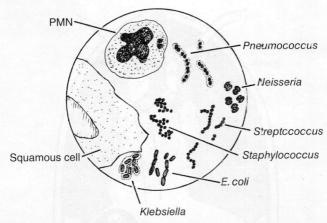

FIG. C.1 **Diagram of sputum Gram stain.** A useful sputum specimen for the identification of a bacterial cause of pneumonia should have 25 or more polymorphonuclear cells (PMNs) and fewer than 10 squamous cells per low-power field.

International Normalized Ratio

The international normalized ratio (INR) was developed to improve the consistency of oral anticoagulant therapy. It is calculated with the mean normal prothrombin time (PT) for a laboratory's system, *not* the PT of normal control material. The relation between PT and INR is as follows:

$$INR = (PT_{patient}/PT_{mean})ISI$$

where $PT_{patient}$ is the patient's PT, PT_{mean} is the mean of the normal PT range (measured by the laboratory), and ISI is the International Sensitivity Index, which is a measure of the responsiveness of the thromboplastin used to measure the PT to a reduction in vitamin K–dependent coagulation factors.

Chest X-ray: Posteroanterior

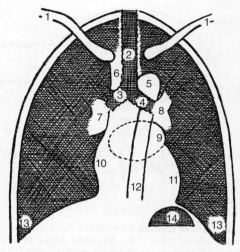

FIG. C.2 Diagram of posteroanterior chest radiograph.

1. Clavicles.
2. Trachea.
3. Right main stem bronchus.
4. Left main stem bronchus.
5. Aortic knuckle.
6. Superior vena cava.
7. Right pulmonary artery.
8. Left pulmonary artery.
9. Left atrium.
10. Right atrium.
11. Left ventricle.
12. Aortic stripe.
13. Costophrenic angles.
14. Gastric bubble.

Chest X-ray: Lateral

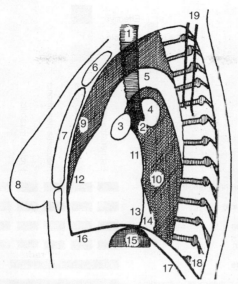

FIG. C.3 Diagram of lateral chest radiograph.

1. Trachea.
2. Left main stem bronchus.
3. Right pulmonary artery.
4. Left pulmonary artery.
5. Aortic arch.
6. Manubrium.
7. Sternum.
8. Breast shadow.
9. Retrosternal space.
10. Retrocardiac space.
11. Left atrium.
12. Right ventricle.
13. Left ventricle.
14. Inferior vena cava.
15. Gastric air bubble.
16. Left hemidiaphragm.
17. Right hemidiaphragm.
18. Costophrenic angle.
19. Scapular shadows.

Antibacterials for UTIs

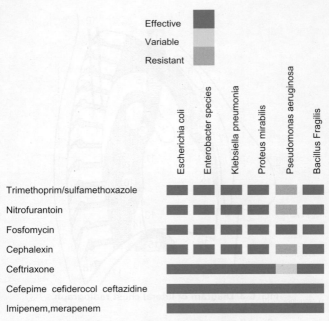

FIG. C.4 **Antibacterials for UTIs.**

Antibiotics for Pneumonia

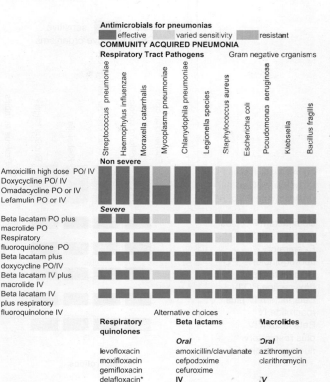

FIG. C.5 **Antibiotics for pneumonia.**

Gram-Negative Infections

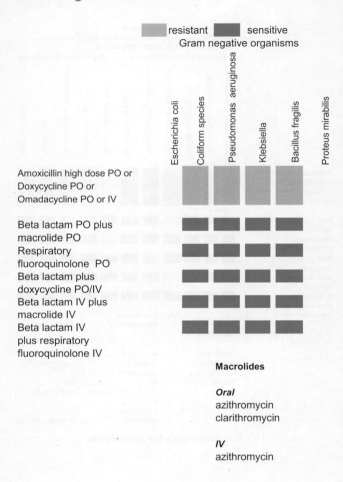

FIG. C.6 **Gram-negative infections.**

Systemic Infections

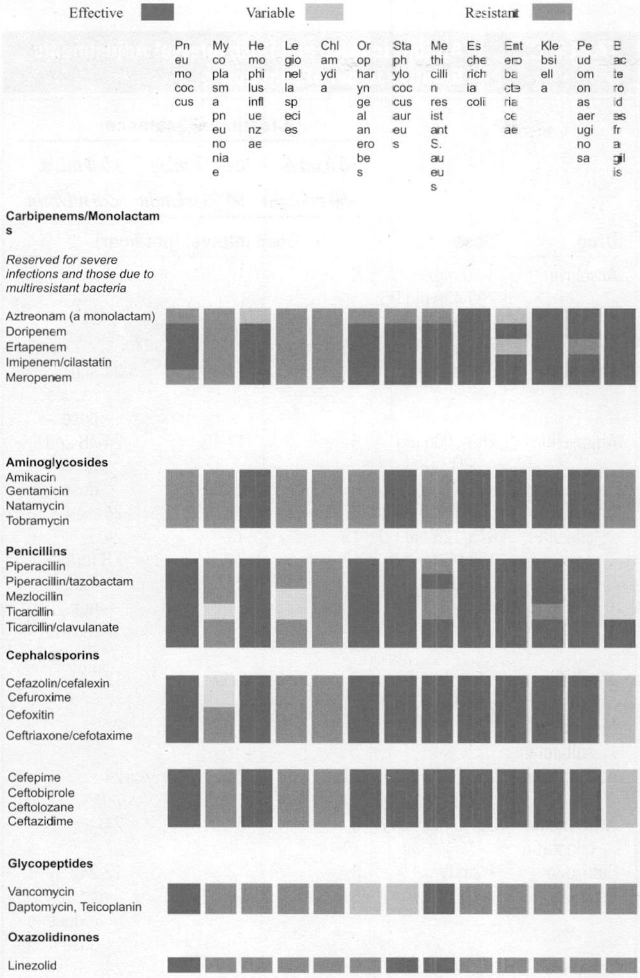

FIG. C.7 Systemic infections.

Antibiotic Dose and Dose Interval Adjustments Relative to Renal Function

TABLE C.1	Antibiotic Dose and Dose Interval Adjustments Relative to Renal Function

		Creatinine Clearance		
		>0.8 mL/s, >50 mL/min	0.8-0.4 mL/s, 50-25 mL/min	<0.4 mL/s, <25 mL/min
Drug	**Dose**	**Dose Interval (per hour)**		
Acyclovir	5-10 mg/kg IV 200-400 mg PO five times per day	8	12	24
Amikacin	5-7 mg/kg IV	8	12-18	24 and reduce dose
Amoxicillin	250-1000 mg PO	8	12-18	24-48 and reduce dose
Amoxicillin/ clavula- nate	500/125 mg PO 875/125 mg PO 1000/62.5 mg PO	8 12 12	12 13 24	24 24 XR formu- lation not recom- mended
Ampicillin	1-2 g IV 250-1000 mg PO	6	6-12	12-24
Ampicillin/ sulbactam	1.5-3 g IV	6	8-12	24
Azithromycin	250-500 mg PO, IV	24	24	24
Aztreonam/ cilastatin	30-40 mg/kg IV	8	8-12	24
Cefazolin	1-2 g IV	8	12	12-24
Cefiderocol	1-2 g IV	8	8	8 and reduce dose
Cefepime	1 g IV	6	8	24
Cefotaxime	1-2 g IV	8-12	12	12-24
Cefoxitin	1-2 g IV	8	12	12-24
Ceftaroline	200-600 mg IV	12-24	12-24	12-24 and reduce dose
Ceftazidime	1-2 g IV	8	12	12-24

TABLE C.1	Antibiotic Dose and Dose Interval Adjustments Relative to Renal Function—cont'd

		Creatinine Clearance		
		>0.8 mL/s, >50 mL/min	0.8-0.4 mL/s, 50-25 mL/min	<0.4 mL/s, <25 mL/min
Drug	Dose	Dose Interval (per hour)		
Ceftizoxime	0.5-4 g IV	8	12	12-24
Ceftriaxone	1-2 g IV	24	24	24
Cefuroxime	1.5 g IV 250=500 mg PO	8	12	24
Cephalexin	250-1000 mg PO	6	8	12
Chloramphenicol	12.5-25 mg/kg PO or IV	6	6	6
Ciprofloxacin	200-600 mg PO or IV	12	12-24	24
Clarithromycin	0.5-1 g PO	12	12	12 and reduce dose
Clindamycin	150-600 mg PO or IV	8	8	8
Cloxacillin	250-1000 mg PO or IV	4-6	4-6	4-6
Daptomycin	6 mg/kg IV	24	24	24 and reduce dose
Delafloxacin	300-450 mg PO or IV	12	12, reduce dose	Not recommended
Dicloxacillin	250-500 mg PO	6	6	6
Doxycycline	100 mg PO, IV	12	12	12
Erythromycin	250-500 mg PO 5-7 mg/kg IV	6-12	6-12	6-12
Famciclovir	500 mg PO	8	24	48
Fluconazole	6 mg/kg PO IV	24	24 reduce dose	24 reduce dose
Gentamicin	5-7 mg/kg IV	24	48	Reduce dose
Imipenem/ cilastatin	500 mg IV	6-8	8	12
Isoniazid	5 mg/kg PO	24	24	24
Itraconazole	100-200 mg PO	12	12	12
Levofloxacin	250-500 mg PO or IV	24	24-36	36-48
Meropenem	0.5-1 g IV	8	12	24

Continued

TABLE C.1	Antibiotic Dose and Dose Interval Adjustments Relative to Renal Function—cont'd

		Creatinine Clearance		
		>0.8 mL/s, >50 mL/min	0.8-0.4 mL/s, 50-25 mL/min	<0.4 mL/s, <25 mL/min
Drug	Dose	Dose Interval (per hour)		
Metronidazole	500 mg PO IV	8	8-12	12
Mezlocillin	4-6 g IV	4-6	6-12	12
Minocycline	100 mg PO	12	12	12
Netilmicin	16-20 mg/kg IV	24	48	Reduce dose
Nitrofurantoin	50-100 mg PO	12	Not recommended	Not recommended
Omadacycline	200 mg IV	24	24	24
Oxacillin	2 g IV	4	4	4
Penicillin G	Variable	4-6	8-12	12-18
Piperacillin	2-4 g IV	4-6	6-12	12
Piperacillin/tazobactam	2-4 g IV	4-6	6-12	12
Rifampin	600 mg PO IV	12	12	12
Teicoplanin	6 mg/kg IV	12	24-36	48-96
Tetracycline	250-500 mg IV PO	12	24-36	48-96
Ticarcillin/clavulanate	1-6 g PO IV	6	8	12-24
Tobramycin	5-7 mg/kg IV	24	48	Reduce dose
Vancomycin	15 mg/kg IV	12-72	2-10 days	Reduce dose

Reference: www.nebraskamed.com/asp Renal dosage adjustment guidelines for antimicrobials

SI Units Conversion Table

SI is the abbreviation for *le Système International d'Unités*. The SI is an outgrowth of the metric system and provides uniform nomenclature for reporting laboratory data among nations. Most laboratory values in the *On Call* series are presented in SI units. Because some laboratories have not yet converted to this system of reporting, the following conversion table for commonly measured laboratory parameters is provided.

Laboratory Test	Previous Reference Intervals	Conversion Factor	Previous Unit	SI Reference Intervals	SI Unit Symbol
Erythrocyte Count					
Women	3.5-5.0	1	$10^6/mm^3$	3.5-5.0	$10^{12}/L$
Men	4.3-5.9	1	$10^6/mm^3$	4.3-5.9	$10^{12}/L$
ESR					
Women	0-30	1	mm/h	0-30	mm/h
Men	0-20	1	mm/h	0-20	mm/h
Hemoglobin					
Women	12.0-15.0	10	g/dL	120-150	g/L
Men	13.6-17.2	10	g/dL	136-172	g/L
Leukocyte Count					
Number fraction (differential)	%	1.00	0.01		
Platelet count	130-400	1	$10^3/mm^3$	130-400	$10^9/L$
Reticulocyte count	10,000-75,000	0.001	$/mm^3$	10-75	$10^9/L$
Number fraction	1-24	0.001	Number per 1000 RBCs	0.001-0.024	1.00
			%	0.001-0.024	1.00
Albumin (serum)	0.1-2.4	0.001	%	40-60	g/L
Alkaline phosphatase	4.0-6.0	10.0	g/dL	0.5-2.0	mkat/L
Amylase (serum)	30-120	0.01667	U/L	0-2.17	mkat/L
Aspartate aminotransferase (AST)	0-130	0.01667	U/L	0-0.58	mkat/L
	0-35	0.01667	U/L		

Bilirubin					
Total	0.1-1.0	mg/dL	17.10	2-18	mmol/L
Conjugated	0-0.2	mg/dL	17.10	0-4	mmol/L
Calcium (Serum)					
Female (<50 years)	8.8-10.0	mg/dL	0.2495	2.20-2.50	mmol/L
Female (xs ≥50 years)	8.8-10.2	mg/dL	0.2495	2.20-2.56	mmol/L
	4.4-5.1	mEq/L	0.500	2.20-2.56	mmol/L
Male	8.8-10.3	mg/dL	0.2495	2.20-2.58	mmol/L
Calcium ion (serum)	2.00-2.30	mEq/L	0.500	1.00-1.15	mmol/L
CO_2 content ($= HCO_3 + CO_2$)	22-28	mEq/L	1.00	22-28	mmol/L
CO (proportion of Hb that is COHb)	<15	%	0.01	<0.15	1.00
Chloride (serum)	95-105	mEq/L	1.00	95-105	mmol/L
Cholesterol (Plasma)	<200	mg/dL	0.02586	<5.20	mmol/L
Complement (Serum)					
C3	70-160	mg/dL	0.01	0.7-1.6	g/L
C4	20-40	mg/dL	0.01	0.2-0.4	g/L
CPK (serum)	0-130	U/L	0.01667	0-2.16	mkat/L
MB fraction	>5 in MI	%	0.01	>0.05	1.00
Creatinine					
Serum	0.6-1.2	mg/dL	88.40	50-110	mmol/L
Urine	Variable	g/24 h	8.840	Variable	mmol/day
Creatinine clearance	75-125	mL/min	0.01667	1.24-2.08	mL/s

Laboratory Test	Previous Reference Intervals	Previous Unit	Conversion Factor	SI Reference Intervals	SI Unit Symbol
Digoxin (Plasma)					
Therapeutic	0.5-2.2	ng/mL	1.281	0.6-2.8	nmol/L
	0.5-2.2	mg/L	1.281	0.6-2.8	nmol/L
Toxic	>2.5	ng/mL	1.281	>3.2	nmol/L
Electrophoresis, Serum Protein					
Albumin	60-65	%	0.01	0.60-0.65	1.00
α_1-Globulin	1.7-5.0	%	0.01	0.02-0.05	1.00
α_2-Globulin	6.7-12.5	%	0.01	0.07-0.13	1.00
β-Globulin	8.3-16.3	%	0.01	0.08-0.16	1.00
γ-Globulin	10.7-20.0	%	0.01	0.11-0.20	1.00
Albumin	3.6-5.2	g/dL	10.0	36-52	g/L
α_1-Globulin	0.1-0.4	g/dL	10.0	1-4	g/L
α_2-Globulin	0.4-1.0	g/dL	10.0	4-10	g/L
β-Globulin	0.5-1.2	g/dL	10.0	5-12	g/L
γ-Globulin	0.6-1.6	g/dL	10.0	6-16	g/L
Ethanol (Plasma)					
Legal limit (driving)	<80	mg/dL	0.2171	<17	mmol/L
Toxic	>100	mg/dL	0.2171	>22	mmol/L
Ferritin (serum)	18-300	ng/mL	1.00	18-300	mg/L
Fibrinogen (plasma)	200-400	mg/dL	0.01	2.0-4.0	g/L

Analyte	Conventional Range	Conventional Units	Factor	SI Range	SI Units
Folate					
Serum	2-10	ng/mL	2.266	4-22	nmol/L
RBCs	140-960	ng/mL	2.266	550-2200	nmol/L
γ-Glutamyltransferase (GGT) (serum)	0-30	U/L	0.01667	0-0.50	mkat/L
Gases (Arterial Blood)					
Po_2	75-105	mm Hg (= torr)	0.1333	10.0-14.0	kPa
Pco_2	33-44	mm Hg (= torr)	0.1333	4.4-5.9	kPa
Glucose					
Serum (fasting)	70-110	mg/dL	0.05551	3.9-6.1	nmol/L
Spinal fluid	50-80	mg/dL	0.05551	2.8-4.4	nmol/L
Haptoglobin (serum)	50-220	mg/dL	0.01	0.50-2.20	g/L
Iron (Serum)					
Female	60-160	mg/dL	0.1791	11-29	mmol/L
Male	80-180	mg/dL	0.1791	14-32	mmol/L
Iron-binding capacity (serum)	250-460	mg/dL	0.1791	45-82	mmol/L
LDH (serum)	50-150	U/L	0.01667	0.82-2.66	mkat/L
LD_1	15-40	%	0.01	0.15-0.40	1.00
LD_2	20-45	%	0.01	0.20-0.45	1.00
LD_3	15-30	%	0.01	0.15-0.30	1.00

Laboratory Test	Previous Reference Intervals	Previous Unit	Conversion Factor	SI Reference Intervals	SI Unit Symbol
LD_4	5-20	%	0.01	0.05-0.20	1.00
LD_5	5-20	%	0.01	0.05-0.20	1.00
LD_1	10-60	U/L	0.01667	0.16-1.00	mkat/L
LD_2	20-70	U/L	0.01667	0.32-1.16	mkat/L
LD_2	10-45	U/L	0.01667	0.22-0.76	mkat/L
LD_3	5-30	U/L	0.01667	0.08-0.50	mkat/L
LD_4	5-30	U/L	0.01667	0.02-0.50	mkat/L
LD_5	0-160	U/L	0.01667	0-2.66	mkat/L
Lipase (serum)	0.50-1.50			0.50-1.50	mkat/L
Lithium ion (serum) (therapeutic)	0.50-1.50	mEq/L	1.00	0.50-1.50	mmol/L
		mg/L	0.001441		mmol/L
		mg/dL	1.441		mmol/L
Magnesium (serum)	1.8-3.0	mg/dL	0.4114	0.80-1.20	mmol/L
	1.6-2.4	mEq/L	0.500	0.80-1.20	mmol/L
Osmolality					
Plasma	280-300	mOsm/kg	1.00	280-300	mmol/kg
Urine	50-1200	mOsm/kg	1.00	50-1200	mmol/kg
Phosphate (serum)	2.5-5.0	mg/dL	0.3229	0.80-1.60	mmol/L
Potassium Ion					
Serum	3.5-5.0	mEq/L	1.00	3.5-5.0	mmol/L
Urine (diet dependent)	25-100	mEq/24 h	1.00	25-100	mmol/d

Protein, Total					
Serum	6.0-8.0	g/dL	10.0	60-80	g/L
Urine	<150	mg/24 h	0.001	<0.15	g/day
Sodium Ion					
Serum	135-147	mEq/L	1.00	135-147	mmol/L
Urine	Diet dependent	mEq/24 h	1.00	Diet dependent	mmol/day
Theophylline (Plasma)					
Therapeutic	10.0-20.0	mg/L	5.550	55-110	mmol/L
Thyroid Tests (Serum)					
TSH	2-11	mU/mL	1.00	2-11	mU/L
T_4	4.0-11.0	mg/dL	12.87	51-142	nmol/L
TBG	12.0-28.0	mg/dL	12.87	150-360	nmol/L
Free T_4	0.8-2.8	ng/dL	12.87	10-36	pmol/L
T_3	75-220	ng/dL	0.01536	1.2-3.4	nmol/L
T_3 uptake	25-35	%	0.01	0.25-0.35	1.00
Transferrin (serum)	170-370	mg/dL	0.01	1.70-3.70	g/L
Triglycerides (plasma)	<160	mg/dL	0.01129	<1.80	mmol/L

Laboratory Test	Previous Reference Intervals	Previous Unit	Conversion Factor	SI Reference Intervals	SI Unit Symbol
Urate (as Uric Acid)					
Serum	2.0-7.0	mg/dL	59.48	120-420	mmol/L
Urine	Diet dependent	g/24 h	5.948	Diet dependent	mmol/day
Urea (serum)	8-18	mg/dL	0.3570	3.0-6.5	mmol/L
Vitamin B$_{12}$ (plasma or serum)	200-1000	pg/mL	0.7378	150-750	pmol/L
		ng/dL	7.378		pmol/L

COHb, Carboxyhemoglobin; *CPK,* creatine phosphokinase; *ESR,* erythrocyte sedimentation rate; *Hb,* Hemoglobin; *LD$_1$ to LD$_5$,* isoenzymes 1 to 5 of lactate dehydrogenase; *LDH,* lactate dehydrogenase; *MB,* muscle brain; *Pco$_2$,* carbon dioxide tension; *Po$_2$,* oxygen tension; *RBCs,* red blood cells; *T$_3$,* triiodothyronine; *T$_4$,* thyroxine; *TBG,* thyroxine-binding globulin; *TSH,* thyroid-stimulating hormone.

The On-Call Formulary

This formulary is a quick reference for information on medications that are commonly taken by patients or prescribed by the student or resident on call.

Antibacterial susceptibility guidelines are presented in Figure D.4. Drugs used in cardiopulmonary resuscitation are described in table format on pages 430-467.

Doses listed are for adult patients with normal renal and hepatic function. Adverse effects in boldface are those that most frequently limit the usefulness of the drug.

ADENOSINE (Adenocard, Adenoscan)

Indications: Drug of first choice for most forms of stable noncomplex supraventricular tachycardia. Effective in terminating tachycardia due to reentry involving the atrioventricular (AV) node.

Actions: An endogenous nucleotide occurring in most cells in the body. Slows conduction through the AV node. Activates vascular adenosine receptors resulting in hypotension.

Side effects: Premature atrial and ventricular contractions, AV block, hypotension, prolonged asystole, cardiac ischemia.

Dosage: 6-12 mg IV rapidly followed by a flush of 10-20 ml normal saline.

ALLOPURINOL (Zyloprim) Xanthine oxidase inhibitor

Indications: Gout, uric acid nephropathy, tumor lysis syndrome.

Actions: Inhibits xanthine oxidase, thus reducing the oxidation of hypoxanthine and xanthine in the formation of uric acid. Has a similar action on some therapeutic drugs with a purine structure, including mercaptopurine and azathioprine, resulting in a decrease in their rate of metabolism.

Side effects: Rash, itching, fever, nausea, diarrhea, **hepatotoxicity**, gout flare-up if you have gout.

Comments: Mercaptopurine and azathioprine levels are increased by allopurinol. Attacks of acute gout may occur shortly after allopurinol is started.

Dosage: 100 to 300 mg PO od.

Better tolerated if taken following meals. Up to 800 mg/day (in divided doses) may be required in severe cases. Reduce the dosage in patients with renal insufficiency.

AMINOGLYCOSIDE ANTIBIOTICS

Indications: Moderate to severe aerobic gram-negative systemic infections. Usually used in combination with another antibiotic. Antibacterial sensitivities should always be done.

Actions: Interfere with the initiation of bacterial protein synthesis in susceptible organisms. Active against aerobic gram-negative bacteria, haemophilus influenza, some anaerobic bacilli, some mycobacteria and methicillin-resistant staphylococci.

Side effects: Use limited because of **renal, cochlear, and vestibular toxicity.** Neuromuscular blockade can occur, particularly in patients with a neuromuscular disorder such as multiple sclerosis or myasthenia gravis and when drug is used in association with other neuromuscular blocking drugs or anesthetics or if given rapidly IV or IP. Serum creatinine level should be measured at the initiation of therapy and every 3 to 4 days during therapy.

Dosage: Once-daily dosing has replaced more frequent dosing for most indications. When an aminoglycoside is used for synergy in enterococcal endocarditis and gram-positive infections, shorter dosing intervals may be required. Elderly patients should be given doses at the low end of the range.

Drug	Trade name	Comments	Usual dosage for systemic infections
Amika-cin	Amikin	Active against many gram-negative organisms resistant to other amino-glycosides. May be less nephrotoxic than genta-micin and tobramycin	5-7 mg/kg once daily IV
Aztreo-nam	Azact-am	Available as Caston for inhalation for cystic fibrosis	1 g q 8 hrs IV One inhalation q8 h
Genta-micin	Gara-mycin	Least expensive. Used since 1971	5-7 mg/kg once daily IV
Netilmi-cin	Netro-mycin	Active against many gram-negative or-ganisms resistant to gentamicin. May be less nephrotoxic than genta-micin and tobramycin	16-20 mg/kg once daily IV
Tobra-mycin	Nebcin		5-7 mg/kg once daily IV

AMINOPHYLLINE (Phyllocontin, Truphylline) Bronchodilator

Indications: Bronchospasm, but no longer considered a first-line agent because in adults it may not improve the bronchodilation achieved with the safer aggressive use of inhaled bronchodilators. Should not be used in chronic obstructive pulmonary disease because of side effects.

Actions: Phosphodiesterase inhibitor that results in smooth muscle relaxation and bronchodilation. Stimulates the respiratory center. Causes cardiac stimulation, diuresis and gastric acid secretion.

Side effects: Tachycardia, **ventricular ectopy**, nausea, vomiting, headaches, **seizures**, insomnia, nightmares.

Comments: Theophylline clearance is decreased by erythromycin, cimetidine, propranolol, allopurinol, and a number of other drugs.

Dosage: Aminophylline loading dose is 5 mg/kg IV over 30 to 45 minutes, up to a maximum of 500 mg, followed by a maintenance dosage of 0.5 to 0.7 mg/kg/h. Maintenance doses in patients with congestive heart failure (CHF) or liver disease and in elderly patients should be reduced to 0.3 mg/kg/h; smokers require a larger dosage of 0.9 mg/kg/h.

AMIODARONE HYDROCHLORIDE FOR INTRAVENOUS INFUSION Antiarrhythmic

Indications: Ventricular tachycardia, cardiac arrest.

Actions: The initial acute effects are predominantly an atrioventricular (AV) intranodal conduction delay and an increase in nodal refractoriness that are caused by calcium channel blockade.

Side effects: **Hypotension, bradycardia** caused by excess AV block; cardiac arrest; cardiogenic shock.

Comments: Use with extreme caution in patients known to be predisposed to bradycardia or AV block.

Dosage: 1000 mg over the first 24 hours of therapy, delivered by the following infusion regimen: loading infusions: 150 mg over the first 10 minutes (15 mg/min), followed by 360 mg over the next 6 hours (1 mg/min); maintenance infusion: 540 mg over the remaining 18 hours (0.5 mg/min).

AMPHOTERICIN B (Fungizone) Antifungal

Indications: Serious fungal infections and leishmaniasis. The fungal infections include aspergillosis, blastomycosis, candidiasis, coccidioidomycosis, and cryptococcosis.

Actions: Binds to sterols in cell membranes, increasing their permeability with a loss of a variety of essential small molecules.

Side effects: Fever, chills, nausea, vomiting, diarrhea, hypotension, **nephrotoxicity**, hypokalemia, hypomagnesemia, thrombophlebitis. The violent chills and fevers have caused the drug to be nicknamed "shake and bake."

Comments: Premedication with antipyretics, antihistamines, antiemetics, and corticosteroids may reduce some of the side effects.

Dosage: Patients should receive a test dose of 1 mg IV in 100 mL D5W over 2 hours. If the test dose is tolerated, another dose of 10 mg can be given on the first day. The dosage can then be increased by 5 mg every day until the desired dosage of 0.5 mg/kg/day is reached. Infusion time should be 4 to 6 hours. Reduce the dosage or dose frequency for patients with renal impairment. Monitor renal function.

ANDEXXA Recombinant factor Xa (see Oral Factor Xa inhibitors)

ANGIOTENSIN-RECEPTOR INHIBITORS (SARTANS, ARBs)

Indications: Hypertension, systolic heart failure, diabetic nephropathy.

Actions: Inhibit the action of angiotensin II resulting in vasodilation in many vascular beds and inhibition of the renin-angiotensin system resulting in a reduction of sodium retention.

Inhibit cardiac and vascular remodeling associated with heart failure, myocardial infarction, and hypertension.

Possess a reno-protective effect independent of blood pressure reduction.

Side effects: **Angioedema, rhabdomyolysis, fatigue,** dizziness, headache.

Comments: Unlike ACE inhibitors ARBs do not inhibit the breakdown of bradykinin and other kinins and therefore their use may be less often accompanied by dry cough and angioedema although they are not free from these adverse effects. Oral ARBs approved for use in systolic heart failure

Often in fixed-dose combination pills with other antihypertensives.

Drug	Trade name	Dose
Candesartan	Atacand	2-16 mg PO once or twice daily
Valsartan	Diovan	40-160 mg PO bid daily (cardiac failure), 80-320 mg PO once daily (hypertension)
Olmesartan	Benecar	20 mg PO once daily
Telmisartan	Micardis	40-80 mg PO once daily

ANGIOTENSIN-CONVERTING ENZYME (ACE) INHIBITORS

Indications: Hypertension, systolic heart failure, and diabetic nephropathy (captopril) and to reduce cardiovascular morbidity and mortality postmyocardial infarction.

Actions: Inhibit the conversion of angiotensin I to angiotensin II resulting in a decrease in arteriolar resistance, an increase in venous capacity, a decrease in cardiac output, cardiac index, and stroke work and a decrease in sodium retention.

Inhibit cardiac and vascular remodeling associated with heart failure, myocardial infarction, and hypertension.

Possess a reno-protective effect independent of blood pressure reduction.

Inhibit the metabolism of bradykinin and other kinins leading to an accumulation of prostaglandins.

Side effects: Rash and altered taste (particularly captopril), cough (particularly with perindopril, ramipril, and fosinopril), **hypotension, angioedema**.

Comments: May cause hyperkalemia if used with potassium-sparing diuretics or potassium supplements. More than a dozen ACE inhibitors are available on the market. Captopril remains the standard. Enaprilat is available for intravenous use with an onset of effect in 15 minutes at the usual dosage of 1.25 to 5 mg IV q6h.

Oral ACE Inhibitors Approved for Use in Preventing Cardiovascular Events Immediately After Myocardial Infarction

Drug	Trade name	Dosage
Captopril	Capoten	6.25-25 mg PO bid or tid
Enalapril	Vasotec	2.5-40 mg PO once daily
Lisinopril	Zestril, Prinivil	2.5-20 mg PO once daily
Perindopril	Aceon	4-8 mg PO once daily
Ramipril	Altace	2.5-20 mg PO once daily

ANGIOTENSIN RECEPTOR BLOCKERS (ARBs)

As effective as Ace inhibitors in reducing blood pressure and equally cardio- and renoprotective.

Less likely to cause cough or angioedema.

Azilsartan	Edarbi	40-80 mg PO once daily
Candesartan	Atacand	8-32 mg PO once daily
Eprosartan	generic	600 mg PO once daily
Irbesartan	Avapro	150-300 mg PO once daily
Losartan	Cozaar	50-100 mg PO once daily or in divided doses

Olmesartan	Benicar	20-40 mg PO once daily
Telmisartan	Micardis	20-80 mg PO once daily
Valsartan	Diovan	80-320 mg PO once daily

DIRECT RENIN INHIBITORS

For use in combination with other antihypertensives but not with an ACE inhibitor.

No proven advantage over an ACE inhibitor.

| Aliskiren | Tekturna | 159-300 mg PO once daily |

Other oral ACE inhibitors include benazepril (Lotensin), cilazapril (Inhibace), fosinopril (Monopril), perindopril (Aceon, Coversyl), quinapril (Accupril), moexipril (Univasc), and trandolapril (Mavik).

ANTACIDS

Indications: Symptomatic relief of pain and discomfort from duodenal peptic ulcer, reflux esophagitis; prophylaxis of stress ulcers and gastrointestinal hemorrhage in critically ill patients.

Actions: Neutralize gastric acid. Aluminum and magnesium preparations are minimally absorbed. About 10% of the calcium in ingested calcium carbonate is absorbed. Sodium bicarbonate is readily absorbed and should be avoided in patients susceptible to sodium overload.

Side effects: All antacids should be used with caution in patients with renal failure. They can result in one or more of the following: aluminum toxicity, hypophosphatemia, hypermagnesemia, hypercalcemia, and sodium overload.

Commonly Used Antacids

Drug	Trade name	Side effects	Dosage
Aluminum hydroxide	Amphojel, Basaljel	Constipation	30-60 ml q1-2h during acute phase, q1-4h and qhs for chronic therapy
Aluminum hydroxide/ magnesium carbonate/ sodium alginate	Gaviscon	Nausea, vomiting, eructation, flatulence	10-20 mL of liquid PO or 2-4 tablets chewed 1-4 times daily after meals and qhs. Contains sodium alginate, a foaming agent aiding dispersion of the antacids.

Drug	Trade name	Side effects	Dosage
Aluminum hydroxide/ magnesium hydroxide	Maalox	Nausea, diarrhea	30-60 ml q1-2h during acute phase, q1-4h and qhs for chronic therapy
Aluminum hydroxide/ magnesium carbonate/so- dium alginate	Gelusil	Nausea, diarrhea	30-60 ml q1-2h during acute phase, q1-4h and qhs for chronic therapy
Calcium carbonate	Tums and many others	Hypercalce- mia	1-4 tablets prn to a maximum of 16 od (regular strength = 200 mg elemental calcium)

ANTIANGINAL DRUGS
Nitrates

Nitrates release nitric acid in vascular smooth muscle leading to vasodilation. Used since 1847.

Drug	Formulation	Dosage	Onset
Nitroglyc- erine	SL tablet (Nitro- stat)	0.3-0.6 mg od up to 1.5 mg od	1-3 min
			1-3 min
	Translingual spray (Nitro- mist)	0.4-0.8 mg tid	60 min
		2-9 mg bid to tid	15-30 min
		0.5-4 inches q	30 minutes
	Extended release	4-8 h	Immediate
	Topical oint- ment	0.2-0.8 mg per day	
	Transdermal patch	12.5- 25 mcg Ti- trate increasing by 5-10 mcg q	
	IV	5–10 minutes	
Isosorbide dinitrate	Oral tablet or capsule	5-10 mg	20-30 minutes
	Extended-re- lease tablet	20-40 mg	Within 2 hrs
Isosorbide mononi- trate	Oral tablet or capsule	10-40 mg bid	10-30 minutes
	Extended-re- lease tablet	50-100 mg od	20-30 minutes

Calcium blockers (see calcium blockers)
Beta-blockers (see beta-blockers)

	Trade name	Action		Dosage	Side effects
Ranola-zine	Ranexa	Inhibition of fatty acid oxidation increasing oxygen supply	Peak effect in 2-5 h Steady state in 3 days	500 mg-1 g bid Usually used together with other agents	Prolonged QT interval dizziness, nausea, headache

ANTICOAGULANTS

See Heparin and Oral and parenteral anticoagulants.

ANTIDIARRHEAL DRUGS

Drug	Trade name	Usual Adult Dosage	Side Effects	Comments
Lopera-mide	Imodi-um	5 mg PO 3 or 4 times per day	Abdominal cramps, distention, dry mouth, sedation, headache Toxic megacolon in colitis	Onset in 2-4 h Less effective if used prn. Also available in combination with simethicone
Diphe-noxylate with atropine	Lomotil	30 mL or 2 tablets or 2 tablets PO per day	Abdominal cramps, distention, dry mouth, sedation, headache toxic megacolon in colitis	Slower onset than loper-amide

Drug	Trade name	Usual Adult Dosage	Side Effects	Comments
Bismuth subsalicylate	Pepto-Bismol Kaopectate	30 mL or 2 tablets or 2 tablets PO every 30 min up to a maximum of 8 doses in 24 h	Darkening of the tongue or stool, tinnitus	
Attapulgite	Kaopectate* Diasor	30 mL or 2 tablets PO every 30 minutes to a maximum of 8 doses per 24 h	Nausea	Acts by absorbing fluid in the gut thus reducing H_2O loss

*The active ingredient of Kaopectate varies from country to country.

ANTIFIBRINOLYTICS

Indications: Prevention and treatment of bleeding caused by excessive fibrinolysis.

Actions: Competitively inhibit the activation of plasminogen and, at high doses, noncompetitively inhibit plasmin.

Side effects: Nausea, vomiting, diarrhea. Increases risk of thromboembolic events. Dizziness, hypotension, particularly with intravenous administration. Rash.

Comments: Trasylol (Aprotinin) is not recommended for general use because of the frequency of anaphylactic reactions on repeat use. It should be administered only in operative settings where cardiopulmonary bypass can be rapidly initiated. The benefit of Trasylol to patients undergoing primary CABG surgery should be weighed against the risk of anaphylaxis associated with any subsequent exposure to aprotinin.

Used mostly to prevent rather than treat bleeding caused by excessive fibrinolysis in patients with hemophilia

Drug	Trade name	Dosage	Comments
Amino-caproic acid	Amicar	4-5 g IV over 1 hour, followed by maintenance infusion of 1-1.25 g/h	Should only be used under a specialist direction
Tranexam-ic acid	Cyklo-kapron	25 mg/kg PO 3-4 times/day. Reduce in the face of renal compromise	Used mostly to prevent rather than treat bleeding caused by excessive fibrinolysis in patients with hemophilia
Trasylol			see comments above

ANTIFUNGAL AGENTS FOR ORAL OR ESOPHAGEAL CANDIDIASIS

Indications: Oral candidiasis can be treated with topical or systemic therapy. Local treatment is generally recommended for reducing the likelihood of the emergence of azole-resistant organisms. Esophageal candidiasis necessitates systemic therapy.

Actions: Bind to sterols in cell membranes, increasing their permeability with the loss of a variety of essential small molecules.

Side effects: All antifungal drugs for systemic therapy are associated with frequent adverse effects, including **GI intolerance, hepatotoxicity**, rash, pruritus, and headaches, as well as with many drug interactions.

Drug		Dosage	Comment
Clotrim-azole	Mycelex	One troche 5 times daily	Not well tolerated—nausea, vomiting
Nystatin	Mycosta-tin	4-6 ml qid or 1-2 pastilles 4-5 times per day	Not well tolerated—nausea, vomiting

Drug		Dosage	Comment
Fluco-nazole	Diflucan	200-400 mg PO daily. Reduce dosage or dose frequency for patients with renal impairment. 400 mg IV od	Drug of first choice
Itracon-azole	Sporanox	Solution: 200 mg PO daily	The solution (not the capsule formulation) is of equal efficacy as fluconazole; fluconazole-resistant cases may respond to itraconazole
Keto-conazole	Nizoral	200-400 mg PO daily. Poorly absorbed, particularly with drugs that reduce gastric acidity	Causes gynecomastia in men
Caspo-fungin	Nizoral, Cancidas	70 mg IV in 1 h, then 50 mg IV daily	Diarrhea, headache, rash, muscle pain. For esophageal candidiasis resistant to other agents
Ampho-tericin	Fungi-zone	0.3-0.7 mg/kg od by slow IV infusion. A test dose is usually given. Use should be restricted to resistant cases because of toxicities	**Anaphylaxis, renal failure, hypotension,** nausea, diarrhea, **hemorrhagic gastroenteritis,** pain at injection site with or without phlebitis

ANTINAUSEANT DRUGS

Drug	Trade name	Dosage	Comments	Side effects
Metoclopr-amide	Maxeran, Reglan	5-10 mg PO, IM, or IV	Stimulates gastric motility	Drowsiness, lethargy

Drug	Trade name	Dosage	Comments	Side effects
Diphen-hydramine	Benadryl	25-50 mg PO, mg IM or IV q4-6h prn		Drowsiness, dizziness, dry mouth, urinary retention
Nabilone	Cesamet	1-2 mg PO bid	A synthetic cannabi-noid used to treat chemo-therapy induced nausea and vomiting	**Halluci-nations, vertigo, confusion, anxiety, panic, diz-ziness, hy-potension**
Prochlor-perazine	Stemetil	5-10 mg IV or IM or 25 mg PR	Antihista-mine with anticho-linergic effects	Drowsiness, dizziness, dry mouth, urinary retention
Prometha-zine	Phener-gan	25-50 mg PO, IM, or PR q4-6h prn or 12.5-25 mg IV q4-6h	Antihista-mine with anticho-linergic effects	Drowsiness, dizziness, dry mouth, urinary retention
Chlorprom-azine	Largactil	For nausea with severe migraine, 0.1 mg/kg IV over 20 min; repeat after 15 min to a maxi-mum of 37.5 mg	Limit use to nausea ac-company-ing severe migraine	CNS depres-sion, hy-potension, **extrapy-ramidal effects**, jaundice

Granisetron (Kytril), Ondansetron (Zofran), and Dolasetron (Anzemet) are serotonin 5-hydroxytriptamine 3 (5-HT_3) receptor antagonists that block the vomiting center and are available to prevent or treat postanesthetic nausea and vomiting and the vomiting associated with chemotherapy and radiotherapy for cancer.

ANTIPLATELET AND ANTITHROMBOTIC DRUGS

Indications: Primary and secondary prevention of thrombotic cerebrovascular or cardiovascular disease.

Actions: Thrombi are formed as a result of platelets adhering to damaged luminal surfaces of arteries. Platelets are activated by a variety of stimuli, including the prostacyclin-thromboxane pathways, and adhere to one another under the influence of fibrinogen and von Willebrand's factor to initiate clot formation. These factors bind to activated glycoprotein IIb/IIIa receptors on the platelet surface. Antiplatelet drugs interfere with platelet activation resulting in decreased tendency of platelets to adhere to one another and to damaged blood vessels' endothelium. Some agents (e.g., aspirin, ridogrel) inhibit the prostacyclin-thromboxane pathways; some (ticlopidine, clopidogrel) interfere with platelet membrane function, inhibiting platelet aggregation; others (e.g., abciximab, tirofiban) act as antagonists at the glycoprotein IIb/IIIa binding sites. Tissue plasminogen activators catalyze the conversion of plasminogen to plasmin the major enzyme responsible for clot breakdown. Intense pharmaceutical development is addressing other potential sites that influence platelet function; thus an ideal agent is yet to be found. They are effective in the arterial circulation, where anticoagulants have little effect.

Platelet Aggregation Inhibitors

Drug	Trade name	Indications	Dosage	Comments
Aspirin (Acetyl-salicylic acid)	Aspirin	Myocardial infarction, unstable angina, stroke, transient ischemic attack	Maximally effective at doses of 75-325 mg PO daily	Used a daily dose of 75-100 mg PO in the prevention of cerebrovascular disease and stroke in patients age 40-59 at high risk of cardiovascular events
Cangrelor	Kengreal	Used as an adjunct to percutaneous coronary intervention (PCI)	30 mcg/kg IV bolus followed immediately by a 4 mcg/kg/min IV infusion	Bleeding events more common than with clopidogrel
Dipyridamole	Persantine	Used as an adjunct to warfarin to prevent prosthetic valve thrombosis	75 mg PO qid	Side effects include GI symptoms and rash
Clopidogrel	Plavix	Acute coronary syndromes	300 mg PO, then 75 mg PO daily	Used in combination with aspirin for acute coronary syndromes; onset of action is 2 h

Platelet Aggregation Inhibitors—cont'd

Drug	Trade name	Indications	Dosage	Comments
Prasugrel	Effient	Acute coronary syndromes	60 mg PO loading dose and then continue at 10 mg PO once daily	Patients taking Effient should also take aspirin (75 mg to 325 mg PO daily)
Ticagrelor	Brilinta	Used in combination with aspirin for acute coronary syndromes	180 mg, then 90 mg PO bid	More rapid onset but shorter duration of action than clopidogrel. No proven advantage over clopidogrel
Ticlopidine	Ticlid	Stroke/transient ischemic attack; acute coronary syndromes	250 mg PO bid with food	Can be associated with fatal agranulocytosis. May be slightly more effective than aspirin in preventing cerebrovascular events. Onset of action is delayed; beneficial effect not seen until after 2 weeks of therapy

Glycoprotein Receptor Antagonists

Inhibit platelet activation and aggregations. Bleeding complications are increased with concomitant heparin therapy.

Drug	Trade name	Indications	Dosage	Comments
Abciximab	ReoPro	As an adjunct in interventional cardiology to prevent cardiac ischemic complications; not recommended for acute coronary syndromes	0.25 mg/kg IV load, then 0.125 mcg/kg/min IV (maximum, 10 mcg/min)	No dosage adjustment required for patients with renal insufficiency
Eptifibatide	Integrilin	As an adjunct in interventional cardiology to prevent cardiac ischemic complications; acute coronary syndromes	180 mcg/kg IV bolus, followed by infusion of 2 mcg/kg	Dosage adjustment required for patients with renal insufficiency
Tirofiban	Aggrastat	As an adjunct in interventional cardiology to prevent cardiac ischemic complications; acute coronary syndromes	0.4 mcg/kg/min IV for 30 min, then 0.1 mcg/kg/min IV	May cause reversible thrombocytopenia. Dosage adjustment required for patients with renal insufficiency

Thrombin Receptor Antagonists

Drug	Trade name	Indications	Dosage	Comments
Vorapaxar	Zontivity	Used in the prevention of cardiovascular events in persons with a history of myocardial infarction or peripheral vascular disease.	40 mg PO followed by 2.5 mg PO daily	Contraindicated in persons with a history of stroke, transient ischemic attacks or intracerebral hemorrhage

Tissue Plasminogen Activators

Thrombolytic agents that catalyze the conversion of plasminogen to plasmin, the major enzyme responsible for clot breakdown. Antidote is aminocaproic acid. Used to treat acute ischemic stroke, acute ST-elevation myocardial infarction, pulmonary embolism associated with low blood pressure, and blocked central venous catheter.

Drug		Dosage			
		Ischemic stroke	Myocardial infarction	Pulmonary embolism	Occluded catheter
t-PA, rt-PA	Alteplase	0.9 mg/kg IV 10% over 1 minute the reminder over 1 h	15 mg IVP bolus over 1-2 minutes, then 50 mg IV infusion over next 30 minutes, and then remaining 35 mg over next 60 minutes	100 mg IV infused over 2 hr	2 mg Cathflo activase into occluded catheter
	Reteplase		10 units over 2 minutes IV repeated in 30 minutes		
	Tenecteplase	0.25 mg/kg IV	30-50 mg IV over 5 sec		

ANTIPSYCHOTICS AND OTHER DRUGS FOR THE COMBATIVE PATIENT

Drug	Trade name	Dose	Side effects	Comments
First-Generation Antipsychotic				
Haloperidol	Haldol	0.25–10 mg PO, IM	Sedation, akathisia, dystonia, neuroleptic malignant syndrome, prolongation of QT interval	Not approved for IV use
Atypical Antipsychotics				
Risperidone	Risperdal	0.5–2 mg PO	Drowsiness, dizziness, lightheadedness, nausea, drooling	Shown to be useful in acute management in Alzheimer disease. Available as a liquid or rapidly dissolvable tablet
Olanzapine	Zyprexa	2.5–10 mg PO or IM	Akathisia, dizziness, **neuroleptic malignant syndrome**	No advantage over risperidone except for the availability of an intramuscular preparation
Ziprasidone	Geodon	20–40 mg PO bid 20 mg IM	Dizziness, restlessness, rash, fatigue	After intramuscular administration of single doses, peak serum concentrations typically occur at 60 minutes post-dose or earlier: the mean half-life (T½) ranges from 2–5 hours. Used to treat schizophrenia and bipolar disorder. The IM form can be used for acute agitation in people with schizophrenia
Alpha-2 adrenergic receptor agonist				
Dexmedetomidine	Igalmi	120 or 180 ug SL	Hypotension, bradycardia	Use limited to schizophrenia and bipolar disorders

ANTIVIRAL DRUGS
Antiviral Drugs for Coronavirus Infection

Drug	Trade name	Dosage	Side effects	Comment
Nirmatrelvir/ritonavir	Paxlovid	Nirmatrelvir 300 mg/ ritonavir 100 mg PO bid for 5 days	Dysgeusia, diarrhea, vomiting, muscle pain, hypertension, headache	Treatment of mild to mod-erately severe coronavirus infection
Fluvoxamine	Luvox	50-100 mg PO od	Headache, nausea, diarrhea, dry mouth, dizziness, increased sweating, feeling nervous, restless, fatigued, insomnia	A serotonin uptake inhibitor used to treat obsessive com-pulsion disorder. Has potential antiinflammatory and antiviral activity used to prevent hospi-tal admissions for adults with coronavirus infection
AntiSARS-Cov2 monoclonal antibodies			**Anaphylactic re-actions,** urticaria, dizziness, nausea, headache, diarrhea	
Bamlanivimab with etesevimab	REGEN-COV		**Anaphylactic re-actions,** urticaria, dizziness, nausea, headache, diarrhea	Usually reserved for patients with compromised immune systems. For current accepted indications check with the FDA. www.fda.gov/drugs. See notes below
Casirivimab with Imdevimab	Actemra			
Tocilizumab	Evushield			
Tixagevimab with cilgavimab				
Bebtelovimab				
Sotrovimab				

Antivirals for Influenza A and B

Current antivirals reduce the symptoms of influenza if started within 48 hrs of the onset of symptoms and are indicated in hospitalized patients at risk of influenza complications. They are effective as prophylactic agents if given within 48 hrs of exposure.

Drug	Trade name	Dosage	Side effects	Comment
Baloxavir marboxil	Xofluza	80 mg PO once daily	Diarrhea, headache, nausea, **hypersensitivity reactions**	As an endonuclease inhibitor distinct from other agents
Oseltamivir	Tamiflu	75 mg PO once daily	**Anaphylaxis**, nausea, vomiting, headache	Inhibits viral transaminase
Zanamivir	Relenza	2 inhalations bid	**Bronchospasm**, nausea, vomiting, diarrhea,	Should not be used in patients with respiratory illnesses
Peramivir	Rapivab	600 mg IM/IV once od	Diarrhea, **neutropenia, Stevens-Johnson syndrome, exfoliative dermatitis,** hallucination	

Antivirals for Hepatitis B

Drug	Trade name	Dose	Side effects
Tenofovir	Viread	300 mg PO od	**Nephropathy, pancreatitis**, hypercholesterolemia weight gain
Entecavir	Baraclude	0.5-1 mg PO od	**Lactic acidosis**, hepatomegaly, steatosis, exacerbation of hepatitis on cessation of dosing

Antivirals for Hepatitis C

The following agents are direct-acting agents targeting viral proteins HCV NS5A inhibitors.

Drug	Trade name	Dose	Side effects
Sofosbuvir/ velpatasvir	Epclusa	400 mg/100 mg PO od	Headache, fatigue, nausea, insomnia, muscle weakness, irritability, **anaphylactic reactions**
Sofosbuvir/ ledipasvir	Harvoni	90 mg/400 mg PO od	**Anaphylactic reactions**, hives, vomiting
Glecaprevir/ pibrentasvir	Mavyret	100 mg/40 mg 3 tablets PO od	Headache, fatigue, anorexia

Antivirals for Herpes Zoster

These agents are effective against the herpes simplex and varicella zoster virus.

Drug	Trade name	Dose	Adverse effects
Acyclovir	Zovirax	800 mg q4h 5 times PO od for herpes zoster. Start within 48 hrs of onset	Anorexia, nausea, vomiting, diarrhea, headache, lightheadedness, swelling of hands and feet
Famciclovir	Famvir	500 mg q8h PO od for herpes zoster. Start within 48 hrs of onset	Headache, nausea, abdominal pain, neutropenia
Valaciclovir	Valtrex	1000 mg q8h Po od. Start within 48 hrs of onset	Anorexia, depressed feelings, fatigue

ANTIRETROVIRAL DRUGS FOR POSTEXPOSURE PROPHYLAXIS

After a needle stick injury with an HIV-infected patient start tenofovir DF 300 mg once a day, lamivudine 150 mg twice a day, raltegravir 400 mg twice a day.

A 28-day course of antivirals is recommended following a needle stick injury with an HIV-infected patient: tenofovir 300 mg PO once daily and lamivudine 150 mg PO bid and raltegravir 400 mg PO bid for 5 days then emtricitabine/tenofovir 200 mg/300 mg PO once daily available as a combined tablet (Truvada) and raltegravir 500 mg PO bid for 23 days.

ANTIRETROVIRAL DRUGS FOR PRE-EXPOSURE PROPHYLAXIS (PrEP)

Pre-exposure prophylaxis (PrEP) is the use of certain antiretroviral medications by HIV-uninfected persons who are at high, ongoing risk of HIV acquisition, beginning before and continuing after potential HIV exposures.

Regimens include: tenofovir disoproxil fumarate/emtricitabine (Truvada) 300/200 mg PO once daily or Truvada 300/200 mg administered "on demand" (two pills taken together 2 to 24 hours before first sexual exposure, followed by one pill daily until 48 hours after last sexual activity). Generic Truvada is much cheaper than the brand name drug.

or

Cabotegravir (Apretude) 600 mg by deep gluteal IM injection every 2 months.

LONG-ACTING ANTIRETROVIRAL DRUGS

Regimens have been simplified with the introduction of long-acting antivirals. The first of these is a combination of cabotegravir (an integrase inhibitor) with rilpivirine (a nonnucleoside)—trade name Cabenuva—and cabotegravir—trade names Apretude, Vocabria. For patients whose HIV has been controlled given as deep gluteal IM injections (total 600 mg) every 2 months. The first inhibitor of the HIV protein capsid, lenacapavir (Sunlenca) was released in 2022. Given orally initially followed by 6 monthly SC injections.

ANTIRETROVIRAL DRUGS

Adverse effects

Nucleoside Reverse Transcriptase Inhibitors (NRTIs)	Confounding adverse effects
Abacavir, ABC (Ziagen)	Hypersensitivity reaction, neuropathy, hypercholesterolemia fever, nausea, diarrhea
Didanosine(Videx, Videx-EC)	Pancreatitis, neuropathy, lactic acidosis, nausea, vomiting, abdominal pain, diarrhea
Entecavir (Baraclude) Used to treat hepatitis B	Headache, fatigue, dizziness, nausea

Emtricitabine (Emtriva) a component of Descovy, Truvada, Atripla, Stribild, Genvoya, Complera, Odefsey, Symtuza, Biktarvy	Hypersensitivity, neuropathy, lactic acidosis rash, skin darkening of palms or soles, diarrhea
Lamivudine (Epivir) a component of Combivir, Trizivir, Epzicom, Triumeq, Cimduo, Delstrigo, Dovato	Lactic acidosis, pancreatitis, nephropathy, neutropenia hematuria, melena
Stavudine, d4T (Zerit, Zerit XR)	Peripheral neuropathy, lactic acidosis, pancreatitis hematuria, melena
Tenofovir (disoproxil fumarate) TDF (Viread) a component of Truvada, Atripla, Stribild, Cimduo, Delstrigo	Nephropathy, pancreatitis, hypercholesterolemia, weight gain
Tenofovir alafenamide, TAF (Vemlidy) a component of Descovy, Genvoya, Odefsey, Symtuza, Biktarvy	
Zidovudine, AZT (Retrovir) A component of Combivir, Trizivir	Macrocytic anemia, neutropenia, lactic acidosis, hypercholesterolemia, steatosis nausea, vomiting
Non-Nucleoside Reverse Transcriptase Inhibitors (NNRTIs)	
Cabotegravir (Cabenuva)	Pyrexia, fatigue, headache, musculoskeletal pain, nausea, sleep disorders, dizziness, and rash
Doravirine (Pietro) a component of Delstrigo	Nausea, diarrhea, dizziness, stomach (abdominal) pain, headache, abnormal dreams, tiredness, skin rash
Efavirenz (Sustiva) a component of Atripla	Hepatotoxicity, suicidal ideation, vivid dreams, anxiety, depression, insomnia, skin rash
Etravirine (Intelence)	Adipogenic effects—redistribution or accumulation of body fat, including central obesity, peripheral wasting, facial wasting, breast enlargement and general cushingoid appearance, skin rash, nausea, fatigue

Nevirapine (Viramune)	Severe hepatotoxicity and skin reactions, **Stevens-Johnson syndrome**, **toxic epidermal necrolysis** and hypersensitivity reactions, nausea, fever
Rilpivirine (Edurant) a component of Complera, Odefsey, Juluca	Osteopenia, which may lead to fractures. immune reconstitution inflammatory syndrome (IRIS), insomnia, headache, nausea, vomiting, dizziness, abdominal pain, drowsiness
Protease Inhibitors (PIs)	
Amprenavir	Hepatotoxicity, nausea, vomiting, diarrhea, epigastric pain, flatulence, paresthesia, headache, rash, and fatigue
Atazanavir (Reyataz) a component of Evotaz	Nephrolithiasis, AV block, hyperglycemia, pancreatitis, immune reconstitution inflammatory syndrome (IRIS)
Darunavir (Prezista) a component of Prezcobix, Symtuza	Diabetes and hyperglycemia. Changes in body fat (lipodystrophy syndrome), immune reconstitution inflammatory syndrome (IRIS), elevated pancreatic amylase, diarrhea, nausea, rash
Lopinavir/ ritonavir(Kaletra)	Hepatotoxicity, cardiac arrhythmia–prolongation of QT interval, abdominal pain, weakness, nausea, diarrhea, vomiting, headache, insomnia
Ritonavir (Norvir) also included to boost other drugs	As a cytochrome P50 inhibitor interferes with the metabolism of a variety of other drugs
Fusion Inhibitor (FI)	
Enfuvirtide (Fuzeon)	As a cytochrome P-450 inhibitor interferes with the metabolism of a variety of other drugs
	Pneumonia, systemic hypersensitivity reactions, nausea, anorexia, constipation, diarrhea, myalgia, depressed mood, weight loss, insomnia

Entry inhibitor
Maraviroc (Selzentry)   Hepatotoxicity, hypersensi-
                                     tivity reactions, postural
                                     hypotension, fever, coryza,
                                     cough, insomnia

Integrase Inhibitors

Bictegravir   Angioedema, Stevens-Johnson
included in Biktarvy   syndrome, urticaria, hepato-
                                     toxicity, neutropenia, lactic
                                     acidosis, nausea, diarrhea,
                                     headache

Cabotegravir (Apretude,   Hypersensitivity reactions,
   Vocabria)   suicidal depression, hepato-
                                     toxicity, asthenia, myalgia,
                                     headache, injection site
                                     reactions following gluteal
                                     IM injections

Cabotegravir and rilpivirine   Hypersensitivity reactions,
   (Cabenuva)   suicidal depression, hepato-
                                     toxicity, asthenia, myalgia,
                                     headache, injection site
                                     reactions following gluteal
                                     IM injections

Dolutegravir (Ivica)   Hypersensitivity, immune
also included in Triumeq,   reconstitution syndrome,
   Dovato, Juluca   depression, hepatotoxicity,
                                     nausea, headache

Elvitegravir (Vitekta)   Suicidal depression, immune
also included in Stribild,   reconstitution syndrome,
   Genvoya   hepatotoxicity, diarrhea,
                                     nausea, rash

Raltegravir (Isentress)   Hypersensitivity reactions, sui-
                                     cidal depression, hepatotoxic-
                                     ity, asthenia, myalgia, headache

gp120 Attachment Inhibitor

Fostemsavir (*Rukobia*)   Prolonged QT interval, immune
                                     reconstitution syndrome,
                                     hypersensitivity reactions,
                                     headache, nausea, diarrhea

Post attachment inhibitor

Ibalizumab (Trogarzo)   Immune reconstitution
                                     inflammatory syndrome,
                                     leukopenia, hypersensitivity
                                     reactions, hyperglycemia,
                                     hepatotoxicity, nephrotoxici-
                                     ty rash, diarrhea, nausea

Capsid inhibitor
Lenacapavir (Sunlenca)   Immune reconstitution inflam-
                                matory syndrome

Long-acting injectable treatment
Cabenuva (cabotegravir + rilpivirine)
Vocabria (cabotegravir)
Isentress HD (raltegravir) 600 mg
Lenacapavir (Sunlenca)

ATROPINE

Indications: Drug of first choice for symptomatic sinus bradycardia. May be beneficial in the presence of AV nodal block or
   ventricular asystole Not effective for intranodal (Mobitz type
   II) block. Second choice (after epinephrine or vasopressin) for
   asystole or bradycardic pulseless electrical activity.
Actions: Anticholinergic (antimuscarinic) agent.
Side effects: Dry mouth, blurred vision, photophobia, **tachycardia**,
   anhidrosis, difficulty in micturition and occasional hypersensitivity reactions.
Dosage: Asystole or pulseless electrical activity: 1 mg IV push. May
   repeat every 3 to 5 minutes to a maximum of three doses (3 mg).
   Bradycardia: 0.5 mg IV every 3 to 5 minutes as needed to a total
   of 0.4 mg/kg (total of 3 mg). Can be given SC or IM.

BENZODIAZEPINES

Drug	Trade name	Dose	Side effects	Comments
Midazolam	Versed	2-5 mg IM	Respiratory depression, sedation, dizziness, cognitive impairment, particularly in elderly patients	Onset after oral administration within 1 h; long half-life of about 100 h
Diazepam	Valium	2-10 mg PO, PR, IM, IV or intranasal	Respiratory depression, sedation, dizziness, cognitive impairment, particularly in elderly patients	Intranasal dosing may result in faster control of seizures in status epilepticus

Drug	Trade name	Dose	Side effects	Comments
Lorazepam	Ativan	0.5-4 mg PO, SL, IM, or IV	Respiratory depression, sedation, dizziness, cognitive impairment particularly in elderly patients	Erratically absorbed after IM injection. Half-life of 10-20 hours

BENZTROPINE MESYLATE Anticholinergic (antimuscarinic)

Indications: Drug-induced extrapyramidal reactions. A drug of choice for terminating acute dystonic reactions. Useful in the symptomatic treatment of Parkinson disease.

Actions: An anticholinergic (antimuscarinic) agent with antihistaminic and local anesthetic properties.

Side effects: **Tachycardia, dizziness**, dry mouth, mydriasis, urinary hesitancy or retention.

Comments: Onset of effect is 2 to 3 minutes after IM or IV injection or 1 to 2 hours after an oral dose. Effects may persist for 24 hours or longer.

Dosage: 1 to 2 mg PO, IM, or IV for acute dystonic reactions. If symptoms return, the dose can be repeated.

β-ADRENERGIC BLOCKERS

Indications: Angina pectoris, secondary prevention of myocardial infarction, treatment of supraventricular tachycardias (SVTs), hypertension, thyrotoxicosis, heart failure, migraine prevention, portal hypertension.

Actions: Competitive antagonism of β-adrenergic receptors in the vascular smooth muscle and the heart, as well as bronchial smooth muscle.

Some act predominantly on cardiac beta receptors cardioselective agents.

Some have additional alpha adrenergic blocking activity useful in blocking unopposed alpha activity hence providing arteriolar vasodilation.

Some have intrinsic beta agonist activity useful in preventing excessive bradycardia with sustained beta blocker therapy.

Side effects: **Hypotension, bradycardia, bronchospasm**, nausea, fatigue, nightmares.

Comments: It is usually useful to start with a low dosage and increase as required, because individual responses vary considerably.

Drug	Trade name	Dosage	Activity
Agents specifically indicated for cardiac arrhythmias			
Esmolol	Brevibloc	0.5 mg/kg/min IV loading dose over 1 min, followed by infusion of 0.05 mg/kg/min (maximum 0.3 mg/kg/min)	Cardioselective
Sotalol	Betapac	80 mg bid. Reduce frequency in face of renal impairment	Noncardioselective
Agents specifically indicated for congestive heart failure			
Carvedilol	Coreg, Carloc, Carvil	3.125 mg bid increasing every 2 weeks to a maximum of 50 mg bid	Noncardioselective with intrinsic alpha blocking activity
Metoprolol sustained release	Toprol XL	25-100 mg once daily with food	Cardioselective
Bisoprolol	Zebeta	5 mg once daily increasing to a maximum of 20 mg once daily	Cardioselective
Nebivolol	Bystolic	5 mg od increasing to a maximum of 40 mg od	Cardioselective
Agents specifically for myocardial infarction			
Atenolol	Tenormin	25-50 mg PO SVTs: 5 mg IV over 5 minutes at 10-minute intervals to a total of 15 mg	Cardioselective

Drug	Trade name	Dosage	Activity
Metoprolol	Betaloc, Lopressor, Teva-Metoprolol	50-200 mg PO bid for hypertension, angina. 1.5 mg/kg/min over 30 seconds followed by 0.15 mg/kg/min increasing to a maximum of 0.3 mg/kg/min	Cardioselective
Propranolol	Inderal	10-80 mg PO bid to qid Aortic dissection: 0.1 mg/kg by slow intravenous push, divided into 3 equal doses at 2- to 3-min intervals; repeat after 2 min if necessary; do not exceed 1 mg/min	Noncardioselective
Other agents *Noncardioselective*			
Nadolol	Corgard	40 mg once daily increasing to a maximum of 240 mg once daily	Noncardioselective
Timolol	Blocadren	10 mg bid increasing to 20 mg bid	Noncardioselective
Labetalol	Trandate, Normodyne	For a hypertensive emergency, 10 mg IV over 1-2 min. May repeat 10-20 mg every 10 min to a maximum dose of 150 mg. Alternatively follow the initial dose with an infusion of 2-8 mg per min.	Noncardioselective with additional alpha blocking activity

Drug	Trade name	Dosage	Activity
Oxprenolol	Trasacor	20 mg PO tid to a total of 480 mg od	Noncardioselective with intrinsic beta sympathomimetic activity
Penbutolol	Levatol	20-40 mg PO od to a total of 480 mg od	Noncardioselective with intrinsic beta sympathomimetic activity
Pindolol	Visken	5 mg PO od to a total of 60 mg od	Noncardioselective with intrinsic beta sympathomimetic activity

Other agents
  Cardioselective

Acebutolol	Monitan, Sectra	100-200 mg PO tid	Cardioselective with beta sympathetic adrenergic activity
Atenolol	Tenormin	25-50 mg PO 5 mg IV over 5 min at 10-min intervals, to a total of 15 mg	Cardioselective
Esmolol	Brevibloc	0.5 mg/kg/min intravenous loading dose over 1 min, followed by infusion of 0.05 mg/kg/min (maximum, 0.3 mg/kg/min)	

BISACODYL (Dulcolax) Laxative

Indications: Constipation.

Actions: Stimulates peristalsis.

Side effects: Abdominal cramps, rectal bleeding.

Comments: Onset: oral ingestion, in 6 to 10 hours; rectal administration, in 15 to 60 minutes. Avoid in pregnancy, myocardial infarction. May worsen **orthostatic hypotension, weakness, and incoordination in elderly patients**.

Dosage: 10 to 15 mg PO qhs prn; 10 mg rectal suppository prn.

BISMUTH SUBSALICYLATE (Pepto-Bismol) Antibacterial, antiinflammatory

Indications: Peptic ulcer disease, diarrhea.

Actions: Acts locally at the ulcer site to promote healing of gastric and duodenal ulcers; has antibacterial activity, including against *Helicobacter pylori*. Neutralizes bacterial toxins and is useful in treating traveler's diarrhea. Salicylate is thought to have an antiinflammatory action.

Side effects: Darkening of the tongue and stools, tinnitus.

Comments: Avoid in patients with **salicylate sensitivity**. Used in combination with an antibiotic in the eradication of *H. pylori*.

Dosage: 2 tablets or 30 mL PO qid; for diarrhea, 2 tablets every 30 minutes, up to a maximum of eight doses per day.

CALCITONIN ANTAGONISTS (eptinezumab, erenumab, fremanezumab, galcanezumab)

Indications: Migraine prophylaxis

Actions: A monoclonal antibody that inhibits calcitonin

Side effects: Hypersensitivity reactions

Dosage: 100 mg IV q 3 months

CALCITONIN SALMON (Salcatonin, Caltine) Hypercalcemia treatment

Indications: Hypercalcemia of neoplastic disease, multiple myeloma, primary hyperparathyroidism, postmenopausal osteoporosis, Paget's disease.

Actions: Decreases bone resorption, thus inhibiting the release of calcium. Increases renal loss of calcium.

Side effects: **Anaphylaxis**, GI symptoms, local inflammation at injection site.

Comments: Onset, 15 minutes; peak, 4 hours; duration, 8 to 24 hours.

Dosage: For hypercalcemia 4 IU/kg every 12 hours SC or IM. May be increased to 8 IU/kg if response is not satisfactory. For osteoporosis nasal spray 200 USP units intranasally od.

CALCIUM CHANNEL BLOCKERS

Calcium blockers decrease systemic vascular resistance. The cardiac responses vary—felodipine, nicardipine, and nisoldipine cause an initial reflex tachycardia while isradipine, nifedipine, and amlodipine have a lesser effect on heart rate and verapamil and diltiazem slow av conduction.

Actions: Inhibit calcium flux through cell membranes. Differ in selectivity of vascular beds

Indications: Angina pectoris, coronary spasm, hypertension, atrial fibrillation, SVTs, left ventricular diastolic dysfunction, subarachnoid hemorrhage, migraine. Felodipine, nicardipine, and nisoldipine are often used to reduce systemic vascular resistance and arterial pressure in the treatment of hypertension.

Side effects: **Hypotension**, flushing, dizziness, constipation, headaches, **peripheral edema**, bradycardia. The edema results from vasodilation and does not respond to diuretics.

Comments: Absorption is highly variable. Absorption of nifedipine and nimodipine is enhanced by grapefruit juice.

Nondihydropyridines: More selective action on cardiac sites, slowing SA/AV nodal conduction, and myocardial contractility.

Drug	Trade name	Dosage	Comments
Verapamil	Isoptin Calan	For rate control or to break SVT, 2.5-5 mg IV over 1-2 min	Should be administered only to patients being monitored
Diltiazem	Cardizem	For rate control or to break SVT, 0.25 mg/kg (usual dosage, 15-25 mg) IV over 1-2 min	Should be administered only to patients being monitored

Dihidropyridines: More selective action on vascular sites with vasodilation and reflex sympathetic tachycardia and an increase in cardiac output. Side effects include headache, **peripheral edema, tachycardia**, dizziness, flushing, tiredness, and fatigue.

Drug	Trade name	Dosage	Comments
Amlodipine	Norvasc	5-10 mg PO once daily	
Clevidipine	Cleviprex	IV infusion 1-2 mg/hr, maximum dose 16 mg/hr	IV use only- t ½ about 1 minute

Drug	Trade name	Dosage	Comments
Felodipine	Plendil, Renedil	2.5-10 mg PO once daily	
Isradipine	Dynacirc	2.5 mg PO twice daily, increasing to a maximum of 20 mg PO per day	
Nicardipine	Cardene	In hypertensive emergencies: 5.0 mg/h (50 mL/h) rate; may be increased by 25 mL/h (2.5 mg/h) every 5 min up to a maximum of 150 mL/h (15.0 mg/h)	
Nimodipine	Nimotop	60-90 mg PO q4h or 1 mg/h IV via continuous infusion, increasing prn to 2-3 mg/h in subarachnoid hemorrhage	In combination with surgery, appears to provide better results than does surgery alone, particularly in patients with mild to moderate neurologic deficits
Nisoldipine	Sular	8.5 mg PO once daily increasing by 8.5 mg PO once daily to a maximum of 34 mg PO once daily	
Diphenyl Pipera- zine			
Flunarizine	Sibelium	10 mg PO qhs	May take 6-8 weeks before benefit is noted

CALCIUM CHLORIDE/CALCIUM GLUCONATE
Calcium supplement

Indications: Symptomatic hypocalcemia, hyperkalemia; adjunct in cardiopulmonary resuscitation (CPR).

Actions: Replaces Ca^{2+} in deficiency states. Decreases cardiac automaticity, raises resting potential of cardiac cells.

Side effects: Administration of Ca^{2+} to patients taking **digoxin may precipitate ventricular dysrhythmias because of the combined effects of digoxin and Ca^{2+}**.

Comments: Note that the chloride is three times as potent as the gluconate:

    10 mL of 10% calcium chloride = 1 gm = 270 mg Ca = 13.5 mEq Ca

    10 mL of 10% calcium gluconate = 1 gm = 90 mg Ca = 4.35 mEq Ca

Dosage: The gluconate is generally preferred except in cardiac resuscitation and verapamil overdose because the **chloride preparation can cause tissue necrosis if extravasated**. See page 238 for doses in cardiac resuscitation and verapamil overdose. See page 415 for use in hyperkalemia and page 387 for use in hypocalcemia.

CAPSAICIN Substance P depletor

Indications: Postherpetic neuralgia.

Actions: Releases and depletes substance P from sensory neurons, rendering the skin insensitive to pain.

Side effects: An extract of jalapeño (Mexican red) peppers that stings and burns on application.

Comments: **Burns mucous membranes**; therefore, care must be taken to wash hands after capsaicin is applied.

Dosage: Available as a 0.025% or 0.075% cream in a petrolatum base. Apply 3–5 times daily.

BETA-LACTAM ANTIBIOTICS
PENAMS (PENICILLINS)
PENICILLINS: NARROW-SPECTRUM Beta-lactamase sensitive

Indications: Infections with many gram-positive bacteria, including non–β-lactamase–producing *Staphylococcus aureus* and *Staphylococcus epidermidis*, *Streptococcus pyogenes*, *Peptostreptococcus* organisms, *Streptococcus pneumoniae*, *Bacillus anthracis*, *Clostridium tetani*, *Enterococcus* organisms.

Actions: Bind to specific protein sites in the bacterial cell wall, inhibiting cell wall synthesis. Not stable against β-lactamase–producing bacteria.

Side effects: Diarrhea, nausea, skin rash, **allergic reactions, anaphylaxis** (0.04%).

Drug	Trade name	Dosage	Comment
Penicillin G Benzylpenicillin	Crystapen Megacillin	500,000-1 million units PO 3-6 times daily; 10 million-20 million units IM or IV daily in divided doses	The most effective penicillin if organisms are sensitive; unfortunately, in the hospital, many infections are due to resistant organisms
Penicillin V (phenoxymethyl-penicillin)	Veetids Pen-Vee-K	250-500 mg PO q6-8h	The preferred narrow-spectrum penicillin for oral use

PENICILLIN: NARROW-SPECTRUM ANTISTAPHYLOCOCCAL Beta-lactamase resistant

Indications: Soon after the first clinical use of penicillin, resistance developed in *Staphylococcus aureus* due to the development of the beta lactamase (penicillinase) enzyme. Newer derivatives were developed that were resistant to this enzyme.

Actions: Effective against beta lactamase producing staphylococci.

Side Effects: Similar to other narrow-spectrum penicillins with the addition of interstitial nephritis.

Comments: Although very useful in treating beta lactamase–resistant organisms, the effect against other bacteria is weaker than other narrow-spectrum penicillins.

Ever resourceful bacteria have developed resistance to these derivatives—so-called methicillin resistance (MRSA), named after the no longer marketed original derivative). These bacteria are resistant to the penicillins and cephalosporins.

PENICILLINS: BROAD SPECTRUM

Indications: Infections due to *Enterococcus faecalis, Listeria monocytogenes, Proteus mirabilis, Borrelia burgdorferi* (Lyme disease), *H. pylori*. Prophylaxis against infective endocarditis after genitourinary procedures.

Actions: Antibacterial spectrum includes some gram-negative bacteria. Bind to specific protein sites in the bacterial cell wall, inhibiting cell wall synthesis. Not stable against β-lactamase–producing bacteria.

Side effects: Diarrhea, nausea, skin rash, **allergic reactions**.

Ampicillin	Ampicin	Prophylaxis in genitourinary procedures: 2 g IV or IM with gentamicin1.5 mg/kg IV or IM immediately before catheterization or 6 hr. later Usual dosage: 250-500 mg PO or IV q6h Higher doses, 150-200 mg/kg/day IV or IM, are required in severe infections	Less well absorbed orally than amoxicillin but available as a parenteral preparation
Amoxicillin	Amoxil	Usual dosage: 250-500 mg PO q8h. For severe infections, doses up to 6 g/day may be required *H. pylori* infection: 1 g amoxicillin with metronidazole 500 mg	Much better absorbed than ampicillin; not available as a parenteral preparation
Amoxicillin/clavulanate	Augmentin	Usual dosage: 250 mg amoxicillin/125 mg clavulanate PO q8h. Severe infections: 500 mg/125 mg PO q8h. Do not substitute two 250-/125-mg tablets to achieve this dose level; the increased amount of clavulanate is associated with more GI side effects	Much better absorbed than ampicillin; not available as a parenteral preparation Clavulanate inhibits penicillinase, extending the antibacterial spectrum

PENICILLIN: EXTENDED-SPECTRUM ANTIPSEUDOMONAL

Indications: This group of penicillins is active against a variety of gram-negative bacilli, including *Pseudomonas aeruginosa*. However, it is inactivated by β-lactamase. Piperacillin and ticarcillin are available in a form combined with a penicillinase inhibitor, which extends the antibacterial spectrum to β-lactamase–producing bacteria.

Actions: The antibacterial spectrum of penicillin has been expanded with the development of a number of semisynthetic derivatives. They bind to specific protein sites in the bacterial cell wall, inhibiting cell wall synthesis. Unfortunately, with this advance, most new penicillins have lost some of their activity against other bacteria.

Side effects: **Allergic reactions, impaired platelet aggregation and bleeding tendencies**, eosinophilia, thrombocytopenia, neutropenia, thrombophlebitis at infusion sites.

Comments: In moderate or severe gram-negative infections, these penicillins are usually used empirically with an aminoglycoside.

Indications: Infections due to *Enterococcus faecalis, Listeria monocytogenes, Proteus mirabilis, Borrelia burgdorferi* (Lyme disease), *H. pylori*. Prophylaxis against infective endocarditis after genitourinary procedures.

Actions: Antibacterial spectrum includes some gram-negative bacteria. Bind to specific protein sites in the bacterial cell wall, inhibiting cell wall synthesis. Not stable against β-lactamase–producing bacteria.

Side effects: Diarrhea, nausea, skin rash, **allergic reactions**.

Drug	Trade name	Dosage	Comment
Carbenicillin	Geocillin	382-764 mg PO qid	
Piperacillin	Pipracil	6-18 g/day IV in 4-6 divided doses	Adverse effects include GI symptoms, diarrhea
Piperacillin/ tazobactam	Tazocin	4-24 g/day IM or IV in 4-6 divided doses	Intramuscular administration is painful; can be mixed with lidocaine 1% (without adrenalin) by deep injection with no more than 2 g/injection
Ticarcillin	Ticar	3 g IV q4h	
Ticarcillin/ clavulanate	Timentin	3g IV q4-6h	

CARBAPENEM and MONOBACTAM ANTIBIOTICS

Indications: Systemic infections caused by multiple drug–resistant gram-negative coliforms and *Bacteroides* organisms. In *Pseudomonas* infections, should be combined with an aminoglycoside.

Actions: Bind to penicillin-binding proteins of cell walls of susceptible bacteria, causing impaired cell wall synthesis and cell lysis. Have the broadest spectrum among the beta-lactam antibiotics.

Side effects: Nausea, diarrhea, vomiting, eosinophilia, rash, seizures. **Local reactions at infusion sites, including phlebitis**.

Comments: Should be reserved for use against severe systemic infections caused by mixed organisms that are resistant to antibacterials with a narrower spectrum of activity. Cilastatin, which is combined in some products, has no antibacterial action but prevents the metabolism of carbapenems and aztreonam by dehydropeptidase in the proximal renal tubular cells and therefore decreases the rate of excretion. Not associated with anaphylactic reactions to penicillin.

Drug	Trade name	Dosage	Comments
Doripenem	Doribax	500 mg IV q8hrs diluted in 500 ml NS or D5W over 1 hour	
Ertapenem	Invanz	250-1000 mg IV q8h to a maximum dose of 50 mg/kg or 4 g, whichever is lower	Do not administer as a direct intravenous injection
Imipenem/ cilastatin	Primaxin	250-1000 mg IV q8h to a maximum dose of 50 mg/kg or 4 g, whichever is lower.	Do not administer as a direct intravenous injection
Meropenem	Merrem	500-1000 mg IV q8h	
Aztreonam/ cilastin	Azactam	90-120 mg/kg/day IV or IM q6h or 8h	This is a monobactam antibiotic

CEPHENS (CEPHALOSPORINS)

There are many products—a limited list only is provided.

- Indications: In spite of the number of cephalosporins, used alone, they are rarely the first choice for the empirical treatment of bacterial infections in hospitalized patients. Combined with other agents, they can be useful in a number of severe infections: sepsis caused by infections with *Escherichia coli*, indole-positive *Proteus* organisms, and *Providencia stuartii* (third-generation cephalosporin with an aminoglycoside).
- Meningitis, epiglottitis, or other serious infection due to *Haemophilus influenzae* (third-generation cephalosporin with vancomycin and with or without rifampin).
- Hospital-acquired pneumonia (third-generation cephalosporin with a macrolide or a fluoroquinolone).
- *Klebsiella pneumoniae* pneumonia (third-generation cephalosporin with an aminoglycoside).

Actions: Like other β-lactam antibiotics, cephalosporins bind to bacterial cell membrane penicillin-binding proteins, thus inhibiting cell wall synthesis and causing cell lysis. They were originally classified as *generations* on the basis of their in vitro activities against gram-negative organisms. With the expanding of this spectrum through successive generations, activity against gram-positive aerobes is weakened.

Side effects: **Diarrhea, allergic reactions,** false-positive glycosuria. About 8% of patients allergic to penicillins have an allergic reaction to first- and second-generation cephalosporins; the overall incidence of allergic reactions to cephalosporins is 4%. This is less likely with third-generation drugs, probably because of the interference with binding caused by the bulky side chains.

Comments: Cephalosporins, particularly the third-, fourth- and advanced-generation parental preparations, are expensive. More advanced generation drugs are effective against methicillin-resistant staphylococci.

Dosage: Dosages and dose intervals vary among products and may have to be altered in the presence of renal impairment (see Table D.1, page 436).

The following list is limited to the derivatives most frequently prescribed.

First Generation (moderate spectrum)

Spectrum: gram-positive bacteria including penicillinase-producing staphylococci

Cefadroxil (Duricef)
Cefazolin (Ancef, Kefzol)
Cephalexin (Keflex and others)

Second Generation

Spectrum: gram-positive bacteria including penicillinase-producing staphylococci

Citrobacter, Enterobacter, *Hemophilus influenzae*, Neisseria and Serratia species

With moderate activity

Cefuroxime (Zinacef, Kefurox)

With anti-Hemophilus activity

Cefaclor (Ceclor)

Cefuroxime axetil (Ceftin)

With anti-pseudomonas activity

Cefoxitin (Mefoxin)

Third Generation

Spectrum: Less active than first- and second-generation against gram-positive bacteria but greater anti-gram-negative activity and greater stability against beta-lactamases.

Cefotaxime (Claforan)

Ceftazidime (Fortaz, Ceptaz, Tazicef, Tazidime)

Ceftizoxime (Cefizox)

Ceftriaxone (Rocephin)

Fourth Generation

Effective against a wide range of gram-positive and gram-negative bacteria.

Cefepime (Maxipime)

Fifth (or Advanced) Generation

Effective against a wide range of gram-positive and gram-negative bacteria including methicillin-resistant staphylococci.

Ceftobiprole (Zeftera)

Ceftaroline (Fosamil)

BETA-LACTAMASE INHIBITORS

Amoxicillin with clavulanic acid (Augmentin)

Tazobactam with ceftolozane (Zerbaxa)

Sulbactam with ampicillin (Unasyn)

Avibactam (Avibactam)

CHLORAL HYDRATE (Noctec and others) Hypnotic

Indications: Insomnia.

Actions: Depression of CNS activity.

Side effects: **Urticaria, erythema multiforme**, vertigo, gastric irritation, rash.

Comments: Do not administer to patients with liver or kidney disease. May be addicting.

Dosage: 0.5 to 1 g PO or rectally (PR).

CHLORPROPAMIDE (Diabinese) Oral hypoglycemic agent

Indications: Type 2 diabetes mellitus.

Actions: Sulfonylurea stimulates insulin secretion and increases the effect of insulin on the liver to increase gluconeogenesis and on muscle to increase glucose use.

Side effects: **Hypoglycemia**, rash, **blood dyscrasias**, jaundice, hyponatremia, edema.

Comments: Has a long duration of action (20 to 60 hours) and is cleared largely by the kidneys. Hypoglycemic reactions may be prolonged in elderly patients and in patients with renal impairment.

Dosage: 100 to 500 mg/day PO in 1 or 2 doses

CITROVORUM FACTOR (leucovorin) Folic acid derivative

Indications: Folate deficiency. Enhances the cytotoxicity of 5-fluorouracil. Diminishes the effect of methotrexate.

Actions: A metabolite of folic acid required as a coenzyme for nucleic acid synthesis.

Side effects: Hypersensitivity.

Comments: Should not be used to treat vitamin B_{12} deficiency anemia because the anemia may respond whereas neurologic sequelae progress.

Dosage: 1 mg PO daily in folate deficiency.

CLINDAMYCIN (Dalacin) Antibiotic

Indications: Serious anaerobic infections with organisms arising in the abdomen or pelvis.

Actions: Inhibits protein synthesis in susceptible bacteria.

Side effects: GI symptoms, rash, hypersensitivity reactions, **pseudomembranous enterocolitis**.

Comments: Parenteral doses are associated with local reactions.

Dosage: PO: 150 to 450 mg every 6 to 8 hours. IV: 600 to 3000 mg in 2 to 4 divided doses.

DAPSONE (DDS, Avlosulfon) Antiinfective

Indications: Leprosy, dermatitis herpetiformis, *Pneumocystis carinii* pneumonia.

Actions: A sulfone that, like the sulfonamides, competes with para-aminobenzoic acid for incorporation into folic acid.

Side effects: **Hemolysis, anemia, widespread allergic rash, fever.**

Comments: Most often used in prevention but can be added to trimethoprim-sulfamethoxazole in the treatment of *P. carinii* pneumonia. Absorption may be interfered with if drug is used with didanosine (ddI).

Dosage: 100 mg PO daily. Reduce dosage for patients with renal impairment.

DEMECLOCYCLINE (Declomycin) Tetracycline

Indications: Occasionally useful in patients with chronic syndrome of inappropriate antidiuretic hormone (SIADH). Not useful as an antibiotic because of its renal effects.

Actions: A tetracycline antibiotic that interferes with the kidney's ability to produce urine that is concentrated.

Side effects: Epigastric burning, nausea, vomiting, **photo-toxicity**, polyuria, and polydipsia.

Comments: Less useful as an antibacterial than doxycycline or minocycline because of its incomplete absorption and its renal effects.

Dosage: 300 to 600 mg PO twice daily.

DESMOPRESSIN (DDAVP injection) Hemostasis agent

Indications: To maintain hemostasis in patients with hemophilia A and factor VIII levels higher than 5% or with mild to moderate von Willebrand disease (type I).

Actions: A synthetic analog of antidiuretic hormone with identical actions on water reabsorption in the renal tubule. Has an additional action to release factor VIII complex and plasminogen activator from endothelial cell storage sites. This action peaks in 1 hour and lasts 8 to 12 hours. It may also have a direct effect on the vessel wall, decreasing bleeding at an injury site.

Side effects: Facial flushing, tachycardia, mild hypotension, water retention, headaches, nausea, abdominal pain, **allergic reactions**.

Comments: Should not be administered to patients with hemophilia B because it has no effect on factor IX. Should not be administered to patients with severe type I or type IIB von Willebrand disease because such patients are less likely to respond and severe thrombocytopenia may develop.

Dosage: 10 mc g/m^2 (maximum dose 20 mcg) by slow IV infusion.

DIGOXIN (Lanoxin) Digitalis glycoside

Indications: CHF. Atrial fibrillation

Actions: Slows AV conduction; increases the force of cardiac contraction; Na+-K+-adenosine triphosphatase (ATPase) inhibitor.

Side effects: **Dysrhythmias**, nausea, vomiting, neuropsychiatric disturbances.

Comments: 80% renally excreted; therefore dosage must be reduced in patients with renal impairment and in elderly patients. Should not be administered to patients with hypokalemia, which can predispose to digitalis-induced arrhythmias.

Dosage: Loading dose: 10 to 15 mcg/kg of lean body weight PO or IV.

Maintenance dose is affected by lean body weight and renal function.

DIURETICS

Thiazides and Related Drugs

Indications: Edema, cardiac failure, hypertension.

Actions: Block Na^+ and Cl^- reabsorption in the cortical diluting segment of the loop of Henle.

Side effects: Electrolyte depletion, hyperuricemia, hyperglycemia, hypercalcemia, pancreatitis, jaundice.

Comments: Drug half-lives differ affecting the choices for diuresis versus hypertension.

Drug	Half-life
Chlorothiazide	45-120 minutes
Hydrochlorothiazide	2.5 hours
Metolazone	8-14 hours
Indapamide	14 hours
Chlorthalidone	45-60 hours

Drug	Trade name	Dosage	Comments
Chlorothiazide	Diuril	500-1000 mg once or twice daily	Despite the long list of side effects, generally well tolerated
Hydrochlorothiazide	Hydro Diuril	12.5-50 mg PO daily	Despite the long list of side effects, generally well tolerated
Metolazone	Zaroxolyn	2.5-10 mg PO daily	
Chlorthalidone	Hygroton	6.25-25 mg PO daily	
Indapamide	Lozol	1.25-5 mg PO daily	

Aldosterone Antagonists

Indications: Edema, ascites, hypertension, hyperaldosteronism.

Actions: Block the action of aldosterone on the renal tubules, resulting in a loss of sodium and water.

Side effects: Hyponatremia, **hyperkalemia**, gynecomastia, confusion, headache.

Drug	Trade name	Dose	Comments
Spironolactone	Aldactone	25-200 mg od	Most effective in hyperaldosteronism; higher doses are required for primary hyperaldosteronism. In hypertension, as potent as thiazides but associated with more side effects. Anti-androgenic effects may cause gynecomastia
Amiloride	Midamor	5-10 mg PO daily	Free from androgenic effects
Eplerenone	Inspra	25-50 mg PO once daily	Gynecomastia has been reported
Triamterene	Dyrenium	100-300 mg PO daily	Free from anti-androgenic effects

Loop Diuretics

Indications: Cardiac failure.

Actions: Inhibitor of Na^+ and Cl^- reabsorption in the ascending loop of Henle.

Side effects: Electrolyte depletion, hyperuricemia, hyperglycemia, anorexia, nausea, vomiting, diarrhea, **hearing loss**.

Drug	Trade name	Dosage	Comments
Ethacrynic Acid	Edecrin	50 mg PO or IV	Ototoxic particularly in association with other ototoxic agents and in renal impairment
Furosemide	Lasix	40 mg PO or IV	The standard loop diuretic well and promptly absorbed from the GI tract
Bumetanide	Bumex	0.5-1 mg PO or IV	No advantage over furosemide and usually more expensive
Torsemide	Demodex	10-20 mg PO or IV	No advantage over furosemide and usually more expensive

DOPAMINE AND DOPAMINERGIC AGENTS

These agents aim to replace dopamine or prevent its degradation. Drugs that replace dopamine are usually given with dopa carboxylase inhibitors to prevent its metabolism. Dopamine receptors are present in a variety of sites particularly in the central and peripheral nervous system and vasculature. Adverse effects are therefore widespread and common.

Adverse effects include ventricular arrhythmia, atrial fibrillation, angina, palpitation, bradycardia, vasoconstriction, hypotension, hypertension, dyspnea, nausea, vomiting, headache, anxiety.

Principal Agents

Dopamine agonists	Trade name	
Levodopa-carbidopa	Sinemet	100 mg/10 mg tablet PO bid increasing to 800 mg/80 mg
Fenoldopam	Corlopam	0.01-0.3 mcg/kg/min. A dopamine D1 receptor agonist primarily affecting renal capillaries reducing peripheral resistance
Dopaminergic agents		
Selegiline	Ensam	6 mg transdermally od
Amantadine	Gocovri	274 mg (2 capsules) PO qhs
Pramipexole	Mirapex	0.125 mg PO tid increasing to max of 4.5 mg PO od
Ropinirole	Requip	0.25 mg PO tid increasing to a max of 8 mg PO tid
Rasagiline	Azilect	0.5-1 mg PO od
Entacapone	Comtan	200 mg PO up to 8 times daily

FERROUS SULFATE Iron supplement

Indications: Iron deficiency.

Actions: Replaces iron stores.

Side effects: **Constipation**, nausea, diarrhea, abdominal cramps.

Comments: Stools may turn black but do not have the typical tarry appearance of melena.

Dosage: 325 mg/day PO tid.

FLUMAZENIL Benzodiazepine antagonist

Indications: Reversal of benzodiazepine sedation.

Actions: Competitive antagonism of benzodiazepine receptors.

Side effects: **Seizures**, nausea, dizziness, agitation, pain at injection site.

Comments: Onset of reversal within minutes. Contraindicated in patients with cyclic antidepressant overdose (risk of precipitating seizures).

Dosage: 0.2 mg IV over 15 seconds. Wait 1 minute. If ineffective, this can be followed by additional doses of 0.2 mg IV every 60 seconds up to a maximum dose of 1 mg. If the patient becomes resedated, this regimen can be repeated again in 20 minutes. No more than 3 mg total should be given in 1 hour.

FLUOROQUINOLONES

Indications: Selection of a fluoroquinolone for the treatment or prevention of an infection should be limited to those conditions that are proven or strongly suspected to be caused by bacteria proven to be sensitive. Several agents have been removed from the market because of severe adverse effects. Rarely indicated as drugs to be used empirically in hospitalized patients, except for the treatment of community-acquired pneumonia (levofloxacin) or in an individual free of chronic disease with an uncomplicated urinary tract infection (ciprofloxacin). A drug of first choice in infections with *Salmonella typhi* and *Shigella* organisms. Used as an agent of first choice with or without rifampin in *Legionella* infections.

Actions: A class of agents modeled after nalidixic acid (a nonfluorinated quinolone) that inhibits bacterial gyrase, an enzyme responsible for developing double-stranded DNA.

Side effects: GI symptoms, depression, allergic reactions, nephropathy, **phototoxicity** (can be particularly serious with levofloxacin, norfloxacin, and sparfloxacin), **prolongation of QT interval** (particularly with moxifloxacin, and sparfloxacin), seizures (ciprofloxacin), **tendonitis and tendon rupture**.

Comments: The emergence of bacterial resistance to the fluoroquinolones is a serious concern, which suggests that their use should be limited. Multiple drug interactions have been reported.

Drug	Trade name	Dosage
Ciprofloxacin	Cipro, Ciloxan	100-750 mg q12h IV: 400-1200 mg/day in 2-3 divided doses. The oral dose is well absorbed, equal in efficacy to the IV dose, and much less costly; 750 mg PO is equivalent to 400 mg IV
Gemifloxacin	Factive	320 mg once daily

Drug	Trade name	Dosage
Delafloxacin	Baxdela	300 mg IV q12hr 450 mg PO q12hr
Levofloxacin	Levaquin	250-500 mg once daily
Norfloxacin	Noroxin	400 mg q12h
Moxifloxacin	Avelox	400 mg once daily
Ofloxacin	Floxin	200-400 mg q12h

GLUCAGON (Dasiglucagon, zegalogue)

Indications: Reversal of severe hypoglycemia due to insulin over-dosage

Action: Promotes breakdown of liver glycogen to glucose and stimulates gluconeogenesis

Dosage: 1 mg IV, IM, SC. If no response, repeat once after 15 minutes. Can be given to conscious patients by nasal device (Baqsimi) 3 mg once.

Side effects: Nausea, vomiting, hypotension, hives, **anaphylactic reactions**.

GLUCOCORTICOIDS

Indications: Glucocorticoids are used principally for their antiinflammatory effect. The choice among the parenteral preparations is influenced mostly by the experience with the particular agents; no important differences have been shown among them.

Actions: Antiinflammatory inhibition of the recruitment of leukocytes and monocyte-macrophages in response to a variety of stimuli, with the subsequent increased vascular permeability, vasodilation, and contraction of various nonvascular smooth muscles, including bronchial smooth muscle.

Comments: *Relative antiinflammatory potency: 0.75 mg of dexamethasone = 20 mg of hydrocortisone = 4 mg of methylprednisolone = 5 mg of prednisolone. Glucocorticoids are efficiently absorbed from the oral route.*

Adverse effects: short-term use can be associated with **anaphylaxis**, **psychotic reactions**, sepsis, venous thromboembolism, fractures, hyperglycemia, hypokalemia, hypokalemia, headache, nausea, and vomiting.

Drug	Trade name	Dosage
Budesonide	Pulmicort, Entocort EC	9 mg PO od
Dexamethasone	Decadron	Bacterial meningitis: 10 mg PO or starting before or with the first dose of antibiotics

Drug	Trade name	Dosage
Hydrocorti-sone	Cortisol, Solu-Cortef	500 mg PO or IV
Methylpred-nisolone	Medrol	Acute asthma: 128 mg PO (eight 16-mg tablets) or 125 mg IV
Prednisone		Acute asthma: 40-60 mg PO
Triamcino-lone	Aristocort	60 mg IM

GLYCOPEPTIDE ANTIBIOTICS

Indications: Serious infections caused by β-lactam–resistant gram-positive organisms and infections caused by gram-positive organisms in patients with a severe allergy to β-lactam antibiotics. Also useful prophylactically in patients at high risk for endocarditis and in patients with life-threatening antibiotic-associated colitis.

Actions: Suppresses RNA synthesis in susceptible bacteria.

Comments: Use should be restricted to reduce the likelihood of the development of resistance in enterococci and staphylococci

Drug	Trade name	Dosage	Activity	Side effects
Teico-planin	Targocid	12 mg/kg/day IV in 1 or 2 divided doses	Effective against methicillin-resistant staphylococci	Marginally less toxic than vancomycin Histamine release related to rate of infusion (*red man syndrome*); **chills, fever, ototoxicity, nephrotoxicity**, phlebitis at infusion site
Tela-vancin	Vibativ	10 mg/kg IV once daily.	Effective against methicillin-resistant staphylococci No more effective than vancomycin	Anaphylaxis, nausea, headache, insomnia, foamy urine. **Nephrotoxicity**, phlebitis at infusion site

Drug	Trade name	Dosage	Activity	Side effects
Vanco-mycin	Vanco-cin	30 mg/kg/day IV in 2-4 divided doses 250-500 mg PO tid or qid	Effective against methicil-lin-resistant staphylococ-ci, *C. difficile* infections	Histamine release related to rate of infu-sion (red man syndrome); **chills, fever, ototoxicity, nephrotoxic-ity, neutrope-nia,** phlebitis at infusion site

HELICOBACTER PYLORI INFECTION TREATMENTS

Drug	Dosage	Comment
Bismuth quadruple therapy		Preferred option but metronida-zole resistance may be an issue
Bismuth sub-salicylate	420 mg PO qid	Available as
Metronidazole	375 mg PO qid	a combined
Tetracycline	375 mg PO qid	tablet- Py-lera
Omeprazole or other proton pump inhibitor	20-40 mg PO bid or tid	
Rifabutin triple therapy		Alternative first-choice option but resistance to amoxicillin may be an issue
Rifabutin	150 mg PO q8h	Available as
Amoxicillin	1 g PO q8h	a combined tablet
Omeprazole	40 mg PO q8h	Talicia
Clarithromycin triple therapy		Where *H. pylori* have been shown to be sensitive to clarithromycin and amoxicillin

Drug	Dosage	Comment
Clarithromy-cin	500 mg PO bid	
Amoxicillin	1 g PO bid	
Omeprazole or other proton pump inhibitor	20-40 mg PO bid or tid	
Or	500 mg PO bid	Available as
Clarithromy-cin	500 mg PO bid	a combined
Amoxicillin	20 mg PO bid	tablet
Vonoprazan		Voquezna Triple Pak or without the clari-thromycin as Voquez-na Dual Pak

H₂-RECEPTOR ANTAGONISTS

Indications: Peptic ulcer disease, gastroesophageal reflux.

Actions: Bind to H_2 receptors, blocking gastric acid production.

Side effects: Diarrhea, headache, dizziness.

Comments: All have similar effects, except that cimetidine reduces the microsomal enzyme metabolism of drugs, including oral anticoagulants, phenytoin, and theophylline.

Oral Dosage for Peptic Ulcer Disease. Intravenous/Intramuscular Dosage for Conditions Caused by Excess Gastric Acid

Drug	Trade name	Dose	Side effects
Cimetidine	Tagamet	800-1200 mg hs or in divided doses qid or bid 300 mg IV or IM q6-8h	Gynecomastia, impo-tence, confusion, di-arrhea, **leukopenia, thrombocytopenia, increase in serum creatinine level**
Famotidine	Pepcid	40 mg hs or 20 mg bid 20 mg IV q12h	Headache, dizziness, constipation, **diar-rhea**
Nizatidine	Axid	300 mg hs or 150 mg bid	Sweating, urticar-ia, somnolence, **elevation of hepatic enzyme levels**

Drug	Trade name	Dose	Side effects
Ranitidine	Zantac	300 mg hs or 150 mg bid 50 mg IV q8h	**Jaundice**, gynecomastia, headache, confusion, **leukopenia**
Combination of ranitidine, calcium carbonate, magnesium hydroxide	Duo Fusion	1-2 chewable tablets od	**Jaundice**, gynecomastia, headache, confusion, **leukopenia** Also contains phenylalanine 2.2 mg and should be avoided in individuals with phenylketonuria

HEPARIN and other antithrombotic drugs

Indications: Prophylaxis and treatment of deep vein thrombosis (DVT), pulmonary embolism, embolic cerebrovascular accident; adjunct in the treatment of unstable angina.

Gradually being replaced by low-molecular-weight heparins because of their more predictable dose response and fewer nonhemorrhagic side effects.

Actions: Enhances the activity of antithrombin III. The heparin–antithrombin III complexes inactivate several coagulation enzymes, particularly thrombin and factor Xa.

Side effects: **Hemorrhage, thrombocytopenia**, urticaria, elevated liver enzymes.

Comments: Monitor activated partial thromboplastin time (aPTT) closely when administering intravenous heparin.

Dosage: For treatment of DVT or pulmonary embolism, 100 U/kg IV bolus (usual dosage, 5000 to 10,000 U IV), followed by a maintenance infusion of 1000 to 1600 U/h; the lower range should be used for patients with a higher risk of bleeding. For prophylaxis, 5000 U SC every 8 hours.

HEPARINS: LOW MOLECULAR WEIGHT

Indications: Prophylaxis and treatment of DVT, unstable angina, myocardial infarction, pulmonary embolism.

Actions: Catalyze antithrombin to neutralize several procoagulant enzymes, including thrombin, factor IIa, and factor Xa.

Side effects: **Hemorrhage**, thrombocytopenia but a lower risk than with unfractionated heparin

Comments: In comparison with standard heparin, low-molecular-weight heparins (LMWHs) have less plasma protein binding, are excreted almost completely by the renal route, and have a longer half-life. The dosage is more predictable, and the kinetic action is not dose dependent. The aPTT is not predictably prolonged and should not be measured in order to monitor the dosage. Newer antithrombotics related to the LMWHs include danaparoid and fondaparinux. Danaparoid is a mixture of nonheparin glycosaminoglycans derived from porcine mucosa, with an action similar to that of LMWHs. Fondaparinux is a synthetic agent that selectively inhibits factor Xa.

Recommended LMWH in the Treatment of Pulmonary Embolus

Drug	Trade name	Dosage
Dalteparin	Fragmin	200 IU/kg by deep subcutaneous injection once daily. For patients with an increased risk of bleeding, 100 IU/kg q12h or 100 IU/kg by continuous intravenous infusion over 12 hr
Enoxaparin	Lovenox	1.5 mg/kg by deep subcutaneous injection once daily or 1 mg/kg SC q12h. Dose should not exceed 180 mg daily
Nadroparin	Fraxiparine	171 IU/kg by deep subcutaneous injection once daily or 86 IU/kg SC q12h Dosage should not exceed 17,000 IU daily
Tinzaparin	Innohep	175 IU/kg by deep subcutaneous injection once daily

Recommended Doses of LMWH and Related Antithrombotics in the Prevention and Treatment of Deep Vein Thrombosis

Drug	Trade name	Dosage	Comment
Dalteparin	Fragmin	200 IU/kg by deep injection SC once daily	For patients with an increased risk of bleeding, 100 IU/kg q12h or 100 IU by continuous intravenous infusion over 12 h 2500-5000 IU SC once daily

Drug	Trade name	Dosage	Comment
Danaparoid	Orgaran	750 IU SC bid. 2250 IU intravenous bolus, followed by 400 IU/h for 4 h, then 300 IU/h for 4 h, then 150-200 IU/h	Principally used for prophylaxis but may be useful in patients with heparin induced thrombocytopenia because of lower risk than heparin
Enoxaparin	Lovenox	1.5 mg/kg by deep subcutaneous injection once daily or 1 mg/kg SC q12h. Dose should not exceed 180 mg daily 30 mg SC bid	
Fondaparinux	Arixtra	2.5-10 mg SC q 24h	Lower risk of thrombocytopenia than with standard low-molecular-weight heparins
Nadroparin	Fraxiparine	171 IU/kg by deep subcutaneous injection once daily or 86 IU/kg SC q12h. Dose should not exceed 17,000 IU daily. 2850 IU SC once daily	
Tinzaparin	Innohep	175 IU/kg by deep subcutaneous injection once daily. 50-75 IU/kg SC once daily	

Other Antithrombotics

See oral and parenteral anticoagulants

HYDRALAZINE (Apresoline) Arteriolar vasodilator

Indications: Hypertension but not used alone because of the reflex cardiac stimulation accompanying the lowering of pressure.

Actions: Arteriolar vasodilator.

Side effects: **Tachycardia, systemic lupus erythematosus (SLE)–like reaction** at higher doses (>200 mg/day).

Comments: Very limited effect on veins, so little postural hypotension results.

Dosage: 10 to 25 mg PO every 6 hours.

IPRATROPIUM (Atrovent) Anticholinergic

Indications: Inhalational aerosol to relieve bronchospasm in chronic obstructive pulmonary disease and asthma.

Actions: Blocks the muscarinic cholinergic receptors in the bronchial smooth muscles

Side effects: Dry mouth, and sedation, skin flushing, and **tachycardia**.

Comments: A quaternary amine and therefore does not cross the blood-brain barrier, which prevents central side effects (anticholinergic syndrome).

Also available in combination with salbutamol (as Duovent).

Dose: 2.5 to 5.0 mg in 3 mL of NS by nebulizer or 180 mcg (2 puffs) by metered-dose inhaler every 4 hours.

ISOSORBIDE DINITRATE (Isordil, Sorbitrate) Vasodilator

Indications: Angina pectoris, CHF.

Actions: Venous, coronary, and arteriolar vasodilator.

Side effects: Headache, **hypotension**, flushing.

Comments: Nitrate tolerance may develop with prolonged, continuous administration.

Dosage: 5 to 30 mg PO 4 times a day.

KETAMINE (KETALAR)

Actions: General anesthesia.

Side effects: **Apnea**, hypertension, postanesthetic delirium (emergence reaction), vomiting, **anaphylaxis**.

Comments: Used to calm delirious patients who are seriously disruptive and a danger to themselves or others. *Should only be used by physicians experienced in administering general anesthetics and in the presence of resuscitation equipment.*

Dosage: 5 mg/kg IM. Onset in 3 to 8 minutes with a duration of 15 minutes to 2 hours.

LABETALOL (Trandate, Normodyne) α_1- and β-Blocker

Indications: Hypertensive emergencies.

Actions: α_1-Blocking action is predominant in acute situations but is accompanied by nonspecific β-blockade.

Side effects: **Postural hypotension, bronchospasm, jaundice, bradycardia, negative inotropic effect**.

Comments: Effect results largely from α₁-adrenergic blocking activity. Contraindications are the same as for *pure* β-blockers.

Dosage: For a hypertensive emergency, 10 mg IV over 1 to 2 min. May repeat 10 to 20 mg every 10 min to a maximum dose of 150 mg. Alternatively follow the initial dose with an infusion of 2 to 8 mg per min.

LEVODOPA-CARBIDOPA (Sinemet) Dopamine agonist

Indications: Parkinson disease.

Actions: Levodopa is converted to dopamine in the basal ganglia. Carbidopa inhibits the peripheral destruction of levodopa.

Side effects: Anorexia, nausea, vomiting, abdominal pain, **dysrhythmias, behavioral changes, orthostatic hypotension,** involuntary movements.

Comments: Side effects are common.

Dosage: Begin with 1 tablet, 100 mg of levodopa/10 mg of carbidopa, PO bid, increasing the dosage until the desired response is obtained, up to a maximum dosage of 8 tablets (800 mg/80 mg) per day.

LIDOCAINE (Xylocaine) Class IB antiarrhythmic

Indications: Prophylaxis and treatment of ventricular tachycardia.

Actions: Lengthens the effective refractory period in the ventricular conducting system. Decreases ventricular automaticity.

Side effects: Nausea, vomiting, **hypotension, confusion, seizures,** perioral paresthesias.

Comments: Lower maintenance doses are required for elderly patients and for patients with CHF, liver disease, and hypotension.

Dosage: For ventricular tachycardia and fibrillation, 1 to 1.5 mg/kg IV. For refractory ventricular fibrillation, an additional 0.5 to 0.75 mg/kg IV push may be administered; repeat in 5 to 10 minutes up to a maximum total dose of 3 mg/kg. This can be followed by a maintenance dosage of 1 to 4 mg/min IV.

MACROLIDE ANTIBIOTICS

Indications: Community-acquired pneumonia.

Actions: Inhibit bacterial growth by inhibiting protein synthesis. Macrolide antibiotics are bacteriostatic. They have been in widespread human and animal use and have been used as growth promoters in animals for food production since the 1950s.

Side effects: The major adverse effects are **GI symptoms** such as nausea, vomiting, abdominal cramps, and diarrhea. High intravenous doses of clarithromycin and erythromycin are associated with **hearing loss** and **prolongation of QT interval.** Allergic reactions, eosinophilia, hepatotoxicity, taste disturbance, and headache are less frequent adverse effects.

Comments: Adverse effects have limited the marketing of some derivatives including roxithromycin, dirithromycin, and telithromycin (acute liver failure). They are not recommended.

Drug	Trade name	Dosage	Side effects
Erythromycin	Numerous	Community-acquired respiratory infections Least expensive	1-2 g PO daily in divided doses, usually q6h Reduce dosage or dose frequency if creatinine clearance <25 mL/min 1-2 g IV daily by continuous infusion or in divided doses q6-8h diluted in 250 mL of saline over 60 min	GI side effects are more likely with erythromycin, largely through the stimulation of motility
Azithromycin	Zithromax	Mycobacterium intracellulare Has greater activity against some genitourinary pathogens: Chlamydia trachomatis, Ureaplasma urealyticum, Neisseria gonorrhoeae, Treponema pallidum	500 mg PO or IV q24hrs 500 mg PO q12h with or without food. Reduce dosage or dose frequency if creatinine clearance <30 mL/min	
Fidaxomicin	Dificid	Clostridiodes infection	200 mg PO bid for 10 days	Has a lower rate of recurrence compared with vancomycin

METRONIDAZOLE (Flagyl) Antibiotic

Indications: Systemic infections with *Bacteroides fragilis*; amebiasis; vaginal infections with *Trichomonas* organisms. Used in combination with amoxicillin for *H. pylori* and *Clostridium difficile* infections.

Actions: Binds to DNA, inhibiting DNA repair and synthesis. Bactericidal.

Side effects: Chest pain, palpitations, metallic taste, hypersensitivity, **vertigo, disorientation**.

Comments: Approximately 80% is absorbed; thus, the oral route is preferred in order to reduce costs.

Dosage: For *H. pylori* infections, 500 mg PO twice daily with amoxicillin, 1 g twice daily. For *C. difficile* infections, 250 to 500 mg PO tid or qid. For systemic anaerobic infections, 15 mg/kg IV, followed by 7.5 mg/kg PO or IV every 6 hours.

Dosage: Usually given as two separate IM injections repeated in 6 months.

NALOXONE HYDROCHLORIDE (Narcan) Narcotic antagonist

Indications: Narcotic antagonism.

Actions: Competitive antagonist at all three classes of narcotic receptors.

Side effects: Nausea, vomiting; **may precipitate withdrawal in narcotic-addicted patients**.

Comments: *Effect is shorter than that of many narcotics.*

Dosage: 0.4 to 2 mg IV, IM, or SC every 5 minutes up to a maximum dose of 10 mg.

Also available in a higher dose as Zimhi (Adamis) 5 mg IM or SC and intranasally as Narcan (Emergent) 4 mg intranasally and Kloxxado (Hikma) 8 mg intranasally.

Nalmefene 0.5 to 1.0 mg IV, IM, SC has a longer duration of action than naloxone derivatives that can precipitate a prolonged period of withdrawal in patients dependent on opioids.

NITROFURANTOIN (numerous brands) Urinary tract anti-infective

Indications: Uncomplicated urinary tract infections.

Actions: Active against *E. coli* and other gram-negative coliforms. Action unknown.

Side effects: **GI symptoms** are relatively common; rare allergic reactions; dizziness.

Comments: Well, absorbed orally; absorption is increased with food.

Dosage: Regular-release product: 50 to 100 mg PO 4 times daily. Slow-release product: 100 mg PO twice daily. A single larger dose (200 mg) given once may be as effective as longer-term therapy.

OCTREOTIDE ACETATE (Sandostatin) Somatostatin analog

Indications: Used mainly in treatment of the carcinoid syndrome and of tumors that secrete vasoactive intestinal peptide. Also used in treatment of bleeding esophageal varices.

Actions: Suppresses the secretion of serotonin, pancreatic peptides, gastrin, vasoactive intestinal peptide, insulin, glucagon, secretin, and motilin. Reduces collateral splanchnic blood flow.

Side effects: Abdominal pain, **transient hypoglycemia, and hyperglycemia**. May decrease glomerular filtration rate and increase intestinal transit time.

Comments: Expensive.

Dosage: For bleeding esophageal varices: 50 mcg IV bolus, followed by 25 to 50 mcg/h IV infusion.

ORAL AND PARENTERAL ANTIHYPERGLYCEMIC AGENTS

INSULIN Hypoglycemic Agent

Indications: Diabetes mellitus.

Actions: Enhances hepatic glycogen storage, enhances the entry of glucose into cells, inhibits the breakdown of protein and fat. Enhances the entry of K^+ into cells.

Side effects: **Hypoglycemia**, local skin reactions, lipohypertrophy at injection site.

Comments: Less immunogenicity with human insulin than with insulin from animal sources.

Dosage: Extremely variable.

Bovine, porcine, and human insulin preparations have different antigenic properties. Bovine insulin is the most immunogenic, and human insulin is the least. Human insulin preparations are associated with fewer adverse reactions (e.g., insulin allergy, antibody-mediated insulin resistance, lipohypertrophy) and should be considered, especially when treatment is intermittent.

Preparation	Onset	Peak	Duration
Regular	½-1 h	30 min-2.5h	6-8 h
Lyspro (NovaLog), Aspart (Humalog) glulisine (Apidra)	<15 min.	1-2 h	4-6 h
Intermediate-acting			
NPH (Isophane)	1-2 h	4-12h	18-26 h
Long-acting			
Detemir (Levemir)	1 h	Flat, Max effect in 5 h	24h
Glargine (Lantus)	1.5 h	Flat, Max effect in 5 h	24h

Preparation	Onset	Peak	Duration
Lente	2-4 h	4-12h	19-26 h
UltraLente	4-10h	10-16h	30-36h
50% NPH, 50% regular (Humulin 50/50)	30-60 min	Dual	10-16 h
70% NPH, 30% regular (Humulin 30/70, Novolin 30/70)	30-60 min	Dual	10-16 h

GLP-1 RECEPTOR AGONISTS

Incretin mimetic hormones or analogues of human glucagon-like peptide-1 that increase insulin secretion when glucose levels are elevated, decrease glucagon secretion, and delay gastric emptying in an effort to lower postprandial glucose level.

Drug	Trade name	Dose	Side effects *All carry the risk of hypoglycemia*
Dulaglutide	Trulicity	0.75 or 1.25 mg SC once per week	**Pancreatitis, renal failure, nausea,** diarrhea, vomiting, abdominal pain, decreased appetite, indigestion, and fatigue
Exenatide extended release	Byetta Bydureon BCise	5-10 mcg SC bid 2 mg once SC once per week	Nausea and diarrhea. The US Food and Drug Administration has warned about serious side effects, including **pancreatitis, renal failure,** and the risk of thyroid malignancy
Liraglutide	Victoza	1.2 or 1.8 mg SC od	**Pancreatitis, renal failure,** nausea, diarrhea, vomiting, decreased appetite, indigestion, and constipation
Semaglutide	Ozempic Rybelsus	0.5-2 mg SC once per week 7 or 14 mg PO once daily	**Pancreatitis, renal failure,** swelling/redness/itching at the injection site, tiredness, nausea, vomiting, diarrhea, constipation

ORAL AGENTS

Drug	Trade name	Dose	Action	Side effects *All carry the risk of hypoglycemia*
Biguanides Metformin	Glucophage	100-250 mg of extended-release tablet PO od with evening meal	Prevent over-production of glucose by the liver; enhance the uptake of glucose by cells.	Diarrhea, nausea, vomiting, flatulence, **lactic acidosis**, agitation, hypersensitivity
Sulfonylureas Glipizide Glimepiride Glyburide	Glucotrol Amaryl Glynase	10-20 mg PO once daily 1-4 mg PO once daily 1.25-20 mg PO once daily	Stimulate beta cells of the pancreas to produce insulin	Nausea, vomiting, diarrhea, tremor, **hypersensitivity**, headache, dizziness
Meglitinides Repaglinide Nateglinide	GlucoNorm Starlix	0.5-4 mg PO tid before meals 60-120 mg PO od in three divided doses before meals	Stimulate beta cells of the pancreas to produce insulin	Weight gain, diarrhea, nausea, joint pain, back pain, headache, runny or stuffy nose, sneezing, headache Weight gain, runny or stuffy nose, sneezing, cough, cold or flu symptoms, diarrhea, nausea

Drug	Trade name	Dose	Action	Side effects All carry the risk of hypoglycemia
Thiazolidinediones Rosiglitazone Pioglitazone	Avandia Actos	4-8 mg PO od with or without food 15-45 mg PO od with meals	Reduce insulin production by the liver	Edema, cold symptoms (stuffy nose, sinus pain, sneezing, sore), **hepatitis** Nausea/vomiting, abdominal pain, edema, **hypersensitivity, hepatitis**
DPP-4 inhibitors Sitagliptin Saxagliptin Linagliptin	Januvia Onglyza Trajenta	50-100 mg PO od with or without food 2.5-5 mg PO od with or without food 5 mg PO once daily	Inhibit dipeptidyl peptidase Reduce glucose production by the liver and increase the release of insulin	Shortness of breath, nasopharyngitis, swelling or fluid retention, an unusually fast increase in weight, tiredness, **pancreatitis, hepatitis** Runny or stuffy nose, sore throat, cough, headache, stomach pain, **pancreatitis, hepatitis stuffy nose** Runny nose, sore throat, cough, weight gain, muscle or joint pain, back pain, low blood sugar
Alpha glucosidase inhibitors			Block breakdown of starches and carbohydrates	

Drug	Trade name	Dose	Action	Side effects *All carry the risk of hypoglycemia*
Acarbose	Glucobay	25-100 mg PO tid with food		Abdominal pain, flatulence, diarrhea, anaphylactic reactions, **hepatitis**, edema
Miglitol	Glyset	25-100 mg PO tid with food		Diarrhea, gas, upset stomach, abdominal pain, skin rash, iron deficiency anemia
SGLT-2 inhibitors Canagliflozin Dapagliflozin Empagliflozin Ertugliflozin	Invokana Farxiga Jardiance Steglatro	100-300 mg PO od 5-10 mg PO od 10-25 mg PO od 5-10 mg PO od	Inhibit sodium-glucose cotransporter. Inhibits glucose reabsorption in the proximal tubule	**Hypersensitivity reactions, volume depletion, aggravation of lower limb ischemia, hypoglycemia, ketoacidosis, urosepsis, bone fractures**

ORAL AND PARENTERAL ANTICOAGULANTS
WARFARIN (Coumadin)

Indications: Prophylaxis and treatment of DVT, pulmonary embolism, embolic cerebrovascular accident.

Actions: Inhibits production of vitamin K–dependent clotting factors (factors II, VII, IX, and X) by the liver.

Actions can be reversed by vitamin K.

Side effects: **Hemorrhage**, nausea, vomiting, skin necrosis, fever, rash.

Comments: The INR was devised to standardize results of prothrombin time measurements. Each manufacturer assigns an ISI value (International Sensitivity Index) for any tissue factor they manufacture. The ISI value indicates how a particular batch of tissue factor compares to an international reference tissue factor. The INR is the ratio of a patient's prothrombin time to a normal (control) sample, raised to the power of the ISI value for the analytical system used.

$$INR = \left(\frac{PT_{test}}{PT_{normal}} \right)^{ISI}$$

Individualize dosage to maintain prothrombin time in the desired range (usually 2.0 to 3.0). Many drugs interact to increase or decrease the effect of warfarin; always look up new medications before starting them in patients taking warfarin to see whether they interact. Fresh-frozen plasma is the treatment of choice to rapidly reverse the effect of warfarin. An alternative is vitamin K.

Dosage: 10 mg daily for 2 days; then an estimated maintenance dosage of 5 to 7.5 mg/day, modified according to the prothrombin time or INR.

DIRECT THROMBIN INHIBITORS

These agents bind to and inhibit thrombin therefore preventing clot formation. Indicated in the prevention of arterial and venous thromboembolism. Most common adverse events are hemorrhages.

Drug	Trade name	Dosage	Comments	Side effects
Oral agents				
Dabigatran	Pradaxa	150 mg bid	Known as direct acting oral anticoagulants (DOAC) Anticoagulant effect can be reversed with idarucizumab	Hemorrhagic events have been reported with its use
Apixaban	Eliquis	5 mg PO bid	Anticoagulant effect can be reversed with andexanet alfa	
Edoxaban	Savaysa, Lixiana	60 mg PO od	Off label use of andexanet alfa to reverse effect	
Rivaroxaban	Xarelto	15 mg PO bid	Anticoagulant effect can be reversed with andexanet alfa	
Betrixaban	Bevyxxa	160 mg PO on day one, then 80 mg PO od	Off label use of andexanet alfa to reverse effect	
Parental agents				
Lepirudin	Refludan	0.4 mg/kg slowly IV then 0.15 mg/kg/hr IV	No specific antidote	
Desirudin	Iprivask	15 mg subcutaneously q12hr	Used to prevent clotting events in hip replacement surgery. No specific antidote	Hemorrhagic events and anaphylaxis have been reported
Bivalirudin	Angiomax	0.75 mg/kg IV followed by 1.75 mg/kg/hr IV	Used to prevent clotting in percutaneous coronary interventions. No specific antidote	

Drug	Trade name	Dosage	Comments	Side effects
Argatroban	Acova	350 mg/kg IV over 5 minutes then 2 ug/kg/min IV	Used to prevent clotting in patients with heparin-induced thrombocytopenia and prophylactically in angioplasty procedures No specific antidote	**Serious hemorrhagic events. Hypotension and chest pain** are the commonest adverse effects

TISSUE PLASMINOGEN ACTIVATORS (THROMBOLYTICS, FIBRINOLYTICS)

Drug	Trade name	Dosage	Comments	Side effects
Tenecteplase	TNKase	0.25 mg/kg IV over 5 seconds (maximum 25 mg)	Longer half-life, greater fibrin specificity, and lesser likelihood of fibrinogen depletion than alteplase	**Hemorrhages,** cholesterol embolism, thromboembolism, arrhythmias
Alteplase	Activase	0.40 mg/kg IV (maximum 40 mg) 0.9 mg/kg, with 10% (0.09 mg/kg) given as an intravenous bolus over 1 minute and the remaining 90% (0.81 mg/kg) given as an intravenous infusion over 60 minutes		**Hemorrhages,** cholesterol embolism, thromboembolism, arrhythmias

THROMBIN INHIBITOR REVERSAL

Drug	Trade name	Action	Dose	Side effects
Idarucizumab	Praxbind	Monoclonal antibody antagonizing dabigatran	2 consecutive IV infusions directly from 50 ml vials or 2 IV rapid injections undiluted.	**Anaphylaxis**, hypokalemia, **seizures**, vomiting, **thrombotic events**
Andexanet alfa	Andexxa	Recombinant Factor Xa reversing rivaroxaban and apixaban. Off label use to reverse edoxaban and betrixaban	400-600 mg IV at a rate of 30 g/min followed by 4-8 mg/min for up to 120 minutes	**Arterial and venous thrombotic events, cardiac arrest,** sudden death, urinary tract infections, pneumonia

PENTAMIDINE (Pentacarinat) Antibiotic

Indications: *P. carinii* pneumonia.

Actions: Interferes with DNA replication.

Side effects: **Hypotension, nephrotoxicity, hypoglycemia, hypersensitivity, leukopenia**.

Comments: Injectable pentamidine is associated with side effects in 60% of patients. Aerosolized pentamidine is well tolerated except for cough, especially in patients who smoke or have asthma.

Dosage: 4 mg/kg per day in 50 to 250 mL D5W given IV over 2 hours. For prophylaxis, 300 mg every 4 weeks by Respirgard II nebulizer.

PHENAZOPYRIDINE (Pyridium) Urinary analgesic

Indications: Urethritis, cystitis.

Actions: Analgesic effect on inflamed urinary tract mucosa.

Side effects: Orange discoloration of urine; nausea.

Comments: Has no antibacterial effect. Do not administer to patients with renal impairment.

Dosage: 200 mg PO 3 times a day after meals.

PHENTOLAMINE (Rogitine Regitine) α-Adrenergic blocker

Indications: Catecholamine crisis in pheochromocytoma.

Actions: Competitively blocks the effects of epinephrine and norepinephrine at α_1- and α_2-adrenergic receptors. Causes arteriolar and slight venular vasodilatation, with a compensatory increase in heart rate and contractility.

Side effects: **Hypotension, tachycardia, angina, cerebral ischemia**, GI symptoms.

Comments: Use with extreme caution in patients with cardiac or cerebrovascular disease.

Dosage: For emergency control of hypertension, 2.5 to 5 mg IV, best given by infusion at a rate of 5 to 10 mcg/kg/min.

PHENYTOIN (Dilantin) Anticonvulsant, antiepileptic

Indications: Seizure disorders.

Actions: Anticonvulsant. Reduces Na^+ transport across cerebral cell.

Side effects: **Hypotension, cardiac dysrhythmias, ataxia**, nystagmus, dysarthria, hepatotoxicity, gingival hypertrophy, hirsutism, megaloblastic anemia, lymphadenopathy, fever, rash.

Comments: At therapeutic doses, the drug is metabolized in the liver at zero order (a fixed, absolute amount per unit time). Relatively small changes in dosage can cause major changes in serum concentrations over the long term.

Dosage: For status epilepticus, 18 mg/kg loading dose IV in normal saline at a rate of 25 to 50 mg/min. For epilepsy 300 mg/day.

PHYTONADIONE (vitamin K₁) Vitamin K

Indications: Vitamin K deficiency, reversal of warfarin effect.
Actions: Essential for hepatic synthesis of factors II, VII, IX, and X.
Side effects: Hematoma formation with subcutaneous or intramuscular administration.
Comments: Avoid intravenous administration because of **hypotension** and **anaphylaxis**. Serious hemorrhage caused by excessive warfarin is better treated with fresh-frozen plasma.
Dosage: 2.5 to 10 mg PO, SC, or IM.

PLICAMYCIN (Mithracin) Parathyroid hormone inhibitor Antitumor antibiotic

Indications: Hypercalcemia caused by neoplasms.
Actions: Lowers calcium level by blocking parathyroid hormone action on osteoclasts.
Side effects: Nausea and vomiting, **nephrotoxicity**, local reactions caused by extravasation, facial flushing.
Comments: **A toxic agent of restricted availability**. Onset of effect is within hours, with a peak effect at 72 hours. Duration of effect of a single injection is 7 to 10 days.
Dosage: 25 mcg/kg per day, with repeat doses given no sooner than 48 hours.

POTASSIUM Potassium supplement

Indications: Hypokalemia.
Actions: Potassium supplement.
Side effects: Nausea, vomiting, diarrhea, abdominal discomfort, hyperkalemia.
Comments: Danger of **hyperkalemia in patients with renal impairment** and those taking ACE inhibitors.
Dosage: Micro-K Extencaps: 8 mmol K⁺. Micro-K 10 Extencaps: 10 mmol K⁺· Slow-K: 8 mmol K⁺; Kay Ciel Elixir: 20 mmol/15 mL. Prevention: 24 to 40 mmol/day. Treatment: 60 to 120 mmol/day or more.

POTASSIUM- AND SODIUM-BINDING AGENTS

These agents are nonabsorbable cation exchange resins that exchange cations in the gut.
Potassium-binding agents used to treat hyperkalemia.
The agents that exchange Na for K carry the risk of hypervolemia. Side effects are nausea, vomiting, and gastric distress. May be given PR in a dose of 30 to 50 g in 150 ml H2O od to bid.

Agent	Trade name	Dosage	Onset	Comments
Sodium polystyrene sulfonate	Kayexalate	15 g PO od to qid	2-6 h	Exchanges Na for K in the gut
Sodium zirconium cyclosilicate	Lokelma	5-10 g PO od	1-2 h	Exchanges Na for K in the gut
Calcium polystyrene sulfonate	Resonium Calcium	15 g PO tid to qid	4-6 h	Exchanges Ca for K in the gut
Patiromer	Veltassa	8.4 g PO od	7 h	Exchanges Ca for K in the gut

Sodium-binding agents used to treat irritable bowel syndrome.

Agent	Trade name	Dosage	Comments
Tenapanor	Ibsrela	50 mg PO bid	Exchanges hydrogen ion for Na in the gut increasing the sodium and water content of the gut

PREGABALIN (Lyrica) Analgesic/Anticonvulsant

Indications: An anticonvulsant to treat neuropathic pain, fibromyalgia, and partial seizures.

Actions: Not clearly understood. Modulates calcium channel function in nervous tissues. Related to the antiepileptic drug gabapentin.

Side effects: **Very common. Dizziness, drowsiness, blurred vision, diplopia, ataxia, edema,** dry mouth, confusion, tachycardia, thrombocytopenia, rash.

Comments Physical dependence can develop; symptoms of insomnia, nausea, headache, and diarrhea may manifest upon abrupt cessation of chronic dosing.

Dosage: 75 mg PO twice a day or 50 mg PO 3 times a day up to a maximum of 300 mg PO per day.

PRIMAQUINE Antimalarial

Indications: Malaria, *P. carinii* pneumonia.

Actions: Unknown.

Side effects: GI symptoms, **methemoglobinemia, leukopenia, hemolytic anemia in patients with glucose-6-phosphate deficiency**.

Comments: Depicted in an episode in the TV series MASH when Max Klinger developed anemia while on primaquine, which confused doctors who thought only blacks were susceptible!

Dosage: Used in combination with clindamycin in the treatment of *P. carinii* pneumonia: 15 to 30 mg/day PO with clindamycin, 600 to 900 mg IV, or clindamycin, 300 to 400 mg PO, every 6 to 8 hours.

PROCAINAMIDE (Pronestyl, Procan) Class Ia anti-arrhythmic

Indications: Atrial and ventricular tachydysrhythmias.

Actions: Reduces the maximum rate of depolarization in atrial and ventricular conducting tissue.

Side effects: **Hypotension**, anorexia, nausea, vomiting, heart block, proarrhythmia, rash, fever, SLE-like syndrome, arthralgias.

Comments: Similar to quinidine except that it does not have an atropinic effect. Cross-allergy to procaine.

Dosage: 1-g oral loading dose, followed by 250 to 500 mg PO every 3 hours; delayed-release preparations can be administered every 6 hours. For life-threatening tachydysrhythmia, 20 mg/min intravenous infusion until the arrhythmia has been suppressed, until hypotension occurs, until the QRS complex widens by >50%, or until a total dose of 17 mg/kg has been given. This can be followed by a maintenance infusion of 1 to 4 mg/min. Alternatively, for refractory ventricular fibrillation or ventricular tachycardia, 100-mg intravenous push doses every 5 minutes up to a maximum dose of 1 g.

PROTAMINE SULFATE Heparin antagonist

Indications: Reversal of heparin anticoagulation.

Actions: Binds to and inactivates heparin.

Side effects: **Hypotension, bradycardia**, flushing.

Comments: Overdosage may paradoxically result in worsening hemorrhage because protamine possesses anticoagulant activity. Derived from proteins in the sperm of suitable species of fish.

Dosage: 1 mg/100 U of heparin IV, slowly, on the basis of an estimation of the circulating heparin. No more than 50 mg should be administered in a 10-minute period.

PROTHROMBIN COMPLEX CONCENTRATE (Octaplex)

Indications: Reversal of warfarin therapy or vitamin K deficiency when rapid reversal is required.

Actions: Contains a mixture of clotting factors II, VII, IX, and X and protein C.

Side effects: Increased risk of **thrombotic events**. Produced from large pools of human plasma; samples may carry the **risk of hepatitis and other viral illnesses** although the manufacturing process ordinarily includes solvent viral inactivation and nanofiltration.

Comments: Reconstitution and administration details are provided in the package insert.

Dosage: Dependent on international normalized ratio (INR) and patient's weight. For adult patients: 40 mL. Maximum rate of infusion, 2 to 3 mL/min. Measure INR 15 minutes after administration. A second dose of 20 mL may be administered if the INR >1.5 and the patient continues to bleed. Maximum dose per episode is 120 mL.

PROTON PUMP INHIBITORS

Indications: Gastroesophageal reflux disease, peptic ulcer, NSAID-induced gastropathy.

Actions: Inhibition of gastric proton pumps, thus inhibiting basal and stimulated gastric acid secretion.

Side effects: Headache, diarrhea, abdominal pain, nausea. Long-term continuous use increases the risk of bone fractures.

Comments: Generally well tolerated. **Many interactions** when co-administered with other drugs (e.g., phenytoin, warfarin, ketoconazole, diazepam).

Drug	Trade name	Dosage
Esomeprazole	Nexium	20-40 mg PO daily
Dexlansoprazole	Kapidex	30-60 mg PO daily
Lansoprazole	Zoton	15-30 mg PO daily
Omeprazole	Losec, Prilosec	20 mg PO daily
Pantoprazole	Protium, Protonix	40 mg PO daily
Rabeprazole	Pariet	20 mg PO daily
Vonoprazan	Takecab	20 mg PO bid

QUININE SULFATE Antimalarial

Indications: Nocturnal leg cramps.

Actions: Unknown.

Side effects: Quinine sulfate may cause **unpredictable serious and life-threatening hematologic reactions including thrombocytopenia and hemolytic-uremic syndrome/thrombotic thrombocytopenic purpura (HUS/TTP) renal failure, in addition to hypersensitivity reactions, QT prolongation, and serious cardiac arrhythmias including torsade de pointes**. The risk associated with the use of quinine sulfate in the absence of evidence of its effectiveness for treatment or prevention of nocturnal leg cramps outweighs any potential benefit.

RIFAMPIN (Rifampicin) Antifungal

Indications: Treatment of tuberculosis and leprosy in combination with other drugs and in the prophylaxis but not the treatment of meningococcal infections. Of limited use in staphylococcal infections.

Side effects: **Hypersensitivity**, rash, urticaria, confusion, GI symptoms, **hepatotoxicity, nephrotoxicity.**

Comments: Resistance develops rapidly so that it is almost always used in combination except in meningococcal prophylaxis.

Dosage: 600 mg PO bid for 48 hrs for meningococcal prophylaxis. Staphylococcal infections: 20 mg/kg/day PO in 1 or 2 divided doses. Intravenous preparation is of limited availability.

SALBUTAMOL (Ventolin, Proventil) β_2-Agonist

Indications: Bronchospasm.

Actions: β_2-Adrenergic agonist.

Side effects: Headache, dizziness, nausea, **tremor, palpitations**.

Comments: Higher doses cause tachycardia. Also available in combination with ipratropium (as Berodural).

Dosage: 2.5 to 5 mg in 3 mL of normal saline by nebulizer every 4 hours as needed. In severe bronchospasm, may be required every 3 to 5 minutes initially or 250 mcg/kg IV over 2 minutes.

Respirator solution: 2.5 to 5 mg in 3 mL of normal saline by nebulizer every 4 hours as needed. In severe bronchospasm, may be required every 3 to 5 minutes initially.

Metered dose inhaler: 180 mcg (2 puffs) up to 4 times daily.

SOMATOSTATIN (Stilamin, Zecnil)

Indications: Used in the control of bleeding esophageal varices.

Actions: Decreases splanchnic blood flow and portal venous pressure.

Side effects: Nausea, vomiting, hyperglycemia, pyrexia. Transient **hypotension and bradycardia**.

Comments: Inhibits the secretion of insulin and glucagon with resulting decrease in blood sugar. Use with caution in diabetics.

Dosage: 250 mcg intravenous bolus over 3 to 5 minutes followed by 250 to 500 mcg/h intravenous infusion.

TETRACYCLINES

Action: Inhibit bacterial growth by inhibiting protein synthesis. Tetracyclines are bacteriostatic. They have been in widespread human and animal use and have been used as growth promoters in animals for food production since the 1950s.

Comments: Resistance has limited their effectiveness against both gram-positive and gram-negative bacterial infections. Resistance to one tetracycline usually implies resistance to the others. They should not be administered to pregnant patients or to children younger than 8 years because they can inhibit bone growth and discolor developing teeth.

Drug	Trade name	Indications	Dosage	Side effects
Doxycy-cline	Vibramy-cin	Mycoplasma pneumonia, Rocky Mountain spotted fever, relapsing fever, Chlamydia infections, Lyme disease, Typhus, Q fever, Psittacosis	100 mg PO, minimally affected by food. 100-200 mg IV daily in 1 or 2 infusions Reduce dosage if creatinine clearance <30 mL/min	Epigastric nausea, vomiting, photo-sensitiv-ity
Minocy-cline	Minocin	Mycoplasma pneumonia, Rocky Mountain spotted fever, relapsing fever, Chlamydia infections, Lyme disease, Typhus, Q fever, Psittacosis	100 mg PO q12h. Reduce dosage if creatinine clearance <30 mL/min	GI symptoms, hypers-en-sitiv-ity, drug-induced SLE
Tetracy-cline	Achro-mycin	Mycoplasma pneumonia, Rocky Mountain spotted fever, relapsing fever, Chlamydia infections, Lyme disease, Typhus, Q fever, Psittacosis	250-500 mg PO q6h on an empty stomach. 250-500 mg IV q12h. Do not ad-minister to patients with renal impair-ment	GI symptoms, photo-sensi-tivity, thrombo-phlebitis associat-ed with intrave-nous use

THIAMINE

Indications: Thiamine deficiency, prophylaxis of Wernicke's encephalopathy.

Actions: Thiamine replacement.

Side effects: Intravenous administration may result in **hypotension** or, in rare cases, anaphylactic shock.

Comments: Consider the oral route even in "emergencies" since it is well absorbed orally. Originally named Vitamin B_1.

Dosage: 100 mg/day PO, IM, or IV for 3 days. For the intravenous route, give slowly over 5 minutes.

TRIMETAZIDINE (Metagard and many others)

Indications: Not approved in North America. Used in stable angina in Europe.

Actions: Inhibits fatty acid oxidation improving myocardial glucose utilization.

Comments: Misused by some Olympic athletes as a performance enhancing drug.

Dosage: 20 mg PO tid.

TRIMETHOPRIM-SULFAMETHOXAZOLE, CO-TRIMOXAZOLE (Bactrim) Sulfonamide, folate antagonist

Indications: Uncomplicated urinary tract infections. Drug of first choice for *P. carinii* infections. Shigellosis.

Actions: The sulfonamide inhibits the incorporation of para-aminobenzoic acid (PABA) into folic acid, and trimethoprim inhibits dihydroreductase, thus reducing the production of tetrafolic acid.

Side effects: GI symptoms, rash, **hypersensitivity reactions**, eosinophilia, anemia.

Dosage: TMP 160/SMX 800 (2 regular-strength tablets) every 12 hours PO. 15 to 20 mg/kg trimethoprim with 25 to 50 mg/kg of sulfamethoxazole every 12 hours IV. Reduce dosage or dose frequency if creatinine clearance <30 mL/min.

TRYPTANS SEROTONIN ($5HT_{1B}$) AGONISTS

Indications: Intermittent treatment to prevent or abort a migraine attack.

Actions: Triptans have a high affinity for serotonin receptors on vascular smooth muscle resulting in vasoconstriction of intracranial vessels agonist actions.

Side effects: Anxiety, dizziness, flushing, sweating, paresthesia, rash. **In rare cases, coronary artery spasm, transient myocardial ischemia, ventricular arrhythmias. See contraindications.**

Contraindications: **Hemiplegic, basilar and ophthalmic migraine, ischemic heart disease, peripheral vascular disease, uncontrolled hypertension. Triptans and dihydroergotamine should not be used within 24 hours of one another.**

Drug	Trade name	Dosage
Dihydro-ergotamine	Migranol Trudhesa	By nasal spray 0.5 mg (one spray) in each nostril, repeated in 15 min, up to a total of 4 sprays (2 mg) Maximum: 6 sprays (3 mg) in 24 h By nasal spray 0.725 mcg in each nostril. Can be repeated after 1 h. Maximum 2.9 mcg OD
Almotriptan	Axert	6.25-12.5 mg PO Maximum: 25 mg in 24 h
Eletriptan	Relpax	20-40 mg PO Maximum: 40 mg in 24 h
Frovatriptan	Frova	2.5 mg PO Maximum: 5 mg in 24 h
Naratriptan	Amerge	1.0-2.5 mg PO Maximum: 5 mg in 24 h
Rizatriptan	Maxalt	5-10 mg PO Maximum: 20 mg in 24 h By nasal spray 2.5 and 5 mg
Sumatriptan	Imitrex PO	25-100 mg PO Maximum: PO 200 mg in 24 h By nasal spray 5 mg and 20 mg SC 6 mg in 0.5 mL
Zolmitriptan	Zomig	2.5-5 mg PO; maximum 10 mg in 24h. By nasal spray 2.5-5 mg; maximum 10 mg on 24h

VAPTANS

Nonpeptide vasopressin antagonists that interfere with the antidiuretic effect of the hormone by competitively binding to V2 receptors in the kidney.

Used in the chronic treatment of hypervolemic hyponatremia associated with congestive heart failure, cirrhosis with ascites, and SIADH. Used in the treatment of autosomal dominant polycystic kidney disease.

Drug	Trade name	Dose	Side effects
Conivaptan	Vaprisol	20 mg IV over 30 minutes then 20-40 mg od by continuous infusion	Erythema and pain at injection site is common
Lixivaptan	Lixar	100-200 mg PO od	Thirst, overcorrection, dehydration, renal impairment
Satavaptan	Aquila	12.5-25 mg PO od	Thirst, arrhythmias, fever, hypo- and hypertension
Tolvaptan	Samsca	15-60 mg PO od	Overcorrection, thirst, dizziness, anaphylactic reactions

WARFARIN (Coumadin) Oral anticoagulant (see Heparin and other antithrombotic drugs)

Index

Pages followed by *b*, *t*, or *f* refer to boxes, tables, or figures, respectively.